Treating Later-Life Depression

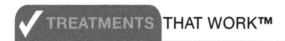TREATMENTS THAT WORK™

Editor-In-Chief

David H. Barlow, PhD

Scientific Advisory Board

Anne Marie Albano, PhD

Gillian Butler, PhD

David M. Clark, PhD

Edna B. Foa, PhD

Paul J. Frick, PhD

Jack M. Gorman, MD

Kirk Heilbrun, PhD

Robert J. McMahon, PhD

Christine Maguth Nezu, PhD

Matthew K. Nock, PhD

Paul Salkovskis, PhD

Bonnie Spring, PhD

Gail Steketee, PhD

John R. Weisz, PhD

G. Terence Wilson, PhD

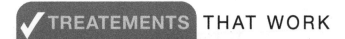
✓TREATMENTS THAT WORK

Treating Later-Life Depression

A Cognitive-Behavioral Therapy Approach

Second Edition

CLINICIAN GUIDE

ANN M. STEFFEN
LARRY W. THOMPSON
DOLORES GALLAGHER-THOMPSON

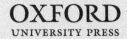

OXFORD
UNIVERSITY PRESS

OXFORD
UNIVERSITY PRESS

Oxford University Press is a department of the University of Oxford. It furthers the University's objective of excellence in research, scholarship, and education by publishing worldwide. Oxford is a registered trade mark of Oxford University Press in the UK and certain other countries.

Published in the United States of America by Oxford University Press
198 Madison Avenue, New York, NY 10016, United States of America.

Library of Congress Cataloging-in-Publication Data
Names: M. Steffen, Ann, author. | Thompson, Larry W., author. |
Gallagher-Thompson, Dolores, author.
Title: Treating later-life depression : a cognitive-behavioral therapy
approach : clinician guide / Ann M. Steffen, Larry W. Thompson,
Dolores Gallagher-Thompson.
Description: 2nd edition. | New York, NY : Oxford University Press, [2022] |
Series: Treatments that work | Revison of: Treating late-life depression /
Dolores Gallagher-Thompson, Larry W. Thompson. 2010. |
Includes bibliographical references and index.
Identifiers: LCCN 2021017567 (print) | LCCN 2021017568 (ebook) |
ISBN 9780190068431 (paperback) | ISBN 9780190068455 (epub) |
ISBN 9780190068462
Subjects: LCSH: Depression in old age—Treatment. | Cognitive therapy.
Classification: LCC RC537.5.G355 2022 (print) | LCC RC537.5 (ebook) |
DDC 618.97/68527—dc23
LC record available at https://lccn.loc.gov/2021017567
LC ebook record available at https://lccn.loc.gov/2021017568

DOI: 10.1093/med-psych/9780190068431.001.0001

Stunning developments in health care have taken place over the last several years, but many of our widely accepted interventions and strategies in mental health and behavioral medicine have been brought into question by research evidence as not only lacking benefit but perhaps inducing harm (Barlow, 2010). Other strategies have been proven effective using the best current standards of evidence, resulting in broad-based recommendations to make these practices more available to the public (McHugh & Barlow, 2010). Several recent developments are behind this revolution. First, we have arrived at a much deeper understanding of pathology, both psychological and physical, which has led to the development of new, more precisely targeted interventions. Second, our research methodologies have improved substantially, such that we have reduced threats to internal and external validity, making the outcomes more directly applicable to clinical situations. Third, governments around the world and health care systems and policymakers have decided that the quality of care should improve, that it should be evidence based, and that it is in the public's interest to ensure that this happens (Barlow, 2004; Institute of Medicine, 2001, 2015; McHugh & Barlow, 2010).

Of course, the major stumbling block for clinicians everywhere is the accessibility of newly developed evidence-based psychological interventions. Workshops and books can go only so far in acquainting responsible and conscientious practitioners with the latest behavioral health care practices and their applicability to individual patients. This series, Treatments *ThatWork*™, is devoted to communicating these exciting new interventions to clinicians on the frontlines of practice.

The manuals and workbooks in this series contain step-by-step detailed procedures for assessing and treating specific problems and diagnoses. But this series also goes beyond the books and manuals by providing ancillary materials that will approximate the supervisory process in assisting practitioners in the implementation of these procedures in their practice.

In our emerging health care system, the growing consensus is that evidence-based practice offers the most responsible course of action for the mental health professional. All behavioral health care clinicians deeply desire to provide the best possible care for their patients. In this series, our aim is to close the dissemination and information gap and make that possible.

The modular cognitive-behavioral therapy (CBT) program presented in this guide is intended to support the personalized treatment of individuals in the second half of life who are experiencing clinical or subclinical depression, with or without accompanying anxiety. The program reflects continuing international scientific and clinical advances in applying CBT to specific age-related problems using individual and group formats. The guide is intended to be used by clinicians from a range of disciplines (e.g., psychology, psychiatry, social work, counseling, marriage and family therapy, nursing, occupational therapy) who are familiar with CBT. Aging-friendly clinical tools are provided for a number of behavioral and cognitive change strategies, including behavioral activation, problem solving, relaxation training, redirecting attention to personal strengths and positive emotional experiences, self-compassion, cognitive reappraisal, healthy habit formation, and communication skills training, among others.

One of the greatest challenges in treatment with aging individuals is the wide variability of life circumstances that accompany depressive symptoms. The culturally responsive practices in this approach target the contexts and drivers of later-life depression, helping clinicians address common concerns of middle-aged and older adults (i.e., changes in brain health, chronic pain, sleep problems, experiences of loss, family caregiving issues). Large-font pages and simplified forms in the client workbook promote learning and retention of adaptive coping skills for clients across a range of outpatient mental health, integrated primary care, and psychiatric partial-hospitalization settings. The appendices in this clinician guide include aging-friendly assessment tools and other resources to support ongoing professional development for work with clients in the second half of life.

Because the processes and techniques that are presented here build upon a treatment protocol with extensive empirical support accumulated over four decades, *Treating Later-Life Depression* will be an indispensable resource for all clinicians who wish to effectively and efficiently help adults in the second half of life reduce depressive symptoms and improve quality of life.

David H. Barlow, Editor-in-Chief
Treatments *ThatWork*™
Boston, Massachusetts

References

Barlow, D. H. (2004). Psychological treatments. *American Psychologist, 59,* 869–878.

Barlow, D. H. (2010). Negative effects from psychological treatments: A perspective. *American Psychologist, 65*(2), 13–20.

Institute of Medicine. (2001). *Crossing the quality chasm: A new health system for the 21st century.* National Academy Press.

Institute of Medicine. (2015). *Psychosocial interventions for mental and substance use disorders: A framework for establishing evidence-based standards.* National Academies Press.

McHugh, R. K., & Barlow, D. H. (2010). Dissemination and implementation of evidence-based psychological interventions: A review of current efforts. *American Psychologist, 65*(2), 73–84.

Contents

The first edition of *Treating Late-Life Depression* was published in 2010 as a treatment of depression (with or without accompanying anxiety) in older individuals. We are happy to offer this second edition, which retains the core of the original intervention while extending its applicability to a wider range of clients and clinical settings. This intervention had its origins in the 1980s and drew heavily from early work on CBT by Aaron Beck, Peter Lewinsohn, and their associates (Beck, 1976; Beck et al., 1979; Lewinsohn et al., 1985, 1986). Over the past four decades, we have also developed and successfully evaluated a number of empirically supported clinical protocols for use with related symptoms and problems commonly experienced by older adults, such as coping with loss and family caregiving.

Since 2010, behavioral health services have continued to evolve in a number of important ways, both within the United States and globally. Mental health integration with primary care has created opportunities to treat clients who are experiencing depressive symptoms in the context of chronic health conditions, using fewer and shorter sessions than is common in traditional psychotherapy. The range of professions and levels of training involved in behavioral health has expanded, with many more master's-level clinicians providing direct services than those at the doctoral level (who are likely to be most active as supervisors and clinic directors). Mental health providers across the disciplines of counseling, nursing, occupational therapy, psychiatry, psychology, and social work are increasingly providing brief interventions as a part of case management and psychoeducational programs, in addition to group and individual psychotherapy. Doctoral-level psychologists and psychiatrists treat the most complex clients, ones who require advanced skills in case conceptualization and treatment planning. Attention to the science-to-practice gap and the treatment gap between those needing and receiving services has led to important developments in dissemination and implementation (D&I) theory, science, and practice. At the same time, the CBTs have matured in response to these advances—there is exciting progress in linking affective and behavioral sciences to the practice of CBT (Hayes & Hofmann, 2018).

Over the past decade, the *Treating Later-Life Depression Workbook* authors have continued to provide direct services to older patients, to supervise clinical trainees, and to train licensed professionals. A special consulting relationship between the Riverside University Health System—Behavioral Health Division, Prevention & Early Intervention Unit and two of the authors (LT and DGT) has provided new insights into the challenges of community mental health center staff and supervisors. These experiences motivated us to revise our treatment recommendations in response to the needs and interests of front-line providers working in culturally diverse communities. As we neared the end of our updates, the COVID-19 pandemic hit. This timing allowed us to send drafts of this second edition to additional clinicians for another round of beta-testing, just as behavioral health services were transitioning to telehealth. Our second edition is both true to the original treatment and responsive to current practice in a range of behavioral health settings.

New in This Edition

Modular Treatment Options

One of the most significant revisions from the first edition is the change to a modular format. This new format of treatment modules reflects important trends in dissemination science and practice (Lyon & Koerner, 2016) and is responsive to clinicians' requests for materials that address variability in client needs and treatment settings. This revised structure allows for more personalized attention to the needs of individual clients. For example, with clients diagnosed as having major depressive disorder (MDD), clinicians can use the original core treatment, which consists of therapy orientation (the *Skills for Getting Started* module), emotional literacy and relaxation training (the *Skills for Feeling* module), behavioral activation and problem solving (the *Skills for Doing* module), cognitive reappraisal (the *Skills for Thinking* module), and termination (the *Skills for Wrapping Up* module). For those with less severe depression and/or comorbid conditions, this second edition includes six new modules to address common issues found in depressed middle-aged and older adults. These resources allow for specialized attention to cognitive aging (the *Skills for Brain Health* module), pain (the *Skills for Managing Chronic Pain* module), sleep (the *Skills for Healthy Sleep* module), caregiving (the *Skills for Caregiving* module), grief and bereavement (the *Skills for Living with Loss* module), and communication within relationships (the *Skills for Relating* module). These modules allow room for clinicians and clients to collaboratively design a treatment package that is in the spirit of personalized medicine. We provide suggestions in Chapter 1 of this clinician guide for treatment planning using this modular approach.

Single-Page Format for Workbook Materials

The didactic materials for clients (now called Learn pages) have been redesigned, moving away from the use of traditional workbook chapters to single pages. This increased flexibility allows clinicians to select pages that fit the needs and abilities of individual clients. This single-page format is especially useful for your work with "oldest old" patients (those aged 80+ years). This age group is growing faster than other aging subgroups and can benefit from clinical strategies to enhance attention and concentration. All Learn pages, along with the between-session worksheets (now called Practice forms), are in a font type and size appropriate for individuals with mild visual and/or cognitive impairments. The transition to single pages also enhances within-session utility, allowing busy clinicians with high caseloads to rely on recognition rather than recall memory when implementing specific change strategies.

Supports for Culturally Sensitive Practice

The original intervention was developed at the Older Adult and Family Resource Center of Stanford University School of Medicine and the Palo Alto Veterans Administration Health Care System. Initially, clients were primarily well-educated non-Hispanic White persons living in the San Francisco Bay area with diagnoses of MDD and an expressed preference for psychotherapy over antidepressant medication. In the years since then, we have worked with a wide range of culturally diverse clients in California and other regions. Based on these experiences, we continue to grow in our understanding of what it means to practice in a culturally humble and responsive manner. This second edition has built-in supports for culturally responsive treatment, including resource sheets in the orientation module (*Skills for Getting Started*) that facilitate discussion of the cultural identities most important for each client. This initial conversation is paired with continued attention to clients' personal values, fostering a strengths-based approach to supporting and building resiliency.

Cognitive reappraisal strategies include an emphasis on the helpfulness of thoughts, in addition to perspective taking, shifting to less extreme language, and examining the evidence; this is considered evidence-based practice with cultural minority clients (Iwamasa & Hays, 2019). Throughout the workbook materials, strategies and case examples reflect client names and practices that are relevant to diverse individuals (e.g., importance of family includes chosen family, inclusion of a range of religious and spiritual traditions, and sensitivity to the realities of low-income clients and those with disabilities). All identifying information has been removed in our case examples.

Applicability to Adults in the Second Half of Life

Within the United States, disparities in access to quality education, nutrition, and health care has led to significant disadvantages for individuals from low-income and/or cultural minority communities. Chronological age, therefore, is less informative than physical and cognitive health and functioning. Some well-resourced 70- and 80-year-olds are healthier and have better daily functioning than some clients in their 50s. This can also be true for racial and ethnic minority clients, LGBTQ+ individuals, and those from rural communities. We have changed the "Late-Life Depression" title of the first edition to "Later-Life Depression" to reflect these realities. Although originally developed for adults aged 65 years and older, this treatment is also appropriate for some middle-aged patients. The second edition's workbook materials and clinician guide have revised language to articulate this focus on the second half of life.

Expanded Resources in Core Modules

As the CBTs continue to develop, the content and language used for change strategies have also evolved. The movement of the CBTs from second-wave interventions (i.e., integrated cognitive-behavioral strategies) to third-wave interventions can be seen in several areas within our core modules. Developments in the affective sciences and emotion-focused CBT have influenced our approach to emotional literacy in the *Skills for Feeling* module, where we have increased the focus on cultivating positive emotions. The influences of positive psychology and positive psychotherapy are evident throughout the workbook, as well as the third-wave CBT emphasis on values-based living and framing therapy goals within clients' values and strengths. Self-compassion research and therapy (Gilbert, 2010, 2017) has grown as a third-wave CBT over the past decade, and we include strategies to build self-compassion in specific modules (i.e., *Skills for Thinking, Skills for Caregiving*). Advances in the psychology of habit formation and change (Verplanken, 2018; Wood & Rünger, 2016) have led us to use the aging-friendly concept of habits more frequently throughout the intervention materials, as well as to emphasize the central importance of repetition in our tips for clinicians. We have done our best to stay rooted in the original efficacy research that provided support for this treatment while also updating materials to be truly state of the art and state of the science of current clinical practice.

Removal of Schema Change Strategies

We have removed schema change strategies in this second edition because of the potential for iatrogenic effects. Current research on interventions for geriatric depression suggests that a therapy focus on schema change may be more harmful than helpful for some clients. Those clinicians who are already trained in cognitive therapy and schema change methods may well decide that this focus is needed for a specific client.

This second-edition guide is divided into three sections to help clinicians navigate the material efficiently. Part I has content related to treatment planning and understanding depression and other concerns in middle-aged and older adults, as well as chapters on assessment, a "CBT 101" primer, and modifications helpful with some aging clients. Part II covers specific recommendations for using the *core* modules that will be relevant for most clients, and Part III includes discussion of how to use the *personalized* modules that are relevant for some clients. Along with including a "Tips for Clinicians" section, each chapter that is linked to a workbook module ends with recommended "Additional Resources for Clinicians" to facilitate continued professional development in that topic area. The appendices have been expanded to support professional practice:

- Appendix A summarizes resources for professional development and training.
- Appendix B provides recommendations for using this treatment in a variety of group settings.
- Appendix C includes guidelines for clinical use of the California Older Person's Positive Experiences Schedule-Revised (COPPES-R), a copy of which is provided in the client workbook.
- Appendix D includes assessment tools that are appropriate for use with your older clients.

We are pleased to be able to share with you these evidence-based strategies and tools for enhancing your clinical practice with middle-aged and older clients!

Acknowledgments

We wish to extend our heartfelt appreciation to the numerous colleagues, fellows, interns, graduate and undergraduate students, and clients with whom we have worked and collaborated in our professional lives over the past 30+ years. Their input has enabled us to develop, refine, revise, and update the materials and strategies included in both the client workbook and clinician guide.

We particularly wish to acknowledge the contributions to our work from Dr. Aaron T. Beck, Dr. Peter Lewinsohn, and Dr. George Kelly; they were instrumental in our early thinking about implementing CBT with older adults. More recently, our colleagues from second- and third-generation forms of CBT have greatly enhanced the content of this revised edition and our application of user-centered design throughout the revision process.

Colleagues who provided their expert consultation and feedback on earlier drafts of this second edition include Dr. Suzanne Meeks (everything!), Dr. Benjamin Mast (brain health), Dr. Beverly Thorn (pain), Dr. Erin Cassidy-Eagle (sleep), Dr. Jason Holland (grief and bereavement), and Dr. Brian Vandenberg (entire workbook). This is a better treatment because of their thoughtful contributions. We wish to recognize the contributions of our colleagues from the Society of Clinical Geropsychology (American Psychological Association Division 12, Section 2), from the Society for Health Psychology (American Psychological Association Division 38), and from Riverside University Health System—Behavioral Health Division, Prevention & Early Intervention Unit (led by Andrea Deaton, MS, LMFT). We are deeply indebted to them for their insights into the first edition of the workbook and willingness to implement early drafts of this second edition. We also wish to thank our two co-authors from the first edition, Drs. David Coon and David Powers, for their many contributions to the evolution of this work.

Finally, our work with clinicians and researchers across the globe has been invaluable in shaping the content and functionality of this second edition. In particular, we'd like to thank Drs. Alma Au and Sheung-Tak Cheng (Hong Kong), Dr. Ken Laidlaw (United Kingdom), Dr. Andres Losada (Spain), Dr. Nancy Pachana (Australia), and Drs. Toni and Bob Zeiss (US Veterans Administration Health Care System, National Office) for their strong encouragement and friendship.

AMS would like to express her deep gratitude to her friends and family and especially her husband, George, for their nurturance, confidence, and love.

LWT thanks the many students and other professionals whose feedback helped shape his perspective and improve his skills for working with older adults. Most of all, he wants to thank his wife for her unwavering support and intellectual companionship throughout the years we've worked together.

DGT is deeply grateful for her parents and grandparents, who valued education and nurtured in her a love of learning and a strong desire to help people in distress. This determination to succeed in her chosen profession was further amplified by the support and encouragement of her devoted husband, who's been a wonderful partner in life (as well as in work!) for the last 40 years.

Master List of Learn Pages and Practice Forms in *Treating Later-Life Depression Workbook*

Module 1: Skills for Getting Started: Planning Your Treatment

Getting Started Learn

Start 1 Learn   Introduction to Skills for Getting Started

Start 2 Learn   How Can This Workbook Help You?

Start 3 Learn   Making This Workbook Work for You[T]

Start 4 Learn   What to Expect from Cognitive-Behavioral Therapy (CBT)[T]

Start 5 Learn   Rules for Our Group

Start 6 Learn   Overview of Clinical Depression[T]

Start 7 Learn   Recognizing Common Signs of Depression

Start 8 Learn   What Is Clinical Depression?[T]

Start 9 Learn   Antidepressant Medications[T]

Start 10 Learn   Your Life Values and Personal Strengths[T]

Start 11 Learn   Celebrating Diversity[T]

Start 12 Learn   Childhood Experiences

Start 13 Learn   What Is the Cognitive-Behavioral Model?[T]

Start 14 Learn   Identifying and Prioritizing Target Problems

Start 15 Learn   Translating Problems into SMART Goals[T]

Start 16 Learn   Measuring Changes Using a Rating Scale

Start 17 Learn   Ways to Think About Progress Toward Your Goals[T]

[T] Pages and Forms with a superscript T are particularly appropriate for telehealth sessions.

Getting Started Practice

Module 2: Skills for Feeling: Recognizing and Managing Strong Emotions

Skills for Feeling Learn

Skills for Feeling Practice

Module 3: Skills for Doing: Values-Based Living and Solving Problems

Skills for Doing Learn

Skills for Doing Practice

Module 4: Skills for Thinking: Self-Compassion and Helpful Thoughts

Skills for Thinking Learn

Skills for Thinking Practice

Skills for Brain Health Learn

Skills for Brain Health Practice

Module 6: Skills for Managing Chronic Pain: Improving Daily Life

Skills for Managing Chronic Pain Learn

Skills for Managing Chronic Pain Practice

Module 7: Skills for Healthy Sleep: Resting Better and Longer

Skills for Healthy Sleep Learn

Skills for Healthy Sleep Practice

Module 8: Skills for Caregiving: Reducing Stress While Helping Others

Skills for Caregiving Learn

Skills for Caregiving Practice

Module 9: Skills for Living with Loss: Bereavement and Grief

Skills for Living with Loss Learn

Skills for Living with Loss Practice

Module 10: Skills for Relating: Getting Along and Communicating Your Needs

Skills for Relating Learn

Skills for Relating Practice

Module 11: Skills for Wrapping Up: Finishing Treatment

Wrapping Up Learn

Wrapping Up Practice

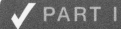

PART I

Introductory
Information
for Clinicians

CHAPTER 1

How to Use This Treatment Approach

The cognitive-behavioral therapy (CBT) program presented in this clinician guide is intended to support your service delivery to clients in the second half of life who are experiencing clinical or subclinical depression, with or without accompanying anxiety. The program reflects continuing international scientific and clinical advances in applying CBT to specific age-related problems. Over the past four decades, the two senior authors of this approach (DGT, LT) have developed empirically supported clinical interventions for older adults that embody the spirit and change strategies of traditional CBT. Many of these efforts have focused on later-life depression, establishing research support for the use of this treatment approach (Coon & Thompson, 2003; Gallagher & Thompson, 1982; Gallagher-Thompson et al., 1990; Thompson, 1996; Thompson & Gallagher, 1984; Thompson et al., 1987, 2001). Our treatment approach is consistent with critical reviews (Braun et al., 2016), meta-analytic studies (Cuijpers et al., 2014, 2016, 2018; Wilkinson & Izmeth, 2016), and the depression treatment guidelines of the American Psychological Association (APA, 2019); all of these support and recommend the use of CBT with depressed older adults.

With the demographic shifts across the globe toward an increasingly aging population, we have packaged this intervention approach to be useful for clients aged 50 to 90+ years. This approach is a modular treatment program (rather than a "lock-step" therapy protocol) and is intended to be used flexibly by you, according to your clients' needs. We expect this treatment to be compatible with individual and group psychotherapy conducted in a variety of settings, including community-based mental health clinics, inpatient services, and home-based programs, as well as being appropriate for briefer interventions within integrated primary care. As licensed psychologists working in the

United States, we are less familiar with the structure of behavioral health service delivery in other parts of the world. We value our international connections to geropsychology colleagues and have attempted to refer to their research and clinical recommendations throughout this guide. It is our hope that the *Treating Later-Life Depression* workbook and this accompanying clinician guide can be useful for clinicians working beyond the United States.

Using a Stepped-Care Model of Behavioral Health Services

We designed this modular intervention program to be relevant across a range of client needs and care settings, employing a behavioral public health perspective that includes attention to stepped care. Within this feedback-informed approach, variability in symptom severity and daily functioning is used to match clients to an appropriate initial treatment that is of the lowest burden possible *while also* likely to result in clinically significant gains. Clients' targeted outcomes are routinely monitored, with more intensive and costly "stepped-up" services provided only if and when the initial treatment does not lead to clinically significant improvements. This stepped-care approach to mental health treatment and preventive interventions is increasingly relevant for a number of community services and health care systems across the globe (van't Veer-Tazelaar et al., 2009), including within the United States (Maragakis & O'Donohue, 2018). Stepped-care behavioral health supports contributions from a wide continuum of providers. Across these levels of training, the goal is for each professional to be working at the top of their own scope of practice. With adequate training and supervision, community peer-support specialists, behavioral technicians, and lower-level clinicians can serve as effective front-line staff to deliver **some** interventions for middle-aged and older adults (Stanley et al., 2016). Peer helpers and bachelor's-level behavioral technicians can be used to implement specific interventions under the supervision of licensed master's- and doctoral-trained therapists (Kraus-Schuman et al., 2015). Master's- and doctoral-level clinicians then work directly with clients experiencing higher levels of symptom severity and functional impairment.

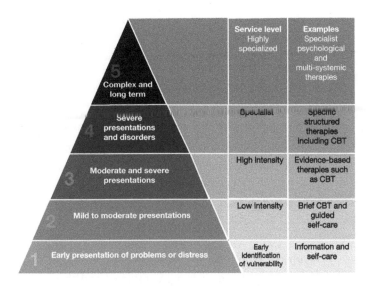

	Service level	Examples
5 Complex and long term	Highly specialized	Specialist psychological and multi-systemic therapies
4 Severe presentations and disorders	Specialist	Specific structured therapies including CBT
3 Moderate and severe presentations	High intensity	Evidence-based therapies such as CBT
2 Mild to moderate presentations	Low intensity	Brief CBT and guided self-care
1 Early presentation of problems or distress	Early identification of vulnerability	Information and self-care

Figure 1.1

Stepped-Care Model of Behavioral Health

Adapted image reproduced with permission by Te Pou (2015)

In keeping with this stepped-care approach to behavioral services, we believe that our treatment approach will be useful across a continuum of client severity, needs, providers, and service settings. As seen in Figure 1.1, we designed this second edition to be appropriate for clients across a range of severity, including levels 2 (mild to moderate symptoms), 3 (moderate to severe presentations), and 4 (severe presentations and disorders). This is an expanded population from the first edition, which was developed as a part of randomized clinical trials with older adults with moderate to severe major depressive disorder (MDD) who were predominantly on level 4 (sometimes 5) of that stepped-care model. Use of some portions of this treatment can be appropriate for case management and time-limited psychoeducational groups, which are on the lower end of the continuum of treatment. Some materials are relevant for inpatient and partial hospitalization, which are all more intensive than individual psychotherapy.

> **Clinician Note**
>
> *If your clinical work is with clients living in long-term care, we'd like to note that we have not evaluated or aimed for this treatment to be used in residential care settings. Because of the need for interventions that explicitly engage and involve staff, we encourage providers to instead utilize specific interventions developed for and within skilled nursing homes. An excellent example of a treatment for depressed older adults that has been created and evaluated specifically for long-term care settings is the BE-ACTIV program developed by Meeks and colleagues (Meeks et al., 2008, 2015, 2019).*

Stepped-care approaches work when clients are evaluated both at the time that treatment is being considered and then also on an ongoing basis during treatment. Treatment is feedback-informed, because the treatment plan is collaboratively adjusted and modified by the provider and client together as symptoms improve, plateau, or become worse. We discuss how this feedback-informed treatment impacts assessment strategies in Chapter 3.

Outline of This Treatment Approach

The workbook that corresponds to this guide (*Treating Later-Life Depression Workbook*) is an integral part of treatment. You will need to have your copy of the workbook available and open while you are reading this clinician guide. When planning treatment for a specific client, you will look over both the didactic "Learn" materials and the between-session "Practice" resources for any modules that are under consideration. Do not, however, become overwhelmed by the volume of available materials! We do not expect that you will use *all* pages in any module with one individual or group; you will most certainly not use all of the modules with any one client. Later sections of this guide address what is needed to implement each specific workbook module, including our recommendations for using specific Learn pages and Practice forms. Thus, this initial chapter is meant to be a guide to general treatment planning; you will need to read specific corresponding chapters for detailed instructions for each module. As you begin the work of customizing treatment for a specific client, assessment is essential, and we provide recommendations in Chapter 3.

Behavioral health clinicians and case managers working in briefer and fewer sessions than is typical for psychotherapy are likely to pick and choose specific Learn pages and Practice forms to fit the needs of specific individuals. The following recommendations for psychotherapy treatment planning have been informed by the clinical research trials conducted at the Older Adult and Family Center of Stanford University School of Medicine and the VA Palo Alto Health Care System. These recommendations are also in keeping with the research literature that has accumulated since then, as well as being shaped by experiences with our clients and our training of professionals from a variety of disciplines. The modules in this treatment are organized into those that we have labeled "core" and others that we refer to as "personalized."

Core Modules (for Most Psychotherapy Clients)

- *Skills for Getting Started* (therapy orientation and goal setting)
- *Skills for Feeling* (emotional literacy, positive and specific negative emotions)
- *Skills for Doing* (behavioral activation and problem solving)
- *Skills for Thinking* (self-compassion and cognitive reappraisal)

Personalized Modules (for Some Psychotherapy Clients)

- *Skills for Brain Health* (preventing and managing cognitive concerns)
- *Skills for Managing Chronic Pain* (psychoeducation and pain management)
- *Skills for Healthy Sleep* (psychoeducation and sleep hygiene)
- *Skills for Caregiving* (for family and informal caregivers)
- *Skills for Living with Loss* (support for healthy grieving)
- *Skills for Relating* (communication and interpersonal effectiveness skills)

Core Module (for Most Psychotherapy Clients)

- *Skills for Wrapping Up* (termination processes and plans)

Middle-Aged and Older Clients with MDD

Individual Psychotherapy

We describe patterns of clinical symptoms and presentation of depression in Chapter 2 of this guide, including MDD. Clients who meet criteria for MDD and who will be seen in individual psychotherapy should receive the core modules in this order: *Skills for Getting Started, Skills for Feeling, Skills for Doing,* and *Skills for Thinking.* Continuous assessment of depression symptoms is indicated, along with periodic assessment of clients' individualized therapy goals. Our experience is that many clients begin to see a lift in their mood at some point while working on *Skills for Doing.* We recommend moving ahead with *Skills for Thinking,* which we believe is useful in preventing relapse or later new episodes of MDD. If clients no longer meet criteria for MDD by the end of *Skills for Thinking,* depressive symptoms are lower, and the client appears to be functioning fairly well in daily life, you can move directly to working on termination in the *Skills for Wrapping Up* module. If the client is still experiencing dysphoria, anhedonia, or functional limitations in daily life, then it is appropriate to consider an additional module that is conceptualized as a contributing factor to maintaining the depression (e.g., brain health, pain, sleep, caregiving, loss, relationships).

The decision to implement a personalized module typically involves a commitment of *at least* three or four sessions (1 month of weekly psychotherapy). As a treatment for depression, progress occurs through active practice and skill development (i.e., between-session use of Practice forms), not from psychoeducation alone (i.e., an over-reliance on Learn pages without integration of skills in daily life). This means that we discourage frequent session-to-session shifts between materials from the various optional modules. A key danger in that strategy is that clinicians believe that they are "covering a lot of ground" while clients feel overwhelmed and confused about what they are supposed to do with that information.

Focus, repetition, and support for building new habits are all key to this approach (Bilbrey et al., 2020b). Regardless of which intervention modules you choose, your work with psychotherapy clients should conclude with the *Skills for Wrapping Up* module to support termination processes and relapse-prevention planning.

Group Psychotherapy

Clinicians trained in this treatment have primarily used an open group format (i.e., individuals enter and leave the group on an ongoing basis) to deliver the program to clients with MDD. This open format appears most compatible with clinical services for moderate to severely depressed individuals, including those in inpatient, partial hospitalization, and outpatient settings. Especially within psychiatric inpatient and partial hospitalization settings, time-limited, structured "closed" groups are not feasible. Instead, group treatment is offered for any patients within the unit who are deemed appropriate. Individuals need access to treatment as soon as possible, and it is not clinically appropriate to make them wait until a new group is ready to begin. The continual influx of new clients helps keep the group focused on skill development rather than devolving into general support. In these types of open-format groups, sections of *Skills for Getting Started*, *Skills for Feeling*, *Skills for Doing*, and *Skills for Thinking* are all appropriate.

There are a variety of ways to effectively integrate behavioral activation into acute inpatient services (Folke et al., 2016). Many inpatient and partial hospitalization programs treating patients with depression find that sleep concerns are so prevalent that there is value in some sleep education. Those settings may choose to use at least some portions of *Skills for Healthy Sleep* within their groups. We make specific recommendations for group treatment in Appendix B. Repetition and support for building new habits are key to this approach, and this is reflected in our recommendations for group content and process. For individuals with MDD who have some access to both group and individual psychotherapy, the termination planning within *Skills for Wrapping Up* is maximally helpful with the support of some individual sessions. Fixed-length closed groups appear less compatible with treating MDD than for clients experiencing milder, subsyndromal depressions.

Middle-Aged and Older Clients with Subsyndromal Depression

Individual Psychotherapy

When middle-aged and older adults have mild to moderate symptoms of depression (e.g., Patient Health Questionnaire-9 [PHQ-9] < 15; Geriatric Depression Scale -Short Form [GDS-SF] < 10; Beck Depression Inventory-II [BDI-II] < 20] and do not meet diagnostic criteria of MDD, there is more choice involved in planning individual psychotherapy. For the majority of these clients, we suggest *Skills for Getting Started* (two or three sessions), *Skills for Feeling* (three or four sessions), and *Skills for Doing* (six to eight sessions), all using the recommendations provided in the chapters of this guide devoted to those modules. If depressive symptoms have abated (e.g., PHQ-9 < 4; GDS15 < 5; BDI-II < 14), then it is possible to move directly to termination planning in *Skills for Wrapping Up* (two to four sessions). Clients may get more benefit from behavioral activation and problem solving than you initially expect, so we advise you to resist the urge to shortchange that module in order to move on to topic-specific content. For all clients, repetition and support for building new habits are key to this approach, so sufficient time in behavioral activation and problem solving is important.

If your clients have had six to eight sessions of behavioral activation and problem solving (i.e., *Skills for Doing*) and are still experiencing clinically significant depressive symptoms, then the strategy for selecting additional module(s) becomes more customized. If your clients have no specialized concerns related to the personalized modules (e.g., pain, cognitive impairment, sleep, caregiving, loss, relating) and are engaged in daily activities but are not experiencing them as pleasurable, then moving on to *Skills for Thinking* is clinically indicated. Repeating some of the material on tracking positive emotions in *Skills for Feeling* may also be helpful in these cases.

There will also be times when your clients have specialized concerns (e.g., pain, cognitive impairment, sleep, caregiving, loss, relating to others) and it will be more effective to move into that personalized module directly after *Skills for Doing*. Difficulties in a personalized module that appear due to cognitive "stuck points" would suggest the advisability of your then using *Skills for Thinking* in a targeted way; focus work in that module on thoughts that are specific to the personalized life domain.

Following *Skills for Doing*, your clients who remain depressed and have specific concerns related to **pain** should next work within the *Skills for Managing Chronic Pain* module, even if they also have additional complaints and issues related to other modules. In other words, **pain concerns take precedence over other areas covered in our program**, due to the strong bidirectional relationships between chronic pain and depression. After four sessions using that module, you can re-evaluate and decide whether the client is now ready to move toward termination. If pain-related cognitions are proving to be a "stuck point" for implementing the suggested pain-management strategies, then move to *Skills for Thinking*, but with a targeted focus explicitly on their specific pain-related cognitions.

We suggest this general approach for your use of the other personalized modules as well. From *Skills for Doing*, you would transition to the module of most pressing concern to a specific client. With some individuals, this most pressing concern is immediately apparent within several sessions of beginning psychotherapy, if it was not already identified at the time of intake. This is especially the case for clients with chronic pain, distressed family caregivers, and individuals who are bereaved. Sometimes, the presenting concerns related to those areas feel so pressing that you and your client will collaboratively decide to move from *Skills for Getting Started* and *Skills for Feeling* directly to one of those areas (e.g., *Skills for Managing Chronic Pain*, *Skills for Caregiving*, *Skills for Living with Loss*). After four to six sessions in that personalized area, you are then more able to implement the strategies in *Skills for Doing* and *Skills for Thinking* using content and examples from that specific life domain. More suggestions for this approach are provided in the chapters of this clinician guide that are devoted to those modules.

For individual psychotherapy, however, we advise clinicians to first implement the behavioral activation and problem-solving module (*Skills for Doing*) **before** making a firm decision to include optional sections for a specific client. Although many of the modules sound interesting to older patients and appear relevant, that additional content may not be **essential** for alleviating the depression. There is a firm evidence base for the effectiveness of behavioral activation with depressed older adults (Solomonov et al., 2019). Our goal is for therapy to progress as efficiently as possible to improve the daily functioning and depressive symptomatology of clients. You want additional sessions focused on optional sections to be very strategically targeted at symptoms and concerns that have not sufficiently improved with behavioral activation. For the same reason, we would not expect any one psychotherapy client or group to actively work on skill development in more than two or three (at the very most!) optional modules. In many cases, your use of one personalized module with clients experiencing subclinical depression will be adequate.

Group Psychotherapy

When middle-aged and older adults have mild to moderate symptoms of depression (e.g., PHQ-9 < 15; GDS15 < 6; BDI-II < 20) and do not meet diagnostic criteria of MDD, there is more choice involved in designing group treatments. For these individuals who may not identify as having mental health concerns or be interested in something labeled as psychotherapy, it is useful to offer time-limited psychoeducational groups that include "Skills" or "Coping" in the titles. We find that 60 to 90 minutes is a good length for such groups that are focused on "Skills for Enjoying Your Life" or "Coping with Caregiving" or another related title. These programs require a full 90 minutes if the group is larger than six to eight members so that all have an opportunity to actively participate at each meeting.

Six weeks is a good length for a group focused primarily on behavioral activation and problem solving. Again, a shorter duration works well with smaller classes of four to six members, which often allows for slightly faster-paced group sessions. Clinicians who wish to include cognitive reappraisal skills, in addition to behavioral activation and problem solving, should consider a longer format and add three or four sessions specifically for that content. It is also possible to offer closed-format groups that are centered on one of the personalized modules, especially caregiving, pain, sleep, or living with loss. These psychoeducational programs can be delivered over a telehealth platform, which makes them accessible to a broad range of individuals, as long as they have access to the workbook. We provide some examples of week-by-week group content in Appendix B.

Treatment Implementation

We understand that clinicians are able to do their best work when they are (1) prepared for the kinds of problems and reactions to expect, (2) provided with strategies to deal with them, and (3) encouraged to employ an individualized case formulation and treatment approach that fits with the needs, strengths, and limitations of individual clients (Pachana et al., in press). Across the chapters of this clinician guide, we aim to provide you with very concrete recommendations for how to use the workbook with your clients. Part I: Introductory Information for Clinicians, in this guide, provides background information about depression, assessment, and modifications to psychotherapy with aging individuals. Later parts of the guide then address what you need to know as you implement specific modules of the workbook.

Prerequisites

The delivery of behavioral health interventions is overseen by state laws and regulating boards. To provide mental health services, an individual must be licensed within the state in which the services are delivered or under the supervision of a licensed clinician. (There are also state-specific laws and regulations for the delivery of telehealth services across state lines.) Once licensure issues are addressed, we find that this approach can be used by a range of clinicians who have completed professional training (or are in the advanced stages of completion) in one of the behavioral health–related specialties, for example social work, counseling, clinical psychology, psychiatry, advanced nursing specialist in psychiatry or another behavioral specialty, and advanced occupational therapy. The critical component here is that in addition to having the requisite interpersonal skills, one must be familiar with foundational attitudes, knowledge, and skills in CBT (Tolin, 2016). In our experience, professionals without training and supervised clinical experience in implementing CBT are typically less effective in using our approach.

After agreeing to try the techniques and experiencing their effectiveness, many initially "CBT-reluctant" professionals become "converts" and proceed with further training with success.

Clinicians should also have knowledge about the problems and issues confronting adults in the second half of life and the general psychological, social, medical, and economic resources available to this population that enable them to accommodate to life stresses. Clinicians should also have some knowledge of how to work with aging individuals, for example regarding the strengths and weaknesses common to this group and how to use this information in maximizing their potential for change. We recognize that most clinicians do not have specialized training in gerontology, and this is *not* required for the effective use of this approach.

Client Access to Workbook

In terms of the timing for clients to purchase their own copy of the workbook, there are a range of options depending upon the clinical setting and your client population. We tend to print out copies of any Learn pages and Practice forms from *Skills for Getting Started* to share with our clients as they are beginning treatment. Once they have continued beyond the content in *Skills for Getting Started*, we then encourage clients to have their own copy of the workbook, which makes it easier for them to find and refer back to after therapy has ended. When treatment is provided via telehealth (e.g., either telephone or video), it becomes especially helpful for clients to have their own copy of the workbook available to use and refer back to. In some clinical settings, it is possible for the clinic to purchase copies of the workbook and prorate the cost over several sessions.

Population/Culture-Specific Adaptations

Numerous clients with depression from diverse racial, ethnic, and cultural backgrounds have been successfully treated in our training and research programs, using the original intervention approach described in the first edition. Adaptations of this approach for use with special populations have been developed for some groups, notably family caregivers who are Hispanic Americans, Asian Americans, African Americans, those of Persian background, and male caregivers. Appropriate translations and back translations of the manuals and instruments for evaluation have been made, and randomized trials have shown the effectiveness of this technique in Latinx, Chinese, Vietnamese, and African American individuals. We refer you to OptimalAgingCenter.com for examples and further information. This work is mentioned here because it suggests that if appropriate translations are made available and are being used by trained professionals who are bicultural/bilingual, there is little doubt that this treatment approach would be effective. It has been well received by numerous ethnic groups. Culture-specific adaptations for diverse older adults are described within the works edited by Iwamasa and Hays (2019) and by Lau and colleagues (2019). Several of the authors in those edited volumes were trained in our center at Stanford University School of Medicine.

Pharmacotherapy for Depression

Historically, pharmacotherapy has been viewed as the first line of treatment for severe depression in middle-aged and older adults, and psychological intervention has been considered an adjunctive treatment. More recent guidelines, however, emphasize combined treatment for severe and treatment-resistant major depression (Reynolds et al., 2019), with antidepressants less likely to be effective for minor or subsyndromal depression (APA, 2019). Clinicians are encouraged to build relationships with geriatric psychiatrists within their local community to serve as resources for referral and consultation.

Risks and Benefits of This Treatment Program

There have been no substantial adverse effects in clients while they were enrolled in treatment programs in our center. Over the years, less than 10% of those receiving CBT or a combination of CBT and pharmacotherapy have required outside consultation because of increasing symptoms (and due to deteriorating medical conditions). The benefits are most often very encouraging, as noted in earlier discussions focused on treatment evaluation. As an overall summary of the clients involved in our research and training programs, approximately 67% of the individuals we have treated with CBT alone have shown substantive improvement, and nearly 60% were classified as being in complete remission with no major clinical symptoms at the conclusion of treatment. The remaining clients either showed no change over the course of 12 to 20 sessions and a 1-year follow-up (12%), became worse during the initial therapy and required more aggressive treatment (roughly 7%), or experienced intermittent improvement and decline over the course of therapy and follow-up (14%).

CHAPTER 2

Depression and Age-Related Issues

This chapter provides an overview of later-life depression and information about common age-related changes and concerns that are often contributing factors. As you prepare to implement this treatment approach, it will be quite helpful for you to have a solid grasp of depression in the context of normative aging, along with understanding common issues for clients in the second half of life.

Depression is a very common psychiatric disorder resulting in poor functional capabilities and low quality of life. In the United States and worldwide, depression is the second leading cause of disability (Kazdin & Blase, 2011). Although a sad mood can be triggered by a number of stressors, depressive symptoms and clinical depression are clearly different from sadness linked to a specific event or having a "low mood" from time to time. This treatment approach is designed to help your aging clients with major depressive disorder (MDD), "minor" or subsyndromal depression, or dysthymic disorder. Although not all clinicians may have diagnosis within their scope of practice, reviewing diagnostic criteria for depression in all adults can be a helpful orientation to your considering key points about depression in later life. It is also important to be able to separate the myths from the facts about later-life depression (Haigh et al., 2018).

Diagnostic Criteria for Depression Regardless of Age

Major Depressive Disorder

According to the fifth edition of the *Diagnostic and Statistical Manual of Mental Disorders* (DSM-5; American Psychiatric Association, 2013), to be diagnosed with MDD the individual must experience, most of the day, nearly every day, for at least 2 consecutive weeks, at least one of these first two symptoms:

- Dysphoric mood either reported by individual (e.g., sad, blue, empty) or observed by others (e.g., sad facial expression, crying);
- Anhedonia, which is a dramatically reduced interest or positive experience of activities that have previously been pleasurable;

and at least four or more of the following symptoms:

- Significant weight loss/gain or change in appetite;
- Insomnia or hypersomnia;
- Psychomotor agitation or retardation;
- Fatigue;
- Feelings of worthlessness or excessive guilt;
- Diminished ability to think or concentrate; and
- Recurrent thoughts of death or suicidal ideation/plans.

In addition, these symptoms must cause clinically significant emotional distress or impairments in social, occupational, or other areas of functioning.

Subsyndromal (Minor) Depression and Persistent Depressive Disorder

We also need to consider *subsyndromal (minor) depression*, which is technically diagnosed as "Other Specified Depressive Disorder" in DSM-5. This is when the individual does not meet full criteria for MDD yet has one of the first two symptoms combined with one to three of the remaining symptoms. Persistent depressive disorder (*dysthymia*) reflects more of a chronic condition; clients must have depressed mood or anhedonia for most of the day, for the majority of days over a period of at least 2 years, along with two (or more) of the other symptoms. Finally, clients may have milder symptoms that do not rise to the level of one of these diagnoses but nevertheless are troublesome and reduce their quality of life.

Aging individuals experiencing clinical or subclinical depression generally fall into two groups: early onset cases (first experiences of depression occur before the age of 60) and late onset (first experiences of depression at age 60 or older; Sachs-Ericsson et al., 2013). Our approach can be used with both groups. Whether chronic/intermittent or occurring for the first time, depression in later life frequently includes psychological distress, impairment in daily functioning, and medical comorbidities. There is an increased risk of all-cause mortality in depressed older adults (Byers et al., 2012; Wei et al., 2019), which is magnified for older adults with cognitive impairment (Georgakis et al., 2016; Kane et al., 2010).

When looking at the prevalence rates of depression, it may be surprising to learn that the prevalence of the most intense level (MDD) is lower in older patients than in younger patients. Rates of subsyndromal depression are much higher than rates of MDD in older patients. Efforts to identify explanatory factors for this have revealed that the findings are complicated and remain controversial for the moment. It remains, however, very important for clinicians to be aware that subclinical depression significantly impacts daily functioning and is responsive to treatment. Meeks and colleagues' (2011) re-analysis of data for older Americans in the National Institute of Mental Health (NIMH) Epidemiologic Catchment Area study showed a high prevalence rate of 31% for subsyndromal depression in older adults. The prevalence of MDD was 6.3%, which is comparable to some estimates of MDD obtained in other studies of younger community samples (Judd & Akiskal, 2002). There is now consensus among clinicians and clinical researchers that depression, however it is considered or whatever diagnostic scheme is used, is a common problem in later life and is responsive to psychotherapy.

You should be aware that the predominant symptom of depression in older adults may be anhedonia (i.e., perceived lack of enjoyment and pleasure on a daily basis) rather than dysphoria (i.e., overt indicators of sadness such as crying, sad facial expressions, or endorsement of the term "depressed" to describe their experience). Because medical and behavioral health providers are more likely to recognize sadness as indicative of depression (Gregg et al., 2013), anhedonic presentations of depression often go under-recognized and undiagnosed.

Newer data-analytic techniques are also providing new insights as to how symptoms of depression are related to each other, and which ones appear most central to the disorder (Fried et al., 2016). As this work continues to progress, we expect to have a better understanding of how these relationships among symptoms may be different for younger versus older adults. Depressive episodes that are a part of bipolar disorder are even more complicated. Because this treatment approach focuses on unipolar depression, we refer clinicians to the work by Reiser and colleagues (2017) on assessment and treatment of bipolar disorder.

Cognitive-Behavioral Therapy Model of Depression in Later Life

Cognitive-behavioral therapies (CBTs) are evidence-based and grounded in a firm understanding of how symptoms develop, are maintained in daily life, and can be improved through systematic application of change strategies. As discussed further in Chapter 4, CBT is deeply humanistic in that you work together with your clients to understand which factors are most important to understand and target for each individual's depression. In your aging clients, there are typically numerous substantive changes in relevant psychosocial and physiological processes that influence strategies used in therapy.

As shown in Figure 2.1, reductions in rewarding daily activities are a primary way that different stressful life events and loss experiences can increase depressive symptoms in aging individuals. There is growing support to indicate that social isolation is particularly important to depression in older adults, leading to a treatment focus on social and interpersonally engaging daily activities (Solomonov et al., 2019). In this model, the most important thoughts related to depression are self-referential, especially self-critical thoughts that continue to perpetuate the downward spiral of social isolation, reduced activity (especially social activities), and anhedonia, thus fueling depression.

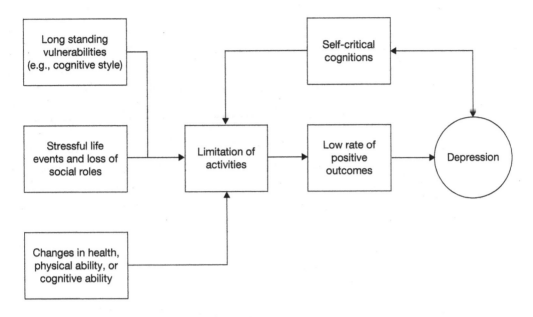

Figure 2.1

Model of Depression in Older Adults

Republished with permission of Annual Reviews, inc., from Fiske et al. (2009). Depression in older adults. *Annual Review of Clinical Psychology,* 5, p. 369; permission conveyed through Copyright Clearance Center, Inc.

Appropriate assessment of your clients' behavioral capabilities is pivotal in the development of an accurate case conceptualization and an effective intervention program. Because of the increased medical and psychosocial changes that occur in the older years, behavioral assessments can be more difficult to complete, but they play an even more important role in developing effective therapy strategies than with younger individuals. Chapter 3 is devoted to assessment issues and techniques.

Ageism and Societal Myths

Societal ageism refers to the ways in which stereotypical attitudes and beliefs about aging influence access to opportunities and resources. From the research literature, we know that ageism is pervasive in Western countries (Levy, 2018) and also evident across the globe (Officera & Fuente-Núñeza, 2018). We do not, however, have to spend a lot of time reading scientific reports to have proof of ageism. All it takes is for you to spend a few minutes browsing through birthday cards in a local store or listening to late-night comedians to see examples of how negative stereotypes about aging are still considered valid, acceptable, and somehow funny. Clinicians and their older clients can, unfortunately, hold negative views of aging that impact mental health and therapeutic interventions. To recognize and counter ageist beliefs in themselves and their clients, clinicians need both knowledge and direct experience with older adults who vary across a range of functioning (Levy, 2018). More than two decades ago, Rowe and Kahn (1998) presented and addressed several common myths about aging. These remain relevant today, and we discuss two that are very relevant for your work with clients in later life. The first one is "to be old is to be sick"; the second, and one that's very relevant for CBT, is "you can't teach an old dog new tricks."

"To Be Old Is to Be Sick"

Not all aging individuals are "sick" or functionally disabled and impaired in their daily lives. A decline in functioning tends to be viewed by clients and family members in "all or none" terms, but aging individuals can usually still perform many of their former tasks in modified form. Although chronic illnesses are more common in adults over the age of 60, they are not synonymous with functional impairment. Despite the high prevalence of conditions such as arthritis, hypertension, heart disease, diabetes, and cancer, aging individuals do not necessarily consider themselves to be in "poor health." Most think of their health more in terms of how these different conditions affect their ability to handle everyday life (rather than focusing on specific medical diagnoses). By age 80, about 28% of older adults report having some problem with activities of daily living (ADLs; e.g., bathing or feeding), and 40% report having difficulty completing some instrumental activities of daily living (IADLs; e.g., paying bills and keeping track of important dates and appointments). Constraints resulting from these limitations can curtail other activities, which lead to individuals with impairments feeling "old" (Haber, 2016). Falling is the most common fear reported by older people and is a good example of the interactions among physical health, behavior, and emotional problems. Fear of falling limits activities and functioning through a cascade of processes. Individuals may feel unsteady on their feet or trip over a floor rug and fall. Once a single fall occurs, they might lose confidence in their ability to avoid falls and to manage well in everyday life. Consequently, they reduce their activities while having increased negative views about themselves and their abilities, thereby reinforcing depressive tendencies.

Other physical changes, such as a higher percentage of body fat, less lean muscle mass, and reduction in the vital lung capacity, are common age-related changes. These can affect quality of life when individuals cannot (or do not) engage in activities they used to enjoy. Decreased activity, however, is more likely due to a sedentary lifestyle than normal age-related changes. About 40% of adults in the second half of life are not active at all and inactivity increases with age, so that by age 75, roughly one in three men and one in two women engage in virtually no physical activity (Uher & Liba, 2017).

By encouraging your clients to learn what their physical limitations actually are, and what they may still be very capable of doing in their current environments (with appropriate training and support), you can make important and concrete differences in their lives. The negative impact of physical health problems can be reduced, and your clients can be supported in building a more active and fulfilling life. Decades of research has conclusively shown that moderate exercise decreases depressive symptoms and likelihood of relapse (Catalan-Matamoros et al., 2016).

It is important for you to take the time to learn about the particular health conditions of your clients and, most importantly, how these are affecting their quality of life. Consultation with clients' primary care providers can help you understand possible areas for improvement in everyday function that could be addressed as part of the treatment program. Aging individuals can still do many of the things they did earlier in life (albeit with some modifications, possibly in frequency and/or intensity). They can also still have meaningful roles (in the family, with friends, as a volunteer, and possibly even still as an employee). There can be a lot of years ahead, and those years can be made more positive by doing a "course" of CBT to learn skills for reducing depression. Doing so now can greatly improve your clients' overall quality of life in their remaining years.

"You Can't Teach an Old Dog New Tricks"

Yes, you can! Overwhelming evidence has proven that aging adults can still learn (Schaie & Willis, 2015) and benefit from psychotherapy for depression as much as younger adults do (Cuijpers et al., 2009). Your firm conviction of this fact will help you be more effective as a clinician. Your aging clients may believe that they can't change; it is your job to help them see that they can, and will, if they engage in the program with you. Remember, the evidence is there to support this position. Often these perceptions of inability to change or learn are based on age-related changes in cognitive processing, as well as changes in sensory-motor function and limitations due to very real medical conditions. In this case, it is easy to become discouraged and look at the glass as "half empty" rather than "half full." We recommend emphasizing that CBT involves learning new things and then asking the client: "*When is the last time you learned something new? What was it?*" (probe for examples, however small). "*Do you think you are able to learn anything else new?*" If the person can't come up with *any* recent new learning, ask: "*Do you think you will be able to learn something new at this point in time?*" Very depressed older clients often say "no," that they are not capable of learning; in these cases it is advisable early on in therapy to set up an "experiment" to determine if this is true. Typically, it is not, and you are able to point that out to your clients based on their personal evidence.

Core Concepts in the Psychology of Aging

Your understanding of the following key concepts will go a long way in the "on-the-spot" decisions that all clinicians have to make during sessions.

Aging Comes with Increased Variability

In later life, chronological age provides only minimal information about an individual's abilities and limitations. You could have a new client who is 75 years old and a long-time marathon runner and senior athlete or a highly functioning business executive. You could also have a 60-year-old client who is severely disabled and heavily dependent on others for daily functioning. With aging comes increased inter-individual variability—*the older we become, the more different we are from others of the same age.* This is true for just about any area you can think of, from education and income, physical health and cognitive functioning, to religious and political preferences.

Along with *inter*-individual variability, there is also *intra*-individual variability. One area of particular strength or limitation does not necessarily tell us about other areas of that individual's life. Different parts of the body age at different rates, and various areas of cognitive and intellectual functioning can be relatively weak or strong. This within-person heterogeneity is true at any specific time, and across time. A decline or improvement in one area of functioning from Time 1 to Time 2 is not necessarily the same pattern that would be seen from Time 2 to Time 3, and so on. All of this variability means that as clinicians we have to assess more than guess.

Aging Involves Both Gains and Losses

Many individuals, including clinicians and their older clients, view the process of aging as mostly a cascade of losses—this is the unfortunate result of societal ageism. Clinicians can inappropriately normalize depressive symptoms in a way that discounts or dismisses the importance of assessment or intervention—for example, "*Of course she is feeling depressed: Look at all of the losses she has experienced in the past few years. I'd feel depressed too if I had all of those. This is just a part of the aging experience.*" This expectation of clinical or subsyndromal depression as normal following loss or other stressful life events can lead you to ignore depressive symptoms and/or not offer treatment. In fact, the majority of aging adults who experience specific loss events are not clinically depressed. Similarly, the belief that significant problems with thinking and memory are normal with age leads to under-assessment, under-diagnosis, and lack of treatment for some reversible cognitive impairments.

When viewed instead through a lifespan developmental framework, aging is recognized as involving *both* losses and gains over time (Freund & Baltes, 2007; Pachana et al., 2015). As many individuals move from adulthood into middle and later adulthood, they come to a better understanding of themselves and their reactions to stressful events. Life experiences can lead to increased emotional literacy and tolerance of strong emotions, interpersonal skills, resilience, and self-acceptance. By the time they have reached 55, for example, approximately 80% of adults will have experienced at least one traumatic life event, yet rates of posttraumatic stress disorder in older adults are quite low (Monson et al., 2016). Even when clinically depressed, your aging clients will have some coping skills and personal resources that are important for you to emphasize and leverage during treatment. As we describe in detail throughout this guide, our treatment approach involves helping you clients identify and use their strengths and resources throughout treatment.

Aging Is One Among Many Facets of Diversity

Clinicians are increasingly aware of the need for cultural humility and sensitivity; there is a strong demand among many communities and clinical services for cultural adaptations of psychological treatments. Our approach reflects and allows for a range of cultural adaptations, balancing culture-specific issues with a focus on intersectionality of personal identities across the lifespan.

As shown in Figure 2.2, we all live and experience our mental health through the combination of a number of personal identities that (1) are held simultaneously, (2) impact exposure to discrimination and access to power/privilege, and (3) are fluid and may change in salience across one's lifetime (Clauss-Ehlers et al., 2019). We are never individuals experiencing problems within a vacuum, but rather we have strengths and challenges that occur in specific contexts. Your clients are never just "people who are aging"; each one is also a person with a specific gender and sexual identity, racial and ethnic background, socioeconomic status, religious and spiritual practices, and so on.

We find the ADDRESSING acronym (Hays, 2016) to be especially helpful as we conceptualize how age and generational influences interact with other personal identities. As shown in Table 2.1, this calls attention to **A**ge and generational influences, **D**evelopmental or other

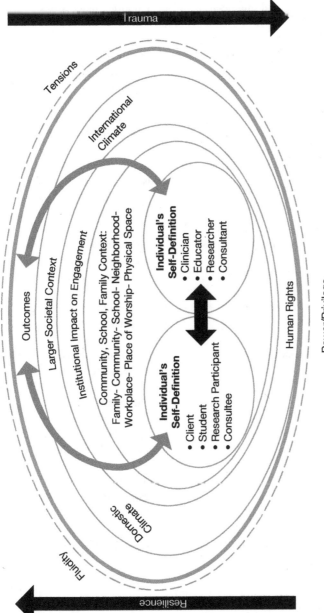

Figure 2.2

Ecological Model of Multicultural Diversity

Table 2.1 ADDRESSING Framework

Cultural influence	Dominant group	Nondominant or minority group
Age and generational influences	Young and middle-aged adults	Children, older adults
Developmental or other Disability	Individuals without disabilities	People with cognitive, intellectual, sensory, physical, and psychiatric disabilities
Religion and spiritual orientation	Christian and secular	Muslims, Jews, Hindus, Buddhists, and other religions
Ethnic and Racial identity	European Americans	Asian, South Asian, Latino, Pacific Islander, African, Arab, African American, Middle Eastern, and multiracial people
Socioeconomic status	Upper and middle class	People of lower status by occupation, education, income, or inner-city or rural habitat
Sexual orientation	Heterosexuals	People who identify as gay, lesbian, bisexual, or other
Indigenous heritage	European Americans	American Indians, Inuit, Alaska Natives, Métis, Native Hawaiians, New Zealand Maori, Aboriginal Australians
National origin	U.S.-born Americans	Immigrants, refugees, and international students
Gender	Men	Women and people who identify as transgender or non-binary

Reproduced with permission of the American Psychological Association from the book by Pamela A. Hays (2016), *Addressing Cultural Complexities in Practice: Assessment, Diagnosis, and Therapy.* Wash., DC: American Psychological Association.

<u>D</u>isabilities, <u>R</u>eligion or spiritual orientation, <u>E</u>thnic & Racial Identity, <u>S</u>ocioeconomic status, <u>S</u>exual orientation, <u>I</u>ndigenous heritage, <u>N</u>ational origin, and <u>G</u>ender identities. Together, these intersecting experiences and identities affect the clinical presentation, course of depression, therapeutic relationship, and collaborative selection of change strategies. In Appendix D of this guide, we provide an ADDRESSING worksheet that you can use to incorporate consideration of multicultural diversity during the process of case conceptualization and treatment planning.

Discussions between you and your clients regarding key identities need to happen early in treatment, using resources we provide in the *Skills for Getting Started* module. This information is then applied to choice of between-session practices. An important aspect of CBT conceptualizations and treatment approaches is the primary focus on person–environment fit. At their core, CBT principles of change are inherently focused on maximizing fit with a specific individual's strengths, limitations, and life circumstances. These facets of CBT will support your work with culturally diverse clients.

Age-Related Changes

Cognitive and Sensory Functioning

For individuals of all ages, there are important associations between depression and cognitive functioning (Wang & Blazer, 2015). Middle-aged and older adults are particularly likely to be aware of, and concerned by, various aspects of their brain health. Cognitive functioning and depression are bidirectionally related: Clinical depression can impair concentration and executive functioning, and neurocognitive disorders can lead to the development of later-life depression. Even in the absence of depression, several common changes in brain health occur with increasing age, and some middle-aged and older adults will present in primary care and behavioral health settings with cognitive concerns and complaints. Thus, there are good reasons for you to learn about and become comfortable discussing issues of brain health with your clients.

Variability in all types of processing, ranging from sensory input to high-level abstract thinking, increases with advanced age. Some individuals in their late 50s and early 60s are already showing signs of mild cognitive impairment (MCI) or even early degenerative dementia, while others in their late 80s or early 90s are still very effective in processing new information. Aging individuals may also evidence substantial variability within themselves. For example, one person may do extremely well on complex cognitive tasks, such as verbal abstract reasoning, and at the same time perform poorly on tasks requiring complex perceptual/spatial reasoning. Another person might perform exceptionally well on spatial reasoning problems but have very limited verbal and spatial memory. When working with clients who show such discrepancies, you may have to introduce modifications in therapy to minimize the effects of specific cognitive impairments and to maximize use of their cognitive strengths. Despite this increased variability (both across persons and within the same person), there are several consistent trends that require special attention by clinicians.

Background on Cognitive Aging

Despite societal myths and misconceptions, there are some realities to how our brains change over time. A basic understanding of cognitive aging will prepare you to share correct information with your clients and counter stereotypes that interfere with expectations for therapeutic progress (i.e., "older adults can't learn new things"). Older adults retain the cognitive abilities needed to function on a day-to-day basis. A seminal work from the Institute of Medicine (Blazer et al., 2015) has provided a careful "state-of-the-art" review of the research literature on normal cognitive aging. These main points, summarized in Box 2.1, reflect gradual changes from early to middle to later adulthood.

There are both age-related changes and areas of stability. Some attentional processes are impacted negatively by age (e.g., selective, divided) and others remain stable across adulthood (e.g., maintenance of sustained efforts). Throughout middle-aged and later years in healthy adults, some facets of memory show modest age-related declines (e.g., working, episodic, prospective, autobiographical, source), while other types of memory do not (e.g., procedural, semantic). This means that when your older clients insist that they still know how to do a well-rehearsed activity such as driving a car, they are factually correct. When older drivers become impaired, for example, it is not commonly due to their forgetting procedural aspects of how to drive (unless they have a neurocognitive disease that impacts memory in a significant way). It is the other complex aspects of driving that are more commonly impacted by age (e.g., reaction times, decision-making), especially medical conditions that are more common in older adults (e.g., limited physical range of motion, reduced sensation of gas and brake pedals due to diabetic neuropathy, or impaired judgment linked to a neurocognitive disorder). In the driving example, healthy older adults demonstrate the ability to accommodate to slower reaction times through behavioral strategies such as limiting nighttime driving, driving within the speed limit, scanning farther down the road, and checking side/rearview mirrors more frequently than younger adults. This is a nice example of "selective optimization with compensation" that is the hallmark of healthy and successful aging (Baltes & Freund, 2003).

Many older adults focus on memory as the most important sign of brain wellness, yet other aspects of cognitive functioning are also central to daily functioning. The role of our frontal lobes in planning, organizing, and decision-making is very important. These are called "executive functions" because they involve key skills that we need to manage daily life and respond to unexpected challenges, just like the chief executive officer (CEO) of a business does. Modest declines in executive functioning have been documented with age, creating some difficulties with particularly complicated tasks (e.g., driving, financial planning, complex medication management). As noted earlier, most healthy older adults develop compensatory strategies for responding to these changes. Aging individuals are also likely to have the benefits of increased social-emotional intelligence and a repository of past successful coping efforts that can be drawn upon. It is usually in the face of comorbid medical and psychiatric difficulties, including depression, that these normal age-related changes create problems in daily life.

Some of the clinical implications of these age-related changes are:

1. More time needed to process and react to new information and changes
2. Increased distractibility; easier to lose one's train of thought and move from topic to topic unintentionally
3. More time needed to switch from one topic or source of information to another
4. More difficulty thinking about and solving complex problems "in one's head"; increasingly important to write things down as a way to think about and process information
5. Memory for past and recent events, along with those planned for the future, is less reliable; need for calendar to track appointments and events, written logs/records of clinically important material
6. Recognition memory and cued recall are retained better than memory as assessed by free recall; using written materials within and between sessions is important.

Slowed Motor Response

Slowing of motor response speed is perhaps one of the earliest and most profound changes observed, starting in young adulthood and continuing through the remainder of the lifespan. Changes within the young adult range are minimal and seldom noticed, except in professional athletes. As individuals move into their mid- to late 60s, slowing of responses is notable in many different daily tasks, and adaptations are often required to maintain effective performance levels.

Decline in Sensory Functioning

Aging individuals often complain of decreased visual acuity. Increased time may also be required to scan and attend to visual details that are important for accurate appraisal of real-life situations. Increased problems in hearing verbal material correctly are extremely common in the later years. Studies indicate that both high and low frequencies are more difficult to detect, which can distort the specific phonemes characterizing some spoken words.

There also appears to be an attentional component that contributes to aging individuals' difficulty in understanding complex verbal material. Older adults may ask others to repeat statements in order to understand what is being said, particularly in situations where there is a high level of background noise (e.g., unstructured social gatherings). Within psychotherapy and primary care sessions, directing someone's attention by using their name first, before providing key information, can be very useful. Alerting the person to pay attention improves comprehension substantially, although your clients may habitually continue to ask you to repeat the information. Your using the client's name in session to focus attention also allows clients some additional time to process information and develop an appropriate response.

Changes in other sensory modalities are not as critical for cognitive processing but nevertheless are important for your clients' general welfare. Decreased ability to taste and smell can change food preferences, which may result in inadequate nutrition and a clear loss of pleasure obtained from eating. Changes in sensory input from the joint and muscle feedback systems and from the vestibular system can influence the ability to adjust posture and maintain optimal balance following rapid movements. Compensatory adjustments in the type and speed of ambulatory movements are often required. Changes of this nature could lead to a decreased quality of life and increased emotional distress for your clients if adequate coping strategies are not in place.

Retained Cognitive Abilities, Including Social Reasoning

Not all cognitive abilities decline during the late-adult years (Blazer et al., 2015). Those that rely heavily on highly over-learned information and that do not require rapid decision-making or complex motor responses show little change and in fact often increase over time—such as social skills and general fund of information. On the other hand, the ability to comprehend and use complex abstract information, either verbal or spatial in nature, decreases in the later years (as noted earlier), and this change is accentuated if complex rapid responding is required.

This general pattern has implications when working with older adults in psychotherapy. As many of us do in social situations, *you might inaccurately judge your clients' ability to understand and deal with complex cognitive material based on their social reasoning capability and social interaction skills.* As many social skills either hold up or increase across time, you might *over*estimate your clients' ability to understand and deal with more abstract materials. In such cases, you can end up setting the level of difficulty for materials presented in session and out-of-session practice too high, resulting in poor performance and increased stress on the part of your aging clients.

Conclusion

Knowledge of healthy aging helps you work collaboratively with your clients to set appropriate expectations for progress, make smart decisions about treatment planning and within-session adaptations, and gauge when termination of treatment is clinically appropriate. Because of the many factors described in this chapter, assessment is very important in your work with aging adults. Clinicians who work with this population of middle-aged and older adults are required to become familiar and comfortable with assessment, and they typically assess across a wider range of functioning than is required for working with younger adults. Chapter 3 of this clinician guide provides an overview of assessment issues and specific recommendations.

CHAPTER 3 — Assessment with Aging Individuals

In this treatment approach, assessment begins early and continues throughout, until termination. We understand that clinicians have limited time available to engage in formal assessment practices, so our recommendations are intended to be as straightforward as possible and useful across different practice settings.

This chapter is organized into four sections. The first three are considered core practices, with the fourth section outlining assessment tools and practices that may be applicable for specific clients. Appendix D includes measures ready for you to use with your clients; these are listed at the end of this chapter. Our suggestions include:

- Basic intake assessment (a 45-minute session)
- Eligibility for treatment and need for additional referrals
- Ongoing practices for feedback-informed treatment
- Optional assessment tools for personalized modules

You may also have a broader range of assessment-related interests and questions that are beyond the scope of this chapter. Fortunately, there are a number of excellent resources on assessment that can inform your clinical work with aging individuals (Knight & Pachana, 2015; Lichtenberg, 2010; Lichtenberg et al., 2015).

Basic Intake Assessment

When scheduling the assessment interview, it is important to remind clients to bring their glasses and/or hearing aids and any other devices or supports needed to be able to respond to your questions. Clients may have other things they need to bring with them for the interview. Individuals with diabetes, for example, may need to bring juice or special food to eat if they experience a drop in blood sugar. Many aging individuals (especially those on multiple medications) need to bring water and their pills with them so that they can remain "on schedule" with their medication regimen. Ask your new clients to bring a list of medications, including the name, dose, time to be taken, and what each drug was prescribed for. It is also important to ask them to bring the name, address, and phone number of their primary care physician (PCP) and any other specialists with whom they have regular contact. This will allow you to ask clients to sign a release of information permitting you to communicate with their medical team. Additional suggestions for interview assessments of older adults are provided by Gerolimatos and colleagues (2014).

Beginning the Intake Session

At the intake, remind clients to use their assistive devices. Ensure that the meeting area is reasonably quiet and free from distraction and has a comfortable workspace (e.g., desk or table for writing) that has sufficient light. Compared to younger clients, many older individuals are less able to balance a clipboard on their lap while completing assessment forms. Keep in mind that evaluation can be threatening, particularly for those with little formal education and/or who are showing evidence of at least mild cognitive impairment. Thus, it is helpful to reassure clients that the reason you are doing this is to enable you to develop a better, more effective plan for their treatment.

Early on, ask your clients how they wish to be addressed and keep in mind how cultural diversity can affect these preferences. Any paper-and-pencil intake forms you use should explicitly ask about sexual orientation, gender identity, and preferred pronouns, and provide options for "Married/Partnered" rather than simply "Married." Such small but important details go a long way toward communicating your sensitivity to the needs of LGBTQ+ clients (Warren & Steffen, 2020). Many clients from ethnic minority groups prefer that you use formal titles such as "Mrs." or "Mr." or "Dr." as a way for you to be respectful, so start formal and wait for their direct invitation before using their first name. If you have a doctoral degree, clients may wish to call you "Dr. So-and-so" and not use your first name (again, as a sign of respect).

Including Family or Other Collateral Sources

Interviews with family members, significant others, friends, and other possible informants are highly recommended if the client grants permission. Obtaining others' evaluations of your client's strengths and weaknesses and general behavioral characteristics can be extremely helpful in your therapy work (Glover & Srinivasan, 2017). If assessments have been completed elsewhere, it will be helpful and save time to review and become familiar with as much information as possible before your first session. If clients wish to bring a family member to the appointment, we generally agree to that; some clients may be unreliable in giving their own history. The family member can often present multiple aspects of the problem, from their perspective, that can be informative for therapy. Ask your clients if they prefer to have the family member in the room or not. Be sure to obtain the client's expressed permission to include the family member in the meeting. This should be documented in your records as well.

In cases where a family member accompanies the client to their first appointment, it is generally fine to begin with the family member there, and then at some point offer clients the opportunity to have an individual, private interview while the family member returns to the waiting room. This is especially helpful prior to beginning the "formal" assessment procedures. Family members are most helpful for obtaining an accurate history but are very distracting once evaluation measures are being administered. If they remain in the room, they often answer "for the client," which is not what you are after.

During the Intake Assessment Session

You have several goals at this point. Importantly, you want to confirm that the client is appropriate for this treatment approach. You will need to determine the extent of interprofessional collaboration that may be indicated for client care, while also starting the process of engaging the client in treatment planning. Assessment of *emotional, cognitive, and functional status, along with personal strengths*, is recommended prior to beginning CBT with aging individuals. This provides a clear understanding of the client's main problems *and* enables you to determine whether or not this individual is a suitable candidate for CBT. It is usually possible to obtain a *brief* psychosocial and psychiatric history, obtain some basic information about medical status, and administer a few screening measures during this initial appointment. Because most clinicians do not have a great deal of time for this, we briefly present recommended measures (i.e., rationale for inclusion, where to find them, scoring, and interpretation) for the essential areas of assessment as shown in Table 3.1. This table also includes several online assessment resources (i.e., completed and scored online or as downloadable PDFs).

Table 3.1 List of Recommended Measures

Assessment Domain	Measure	Where to Find
Depression	Geriatric Depression Scale-Short Form (GDS-SF)	Appendix D https://web.stanford.edu/ ~yesavage/GDS.html
	PHQ-9	https://www.phqscreeners.com
Anxiety	GAD-7	Appendix D https://www.phqscreeners.com
Therapeutic Alliance	Agnew Relationship Measure-5 (ARM-5)	Appendix D
Suicide Risk	No Prior History	http://cssrs.columbia.edu/
	Columbia Suicide Severity Rating Scale: Screen Version-Recent (C-SSRS-Screener-Recent-with Triage)	
	Prior History	
	SAFE-T Protocol with C-SSRS (Columbia Risk and Protective Factors) Lifetime/Recent	

Table 3.1 Continued

Assessment Domain	Measure	Where to Find
Health	PROMIS Scale v1.2 Global Health	https://www.healthmeasures.net/
Functional Impairment	Instrumental Activities of Daily Living (IADL)	http://www.acsu.buffalo.edu/ ~drstall/iadl.html
Cognitive Impairment	Mini-Cog	https://mini-cog.com
	AD8	Appendix D
Elder Abuse Risk	Elder Abuse Suspicion Index (EASI)	Appendix D
Alcohol Abuse Risk	Short Michigan Alcoholism Screening Test-Geriatric Version (SMAST-G)	Appendix D
Strengths	Personal Strengths and Values	Workbook; Start 5 Practice
Positive Events	California Older Person's Positive Experiences Schedule-Revised (COPPES-R)	Scoring information and instructions provided in Appendix C; COPPES-R provided in workbook. An online administration and scoring tool is available at www.optimalagingcenter.com
Pain Interference	PROMIS Adult Short Form v1.0—Pain Interference 6b	https://www.healthmeasures.net/
Sleep Anxiety	Glasgow Sleep Effort Scale	Appendix D
Caregiving	Caregiving Intake Assessment Interview	Appendix D
	REACH II Risk Appraisal Measure (RAM)	Appendix D
	Caregiver Abuse Screen (CASE)	Appendix D
	Neuropsychiatric Inventory Questionnaire	NPItest.net
	Caregiver Self-Assessment Questionnaire	https://www.healthinaging.org/tools-and-tips/caregiver-self-assessment-questionnaire

(continued)

Table 3.1 Continued

Assessment Domain	Measure	Where to Find
Grief	Traumatic Grief Inventory-SR (TGI-SR)	Appendix D
	Brief Unfinished Business in Bereavement Scale (Brief UBBS)	Appendix D

<u>**Online Assessment Tools**</u>

American Psychiatric Association's site of downloadable measures to assess a range of symptoms and problems: https://www.psychiatry.org/psychiatrists/practice/dsm/educational-resources/assessment-measures

Mental Health America's site of screening tools that can be completed and scored online: https://screening.mhanational.org/screening-tools

Assessment of Depression

Detailed information about the assessment of psychopathology via self-report scales can be found in several excellent reviews (Brown & Astell, 2012; Edelstein & Segal, 2011; Hinrichsen, 2020; Lutz et al., 2018), including recommendations for working with culturally diverse older populations (Samarina et al., 2021). We recommend use of one of these two depression scales in your practice: the Geriatric Depression Scale—Short Form (GDS-SF; Sheikh & Yesavage, 1986) and the Patient Health Questionnaire-9 (PHQ-9; Kroenke et al., 2001). Both have their own pluses and minuses and may have different uses for clinicians in different settings. Both are sensitive to change over time and thus are useful tools to routinely monitor treatment response.

GDS-SF

The GDS was designed specifically for use with older adults and is available in multiple languages and at no cost. Versions containing 30 or 15 items are available as either paper-and-pencil hard copies or as apps for the iPhone and Android (30-item version: Yesavage et al., 1983; 15-item short form: Sheikh & Yesavage, 1986). Compared to other depression scales, most somatic items have been removed, and all forms of the GDS use a simple "yes/no" response format. These features are advantages for two reasons: (1) the response format allows the GDS to be completed even by those with mild cognitive impairment and (2) lack of somatic items means the GDS taps into the psychological aspects of depression in detail and does not overestimate depression in clients with chronic health conditions. There are not, however, any items that screen for suicidal wishes or behaviors, so it is important to screen separately for that. Because of its strong psychometric qualities and clinical utility (Friedman et al., 2005; Mitchell et al., 2010; Pocklington et al., 2016), the GDS-SF is an excellent fit in community practice and primary care settings. It takes most older clients 2 to 5 minutes to complete (Smarr et al., 2011). We provide a user-ready copy of the GDS-SF in Appendix D. Items are scored 1 when the response is in the direction of indicating depression; total scores of 5 or more are indicative of depression and the need for further evaluation. Further information, including scoring and interpretation, is available at https://web.stanford.edu/~yesavage/GDS.html.

PHQ-9

The Patient Health Questionnaire (PHQ) includes a nine-item scale to assess the frequency of a wide range of depressive symptoms (PHQ-9), using a multiple-choice response format. It contains a suicide screening question as well as a question on how endorsed symptoms have affected the client's functioning, making it more in alignment with typical DSM-5 criteria. It is commonly used as a screening tool in health care settings. This scale is copyrighted by Pfizer, Inc., but is a public-domain resource, with no fees or permissions needed by clinicians to use or photocopy the measure (https://www.phqscreeners.com). The PHQ-9 has been translated into multiple languages and validated for international use. There is an ultra-brief two-item version (PHQ-2) used to screen for depression in some medical settings, but we recommend the nine-item scale for behavioral health clinicians working with clients being considered for treatment. The PHQ-9 has nine items, each of which is scored 0 to 3, providing a total score that ranges from 0 to 27. Scores of 5, 10, 15, and 20 represent cut points for mild, moderate, moderately severe, and severe depression, respectively.

Assessment of Anxiety

Anxiety frequently co-occurs with depression in aging individuals. About half of those with depression report symptoms of anxiety, including physiological (e.g., upset stomach and heart fluttering, which are identified as signs of tension rather than due to medical causes) and psychological (e.g., worry, fear, and mental tension). Depression that includes co-occurring anxiety symptoms is often more chronic and difficult to treat, with more somatic symptoms and social and functional impairments, and higher suicide risk (Petkus et al., 2013). For these reasons, we recommend that all clients be screened for anxiety as a part of planning depression treatment. Current cohorts of aging individuals do not generally use "anxiety" or "anxious" as terms to describe their experiences and symptoms; instead, age-appropriate adjectives include terms such as "tense," "tension," "nerves," "nervous," "jittery," and "worried." This choice of wording is reflected in our recommendation of the Generalized Anxiety Disorder seven-item scale (GAD-7).

Similar to the PHQ-9, the GAD-7 is copyrighted by Pfizer, Inc., but it is a public-domain resource, with no fees or permissions needed by clinicians to use or photocopy the measure (https://www.phqscreeners.com). It is used to screen for anxiety symptoms, with individuals selecting a severity rating for each item in the past 2 weeks. The GAD-7 has demonstrated strong psychometric properties in primary care and community settings and for use with older adults (Wild et al., 2014). Seven items, each of which is scored 0 to 3, provide a total severity score of 0 to 21. Scores of 5, 10, and 15 represent cut points for mild, moderate, and severe anxiety, respectively. Scores of 10 or greater suggest need for further evaluation.

Assessment of Suicide Risk

We recommend a brief formal evaluation of suicide risk at the beginning of your intake session for very important reasons. If a client is currently at moderate to high risk, you want to know this as early in the session as possible. *Addressing this risk will require the full session and will take priority over any other part of your assessment process.* You likely know at the start of your intake session that your client is experiencing some symptoms of depression, but you may not yet have clear information about their suicide risk. Sometimes clients are reluctant to bring up suicidal thoughts during the first contact with you because they do not wish to be turned away from therapy. Strong risk factors for suicidality include status as an older White male, along with change in functional abilities and onset of new disabilities, which are common concerns that bring older adults into treatment for depression (Lutz & Fiske, 2018). Global suicide rates for older adults are high (Sachs-Ericsson et al., 2016), and you have a responsibility to directly assess suicidal thoughts and behaviors using validated screening tools (Dennis & Brown, 2011).

Toward the start of your intake session, you can say something like:

We will spend our session today in several different ways. I want to hear more about the problems you are having that led you to consider treatment for your depression. There are also several areas of life that I'd like us to talk through, using questions that I ask all clients. So that is how we will start. Sometimes people feel so bad that they wish they were dead or have thoughts about ending their life.

Then launch immediately into a formal structured suicide risk assessment measure.

Columbia Suicide Severity Rating Scale: Screen Version-Recent

This scale is from the Columbia Lighthouse Project and has several different versions plus online trainings for professionals (http://cssrs.columbia.edu/). Of the screening tools they provide, we suggest the Columbia Suicide Severity Rating Scale: Screen Version-Recent (C-SSRS-Screener-Recent-with Triage) for use with most clients without a known history of suicidal ideation or behaviors. This version includes questions about suicidal ideation in the past month and suicidal behaviors across the individual's lifetime. When clients endorse specific items, follow-up questions are asked to determine current level of risk. Printing this scale in color allows you to use their triage colors to evaluate current risk as low, moderate, or high. In clients at low risk, this screener takes less than 5 minutes to complete together.

SAFE-T Protocol with C-SSRS Lifetime/Recent

When you already know that the person you are assessing has a previous history of suicidal ideation and/or behaviors, or you have determined using a screener that a client is at moderate or high risk, then we suggest use of the SAFE-T Protocol with C-SSRS (Columbia Risk and Protective Factors) Lifetime/Recent, also available at the Columbia site (http://cssrs.columbia.edu/). This version provides you with clinically rich information that helps you begin the work of risk reduction.

Treatment Decisions Related to Suicidal Risk

You are likely to use our treatment approach with clients who have some current or past history of suicidal ideation. However, when the process we have described leads to your evaluating a client as at a moderate to high risk for suicide, then you would *not* begin therapy with our treatment approach. Instead, it is important to target the suicidal symptoms directly in therapy using an evidence-based treatment for suicide risk reduction (Dennis & Brown, 2011). Although considered appropriate in the past, treating depression and seeing a reduction in other depressive symptoms is no longer considered evidence-based practice for treating suicidality.

In the United States, the Joint Commission is responsible for accrediting hospitals and acute-care settings. In their National Patient Safety Goal 15.01.01 for patients in psychiatric hospitals as well as those being treated for emotional or behavioral disorders in general hospitals, the Joint Commission lists three specific treatments as effective and recommended: Cognitive Behavioral Therapy for Suicide Prevention (CBT-SP: Bryan & Rudd, 2018; Wenzel et al., 2009), Dialectical Behavior Therapy (DBT; Linehan, 2015), and Collaborative Assessment Method for Suicidality (CAMS; Jobes, 2016). Clinicians who are already fully trained in DBT can use that approach for managing suicidality in aging individuals. Similarly, if you are already trained and functioning as a CBT clinician, then using one of the CBT protocols developed specifically for suicidality is appropriate (CBT-SP: Bryan & Rudd, 2018; Wenzel et al., 2009). For all other clinicians, we suggest using the CAMS in light of the detailed guidance available through the CAMS workbook (Jobes, 2016) and the professional training site (https://cams-care.com). If your training and experience have not prepared you to work with suicidal individuals, consult with your clinical supervisor and/or follow whatever protocol is in place at your facility or agency for handling clients who are acutely suicidal

When the client's suicide risk is assessed as low on the basis of your screening assessment, you can continue to evaluate eligibility for treatment using our approach.

Medical History, Medications, and Functional Impairments

Older clients typically have a number of medical problems that need to be considered when developing therapeutic goals. Many clients' psychological distress can be due to some aspect of their physical condition, medications they are taking, and/or medical interventions they must undergo. It is extremely useful to become aware of your clients' medical status, diagnoses, functional limitations associated with these diagnoses, and current medications prescribed. As a part of your intake assessment, record all medications, including name, dose, time to be taken, and what each drug was prescribed for. For most clients, it will be useful to forge an alliance with their PCP, and consider consulting with other medical specialists who might be involved in their care. Some of your aging clients may be followed by a multidisciplinary or interdisciplinary team comprising allied health professionals as well as medical specialists (Decaporale-Ryan et al., in press; Steffen et al., 2015; Steffen & Zeiss, 2017). In this instance, it is helpful to consult with other professionals in the team, which might include physical and occupational clinicians, neuropsychologists, social workers, and nurse specialists.

PROMIS Scale v1.2 Global Health

The HealthMeasures resource is supported by the National Institutes of Health to provide state-of-the-art assessment tools in the areas of physical, mental, and social health. We suggest that you use their Global Health scale, which can be completed via self-report by clients ahead of the intake assessment session. The 10 items capture a broad range of concerns, including quality of life, physical health, pain, fatigue, social activities, and functional limitations. All of the scales are available to download and use (https://www.healthmeasures.net/). Clinicians can obtain this scale by selecting the following options: Age = Adult, Category = Global & Multiple, Measure Type = Fixed Length Short Form, System = PROMIS.

Instrumental Activities of Daily Living

When clients appear to be significantly impaired in their ability to care for themselves or take care of everyday activities of daily living (ADLs), there probably is a designated "caregiver" who provides this care. It is recommended to have that person complete one or more of the scales assessing functional dependence/independence, such as the Instrumental Activities of Daily Living scale (Lawton & Brody, 1969; download free from http://www.acsu.buffalo.edu/~drstall/iadl.html), to provide information that is relevant for treatment planning.

Screening for Cognitive Impairment

Assessing cognitive functioning is critical due to the significant impact it can have on clients' overall functioning and ability to participate in, and benefit from, CBT. Many clinicians find themselves uncertain as to how to work with someone with suspected, but not diagnosed, cognitive limitations. With cognitive limitations come additional concerns about individuals' capacity for decision-making (Moye et al., 2013) as well as risk for being a victim of elder abuse. Fortunately, there are some excellent no-cost resources available to guide clinicians through these often murky waters. We suggest using either the Mini-Cog© or the AD8 to screen for cognitive impairment and the EASI as a screener for elder abuse. Additional suggestions for administration of cognitive screeners and brief assessments via telemental health sessions are available in the professional literature (Castanho et al., 2014; Zietemann et al., 2017).

Mini-Cog

The Mini-Cog is a very brief (3-minute) screening test to help detect cognitive impairment in aging individuals; it has been effectively used in a range of health care and community settings (Holsinger et al., 2012). It consists of two components, a three-item recall test for memory and a simply scored clock-drawing test. Points from these two elements are added for a total score that ranges from 0 to 5. A total score of 3 or higher suggests a lower likelihood of a neurocognitive disorder but does not rule out some degree of cognitive impairment. An important limitation is that this measure captures a client's abilities at the time of assessment but does not ask about change over time. The Mini-Cog is available for use by clinicians free of charge and can be downloaded from the website that also includes instructions for administration, scoring, and interpretation (https://mini-cog.com). Due to the clock-drawing component, it can be administered in telehealth sessions that use video, but not via telephone.

AD8

The AD8 (Galvin et al., 2005) is a questionnaire that asks eight questions about observed changes in cognitive functioning (memory, orientation, and executive functioning) over the past several years. Responses are yes, no, or I don't know. It takes no more than 3 minutes for most individuals to complete. There are several advantages to the AD8. You can ask clients to complete it on their own, prior to the intake assessment, and then review and discuss together. It can also be used as an informant-based assessment in which you ask someone other than the client (usually a spouse/partner, child, or non-family caregiver) to assess whether there have been changes in the past few years in certain areas of cognition and functioning. Because of the nature of yes/no response choices, it is appropriate for administration in both videoconference and telephone sessions. When two or more items indicate a change, then further evaluation is suggested. We provide a copy of the AD8 in Appendix D.

Cognitive Assessment Referrals and Additional Resources

As screening tests, neither the Mini-Cog nor the AD8 is a substitute for a complete diagnostic workup. When your initial assessment of a client raises concerns about cognitive functioning, then referral to that client's PCP is indicated (or to a geriatrician, if the client does not have a PCP). For additional information about screening and referrals for cognitive concerns, there are some excellent resources provided within the KAER Toolkit developed by the Gerontological Society of America (https://www.geron.org/images/gsa/kaer/gsa-kaer-toolkit.pdf). KAER stands for the steps involved in this approach: **K**ickstart, **A**ssess, **E**valuate, and **R**efer. The appendices within the KAER Toolkit include handouts to use with clients and family members and step-by-step guidance for staying within your own scope of practice while connecting clients to additional resources. We provide additional suggestions and resources for working with cognitively impaired clients in Chapter 11 of this guide and within our *Skills for Brain Health* module of treatment.

Risk for Elder Abuse

The Elder Abuse Suspicion Index (EASI-sa; Yaffe et al., 2012) is a self-report measure developed to screen for elder abuse in primary care. Use of this scale can help you determine whether it might be reasonable to propose a referral for further evaluation by social services, adult protective services, or equivalents. This can be administered as a paper-and-pencil self-report measure or during an interview. All six questions should be asked; a response of "yes" on one or more of Questions 2 through 6 may establish concern. We provide a copy of the EASI-sa in Appendix D.

Alcohol and Other Substance Misuse

Alcohol or other substance abuse or misuse can be a source of numerous problems, including behavioral disturbances, cognitive problems including delirium, and affective changes (Blow & Barry, 2012). Brief assessment for alcohol problems is recommended whenever depression is present, as alcohol can be used to self-medicate, and problems with it can be more difficult to detect in older adults. Many older problem drinkers are widowed or divorced, retired, and not driving as frequently, so the probability of their problem being detected by others is reduced. We recommend using the Michigan Alcoholism Screening Test— Geriatric version (MAST-G). The Short MAST-G (SMAST-G; Blow et al., 1998; Blow & Barry, 2012) is a 10-item self-report scale using yes/no responses. This scale asks about thoughts and behaviors related to possible alcohol abuse. These "face valid" items seem to encourage honest responses on the part of older adults. Both clinicians and clients find that this is a respectful way to screen for alcohol-related concerns. Responses of "yes" are scored as 1 and then totaled. Two or more "yes" responses indicate a possible alcohol misuse problem. We provide a copy of the SMAST-G in Appendix D.

Aging individuals who are depressed may inadvertently misuse medications. "Street drugs" are less often used by aging individuals, although as the baby boomer generation ages, we are likely to see increasing rates of cannabis misuse in depressed clients. More commonly, errors in complying with often complex medication regimens can result in unexpected negative side effects such as cognitive confusion, difficulties concentrating, and changes in mood. Most emergency department visits by older adults that involve substances are due to accidental misuse of prescription and over-the-counter medications (Arnold, 2008). In addition, some aging individuals consciously abuse prescription medications such as painkillers and anti-anxiety medications. This complex topic is beyond the scope of this guide, but we mention this to sensitize you to the importance of collecting information about what medications are being taken on a regular basis. This helps you be alert to possible problems in this area, which then require referral to a medical professional for appropriate evaluation and treatment.

Strengths Assessment

The CBT conceptual model and treatment approach both emphasize the importance of attention to clients' personal strengths and competencies. As we note throughout this guide, a key role of the clinician is to help remind clients of their personal strengths, which have been demonstrated through past successful coping efforts. These strengths are then used as the foundation of further skill development. For all of these reasons, it is important to include attention to personal strengths and values as a part of your early work with clients. Once you begin therapy, we recommend using <u>Start 10 Learn: Your Life Values and Personal Strengths</u> and <u>Start 5 Practice: My Values and Strengths</u> from the workbook for a strengths-based assessment.

Eligibility for Treatment and Need for Additional Referrals

Eligibility for Treatment

Taken together, the results from these assessments will typically enable you to decide if this is a suitable client for CBT—that is, someone who is likely to benefit, given the profile of people who have benefited in previous research studies. Here is a checklist that we use in our practice to help us decide on the next steps in the process:

- ✓ Are the intensity and severity of the depression manageable on an outpatient basis? Most importantly, is the client expressing strong suicidal ideation, or wishes, and/or a definite plan that appears imminent, such that immediate hospitalization or another form of urgent care is needed?
- ✓ Can the client adequately process information?
- ✓ Is the client physically well enough to attend sessions on a regular basis?
- ✓ Are there family conflicts and strains likely to interfere with the client's participation in treatment (e.g., are there lots of family crises that the client feels must be attended to first?)
- ✓ What other problems have you detected in addition to depression?
- ✓ Is concurrent treatment (e.g., pharmacotherapy) indicated?

Referrals for More Extensive Evaluation

Referrals may be indicated if there are questions/concerns raised during the intake process that require additional expertise. For example, if there are concerns about the interaction of depressive symptoms with medical issues and/or medications, asking the client to see their PCP for further clarification and your own follow-up with the PCP will be informative for treatment planning. In any case, usually CBT can proceed at the same time as these additional evaluations are taking place as long as there is a mechanism for sharing information learned. For this, a signed informed consent allowing you to communicate with the specialists, PCP, or team members is usually required (unless you are in a health care system with shared electronic medical records, in which case all providers can access all medical records of a given patient).

Assuming the decision (by both parties) is to move forward, end the session by setting up the first CBT appointment. Writing it down for the client, along with giving your card, can help to facilitate memory and compliance.

Ongoing Practices for Feedback-Informed Treatment

There is a firm expectation that you use a planned and individualized assessment approach to routinely monitor a client's progress toward their own unique targeted outcomes. This is assessment with a little "a," involving procedures that take no more than 5 minutes and are easy to use routinely. Feedback-informed treatment provides encouragement, helps maintain focus, and allows you to make adjustments to treatment depending upon that information (Prescott et al., 2017). The research evidence supporting routine outcome monitoring is now so clear that this can be considered a part of ethical practice of psychotherapy (Muir et al., 2019).

Clinicians who have less experience in using standardized scales are sometimes reluctant to "bother" clients with formal assessment tools, especially when this involves repeated administration. Now is the time for us to relieve you of those concerns. We know from both the published scientific literature and our own clinical experiences that adults of all ages value the periodic opportunity to "see where they are at" in their depression treatment. Your clients are as interested in discussing patterns of change in their depression as cancer patients are interested in the results of the latest scan or tumor marker blood test. Medical patients who are working hard at managing their weight or blood sugar need the feedback provided by weekly weigh-ins or daily blood sugar readings. Those data help answer the question as to whether current efforts at engaging in healthy behaviors are working. The ability to see numbers change on a form or graph can be very encouraging! It is also critically important to monitor symptoms and evidence of change to identify when patients are *not* improving, or are in fact getting worse. Thus, routine outcome monitoring is a foundational component of this treatment approach. Because CBT for later-life depression is aimed at reducing depressive symptoms *and* improving quality of daily life, assessment across the course of treatment will focus on several different strategies.

Weekly Depression Assessment

Whether you have selected the GDS (long or short form) or the PHQ-9 to measure depressive symptoms during intake, you will then also use that same scale to monitor therapy progress. Some clinics already have routine assessment procedures using electronic devices (e.g., tablets); if that is the case for your clinic, you are already set! If your clinic has a procedure for checking clients in and collecting payment prior to each session, then have that staff member provide the scale on a clipboard for clients to complete and hand back to that staff member. This allows you to have that information as you begin the session. If your practice setting does not include reception staff, then we suggest that you have a table holding several clipboards with the scale. A sign on the wall, right above that table, can direct clients to take and complete the weekly form, which they will hand to you at the beginning of session. Telehealth sessions can begin with you assisting the client in completing the scale; display the items by sharing your screen and/or by reading each item aloud. You can score that measure in front of the client at the beginning of the session and discuss the pattern of scores (e.g., same, lower, higher) from previous weeks. You will also record the score in that session's progress note. Rather than focusing on week-by-week changes, you should focus on general patterns of scores over multiple weeks.

Ongoing Assessment of Individualized Treatment Goals

CBT also has a strong focus on identifying and routinely assessing individual-level (i.e., idiographic) concerns and treatment goals. In this treatment, you will help your clients track weekly (or each session) progress on personal treatment goals that have been developed collaboratively. After completing the *Skills for Getting Started* module, the first Practice form of each module provides clients and clinicians a structured way of doing this. By reviewing and rating their therapy goals regularly (and toward the beginning of sessions), aging clients are better able to sustain focus and less likely to get distracted by problems of the week. You can develop and use single-item ratings to capture what is most important for the individual client (e.g., *"On a scale from 1 to 10, how connected did you feel with at least one person over the past week?" "As you think about the past week, how strong is your belief that your life is meaningful, from 1 to 10?"*). This culturally sensitive and flexible approach fits well with the personal goals of individual clients. Tracking these personal goals on an ongoing basis helps you and your clients stay on track with change strategies (even when the change is increased acceptance of life's ups and downs!). Most older adults have experience with an illness or recovery from surgery in which they have been asked to use a 1-to-10 pain scale to rate their level of pain. Thus, single-item ratings in session are familiar, and the use of 1-to-10 scales makes intuitive sense.

Periodic Assessment of the Therapeutic Alliance

In contrast to routine symptom and goal-focused assessment, which is typically done either before or at the very beginning of a therapy session, periodic assessment of your clients' views of the therapeutic relationship is typically done right after a session has ended. In Appendix D, we provide a client-ready copy of the five-item version of the Agnew Relationship Measure (ARM-5; Cahill et al., 2012). Asking for (and being nondefensively receptive to) client feedback regarding the therapy relationship is a vital part of evidence-based practice (Tolin, 2016). At minimum, we suggest that you plan to do this at least once in the early phase of treatment (i.e., after session 3 or 4), several times in the middle phase of treatment (i.e., after sessions 10 and 16), and as you are beginning to move toward termination. This measure is best collected immediately after a therapy session has ended; clients can be provided with a copy of the ARM-5 on a clipboard and asked to complete it in the waiting room before leaving the clinical setting. Clients being treated via telehealth can be mailed the ARM-5 with a stamped return envelope. This allows some privacy and increases the likelihood of honest reporting of clients' current views of the therapy relationship. Their responses can then be discussed and processed in the following session and can be used to make any needed adjustments to the working relationship.

Optional Assessment Tools for Personalized Modules

Throughout this treatment approach, there will be occasions in which additional measures will be useful clinically. In this section, we highlight those assessments that we have included in Appendix D and the client workbook.

Measures to Enhance Daily Functioning

California Older Person's Positive Experiences Schedule-Revised (COPPES-R)

Most depressed older adults significantly reduce their frequency of engagement in everyday positive activities due to feeling down and uninvolved in life. Some would like to do more of what they think will make them feel better but are unsure about where to start and how to get going. In either case, it is helpful for clients to reflect on the kinds of activities they would probably enjoy doing at this point in their lives, emphasizing small things (watching a favorite TV show, enjoying a special cup of tea, talking on the phone with a friend) that can be done with minimal resources. Often clients cannot think of things on their own that are do-able and that improve mood, and so they benefit from completing the COPPES-R (Rider et al., 2016) to help "prime the pump." This measure contains 46 items covering a broad range of simple everyday activities, such as "listening to sounds of nature." Chapter 8 discusses how to use the COPPES-R as a part of the *Skills for Doing* module. Full instructions for administration and interpretation are provided in Appendix C of this clinician guide, with an online administration and scoring tool provided at www.optimalagingcenter. com. The actual COPPES-R scale is provided in the client workbook.

PROMIS Adult Short Form v1.0—Pain Interference 6b

This scale measures an individual's perspective of how pain influences daily life and engagement with social, cognitive, emotional, physical, and recreational activities. The advantage is that this measure is not disease-specific, so it can be used with clients experiencing pain due to a number of different conditions. Items utilize a 7-day recall period ("the past 7 days"). This scale is available to download and use (https://www.healthmeasures.net/). You can obtain this scale by selecting the following options: Age = Adult, Category = Pain, Measure Type = Fixed Length Short Form, System = PROMIS.

Glasgow Sleep Effort Scale (GSES)

This self-report scale (Broomfield & Espie, 2005) allows clients to describe how much effort they are devoting to sleep; this is a common issue for individuals with insomnia. There are seven Likert-type items, and a higher total denotes greater sleep effort.

Measures of Caregiving Issues

Caregiving Intake Assessment Interview

Chapter 14 provides detailed instructions for how to use the *Skills for Caregiving* module with your clients. When working with clients who are family caregivers, there are a number of important domains to assess prior to engaging them in treatment around caregiving issues. Appendix D includes a structured interview specific to caregiving concerns.

REACH II Risk Appraisal Measure (RAM)

The RAM (Czaja et al., 2009) is a brief screening measure that systematically identifies needed areas of support for family caregivers of clients with dementia. Six areas with known relationships to caregiver risk and adverse outcomes are included: depression, burden, self-care and healthy behaviors, social support, safety, and client problem behaviors. Indicators allow clinicians to differentiate between moderate and high risk.

Caregiver Abuse Screen (CASE)

The CASE, a brief self-report abuse screen (Reis & Nahmiash, 1995), can be used with family caregivers. The items are worded in a way that minimizes defensiveness and provides a nice way to initiate conversations about concerning neglectful and abusive behaviors. Rather than using a cutoff score, caregivers should be queried about any "yes" response for more details to determine need for intervention, including mandated reporting.

Neuropsychiatric Inventory Questionnaire (NPI-Q)

The NPI-Q (Kaufer et al., 2000) is a self-administered question-naire that can be completed by caregivers about their family member with dementia. Most caregivers are able to complete this in 5 to 10 minutes. There are 12 domains of problems; caregivers first respond "yes" (problem is present) or "no" (problem is absent). If "yes," then the caregiver rates both the severity of the symptom present within the last month and the impact on them in terms of caregiver distress. This results in a total severity score and a caregiver distress score. The NPI-Q can be found at NPItest.net.

Caregiver Self-Assessment Questionnaire

This 18-item, caregiver self-report measure was devised by the American Medical Association as a means of helping physicians assess the stress levels of family caregivers accompanying chronically ill older adult patients to their medical visits (Epstein-Lubow et al., 2010). Caregivers are asked to respond either "yes" or "no" to a series of statements, such as "During the past week or so, I have felt completely overwhelmed" and "During the past week or so, I have felt strained between work and family responsibilities." This tool is available to download as a PDF and print out, or caregivers can complete it interactively online. The online version is then scored and interpreted, with recommendations provided to caregivers. It is available at

https://www.healthinaging.org/tools-and-tips/caregiver-self-assessment-questionnaire.

Measures of Grief

Traumatic Grief Inventory-SR

In Chapter 15, we describe how to use the *Living with Loss* module with clients who are experiencing distress following a range of losses. Use of this 18-item self-report measure can help you evaluate if clients are experiencing a grief reaction that requires specialized treatment for complicated grief. The responses vary from 1 (never) to 5 (always). All items are summed, and a total score of 54 or greater can be used to indicate clinically significant grief that merits specialized intervention (Boelen et al., 2019).

Brief Unfinished Business in Bereavement Scale (Brief UBBS)

As noted in the previous paragraph, in Chapter 15, we describe how to use the *Living with Loss* module with clients who are experiencing distress following a range of losses. The Brief UBBS (Holland et al., 2020) is a psychometrically validated scale that can be used to identify unresolved issues with the deceased, including both unfulfilled wishes and unresolved conflict. We provide the brief version of the scale in Appendix D. Average the ratings for a total UBBS (UBBS total score of 3.9 or higher is indicative of problematic levels of concerns). For the Unfulfilled Wishes subscale, average items 1, 3, 5, and 7 (a subscale score of 4.8 or higher is indicative of problematic levels). For the Unresolved Conflict subscale, average items 2, 4, 6, and 8 (a subscale score of 3.4 or higher is indicative of problematic levels).

Clinicians with less experience using standardized assessment tools routinely in clinical practice sometimes worry that they will overwhelm their clients, will become overwhelmed themselves, or both. As described in Chapter 2, individuals become more different from each other as they age, and it is our professional responsibility to "assess more than guess." This process of conducting a careful intake assessment, followed by routine monitoring of targeted outcomes for each client, is often very interesting to clients. They benefit from your feedback about their responses, so be sure that you are sharing this information (and in a way to enhance clinical effectiveness). Your use of standardized assessment strategies can also increase clients' confidence in the therapeutic relationship and lead to a stronger alliance.

CHAPTER 4

Cognitive-Behavioral Therapies 101

Some clinicians will use this treatment approach (i.e., workbook plus clinician guide) as a part of their ongoing CBT practice. Others will be interested in using the workbook and guide but have less background in behavioral and cognitive therapies. This chapter is intended to serve as a brief orientation to the CBTs across problem areas and populations, with recommendations for further professional development. Chapter 5 describes common modifications for middle-aged and older clients with depression.

Concepts That Unify Behavioral and Cognitive Therapies

There is no one CBT intervention, creating some confusion about what CBT is and what holds all of these approaches together. CBT theory and practice continue to evolve in a number of important ways (Karpiak et al., 2016). At its heart, CBT is a theoretical orientation to behavioral health and wellness that prioritizes scientific evidence while also being deeply humanistic in emphasizing transparency and collaboration between clients and clinicians throughout treatment. Due to the attention given to learning and developing skills, CBTs are very compatible with the stepped-care approach to behavioral health service delivery that we described in Chapter 1. Evidence-based CBT interventions have been developed for a range of delivery formats (e.g., bibliotherapy; internet; phone apps; telehealth; outpatient individual, couples, family, and group treatments; inpatient individual and group treatments) and for clients across the lifespan. With appropriate oversight and supervision by licensed behavioral health providers, some CBT interventions can be implemented by a range of behavioral health professionals with varied levels of training. The essence of CBT is seen in its biopsychosocial case conceptualization.

CBT Conceptual Model

Instead of thinking about CBT in terms of specific therapy strategies, we encourage you to see CBT as an orientation to treatment that uses a biopsychosocial conceptualization of problems and principles of change. Thus, the cognitive-behavioral model is first and foremost an approach to understanding each individual's symptoms and problems (i.e., individualized case conceptualization). This CBT model (i.e., theoretical orientation) focuses on a number of important questions for our work with clients:

- How did their problems develop?
- Once developed, what has led to these problems continuing into the present?
- How do cultural factors influence presenting problems and the therapy process?
- What should we assess?
- What focus should treatment take?
- After treatment ends, how do earlier changes stick over time?

As shown in Figure 4.1, four primary domains are emotional, physiological, behavioral, and cognitive, with the bidirectional arrows reflecting that each domain influences the others. Environment, a key additional consideration in this model, refers to the physical settings, interpersonal relationships, social settings, and cultural contexts of the client's experiences. Clients and their problems are considered in the context of their own unique learning history, along with their current social, cultural, and physical environments. Specific problems, for example, may be evident in close personal relationships but not manifested in professional relationships or at work. Rather than viewing all concerns as global and generalized across all of life, there is attention to how specific environments either support healthy functioning or are more likely to trigger problematic emotional, cognitive, behavioral, and physiological responses.

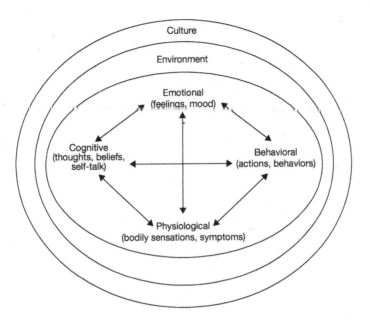

Figure 4.1

CBT Conceptual Model

The work of conceptualizing your client's presenting concerns involves considering how different situations and facets of their cultural, social, and physical environments impact the four areas. In this way, the CBT conceptual model is not simply intrapersonal but also transactional in nature. Presenting concerns, along with personal strengths and competencies, make sense in light of these interacting influences. There are a range of possible ways to implement a strengths-based perspective in CBT interventions with your clients (Padesky & Mooney, 2012).

This model's emphasis on personal learning history, focus on the role of environmental/societal contexts, and attention to personal strengths are some of the reasons that CBT works well with individuals from diverse cultural backgrounds (Iwamasa & Hays, 2018). We encourage clinicians to become familiar with the central CBT conceptual model before helping clients understand it in the *Skills for Getting Started* module. You will be applying this framework with clients, within the interventions you select and the language you use within sessions (Petrik et al., 2013).

Six "Think" Rules of CBT

In the 1980s, Kanfer and Schefft (1988) described six "think" rules that continue to work very well as an overview of what the CBTs all have in common:

1. *Think Behavior*—Work with clients to define problems and goals as specific behaviors instead of general or abstract concepts.
2. *Think Solution*—Encourage clients to consider what they can try before the next session to make the situation better.
3. *Think Positive*—Have clients identify their personal strengths and the positive aspects of any event or change effort, while validating their concerns and difficulties.
4. *Think Small Steps*—Assist clients in breaking larger goals into smaller pieces to increase likelihood of success and reward efforts.
5. *Think Flexible*—Spend time in session helping clients prepare for the unexpected and develop backup plans.
6. *Think Future*—Keep therapy focus on future events rather than the past and facilitate planning and rehearsal.

Developing and Maintaining a Therapeutic Relationship

We wish to echo Tolin's (2016) observation that as CBT clinicians, we are all aiming for good therapy relationships, good conceptualizations, and good technique (Figure 4.2).

Research on the importance of the therapeutic relationship has focused on three components of alliance between the client and clinician: (1) agreement on therapy goals, (2) agreement on therapy strategies, and (3) a warm, trusting relationship. The CBTs have a leg up on many other therapy approaches because of the strong emphasis on collaboratively and explicitly working with clients to develop agreement on therapy goals and the selection of specific change strategies. The CBTs also have a long history of emphasizing the importance of a warm collaborative therapy relationship (Okamoto et al., 2019). In fact, the largest research study in the United States evaluating the effectiveness of CBT for depression with younger and older veterans highlighted this.

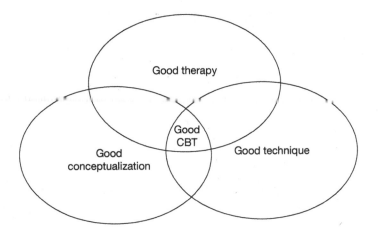

Figure 4.2

Good CBT

Client ratings of therapeutic alliance, especially agreement on the goals and strategies of therapy, were especially important predictors of positive therapy responses of older, compared to younger, veterans with depression (Karlin et al., 2015).

Using the *Skills for Getting Started* module, you will help your clients develop concrete and specific therapy goals. These goals will then be reviewed at the time of starting each new module in order to track therapy response and ensure continued focus on these goals. The structure of each therapy session, discussed later in this chapter, also facilitates the development of a strong therapeutic relationship. The collaborative nature of agenda setting emphasizes teamwork and the sense that "we are working on this together." A special feature of each CBT session is the end-of-session feedback, during which you specifically ask clients for feedback about what worked in that session and whether there was anything that you said or did that was upsetting or didn't work. This routine solicitation of feedback in CBT sessions (along with your nondefensive and curious responses to negative feedback) helps to prevent and heal ruptures in the therapeutic alliance, leading to stronger, warmer, and more effective therapeutic relationships (Castonguay et al., 2010).

As commonly found in other CBT interventions, when working with individuals or with closed/structured groups, your therapy for later-life depression will have four phases:

- The first phase is loosely referred to as "socializing the client into therapy" and usually takes two or three sessions. Using the resources in the *Skills for Getting Started* module, you elicit several primary complaints and work collaboratively with your clients to develop therapy goals to address these. You also educate your clients about the techniques used in therapy and what to expect. You place emphasis on describing clients' roles and responsibilities during the course of individual or group therapy.
- The second phase is the longest and focuses on helping your clients acquire the emotional, behavioral, and cognitive skills needed to meet their specific therapy goals.
- The third phase focuses on termination and how to maintain the gains obtained in therapy. Using resources from the *Skills for Wrapping Up* module, your clients will develop a "Maintenance Plan" to remind them of which skills can be most helpful in various stress-producing situations that are likely to occur. We also recommend that, for your individual psychotherapy clients, sessions be spaced further apart to strengthen self-efficacy and help your clients become less reliant on you and therapy sessions.
- In the final, fourth phase, having a few booster sessions at intervals of several months after therapy has ended can facilitate your clients' continued use of skills and thus lower the risk of relapse. It is also possible to build in and schedule individual booster sessions for clients who have completed a closed/structured group treatment; our experience does suggest that not all clients return for group booster sessions due to the complexity of scheduling a group of individuals.

Early Phase of Therapy

A number of tasks must be accomplished during the first few sessions if therapy is to be successful. These tasks can be grouped into three parts: (1) the initial clinical assessment, described in Chapter 3, (2) engaging your clients in therapy and enhancing motivation for compliance, and (3) collaboratively developing a case conceptualization, which provides the initial focus for clients' work within either individual or group treatment. When you are proactive in engaging and working collaboratively with your clients, you will enhance your work with clients from a variety of cultural backgrounds. Meta-analyses support this, showing that well-conducted therapy is equally effective for clients across a range of racial and ethnic groups (Ince et al., 2014). You will typically focus on all three of these tasks throughout the early phase, using *Skills for Getting Started* and the recommendations we discuss in Chapter 6 of this guide. You will work with your clients to identify a small number of problems (two or three at the most) and develop specific treatment goals that are observable and measurable.

Activities in the second component can be summarized as the "5 Es" for effectiveness:

- EASE your clients into a therapy mode. The process of psychotherapy is usually a unique experience for older individuals. They must acquire a new way of thinking and behaving as they become familiar with the expectations and procedures involved in CBT.
- ELICIT several target complaints (usually two or three at the outset), which are then used to develop specific treatment goals. You and your clients will work together to choose goals that can be attained within a relatively short period of time, depending on the usual practice parameters in your setting. Once established, goals should be prioritized so that items placed on session agendas have maximal relevance for your clients.
- EXPLAIN the CBT approach in a straightforward manner to help your clients understand how thoughts, feelings, and behaviors affect one another. It is also important that your clients indicate they understand this approach and want to participate.
- EMPHASIZE the importance of home practice; the empirical data clearly show that out-of-session practice facilitates the effectiveness of the therapy.
- ENCOURAGE your clients to continue in therapy by developing a strong empathic relationship and engendering a positive attitude about therapy outcomes.

The third component, formulation of a case conceptualization, continues throughout the first few sessions and is necessary to maximize the effectiveness of treatment. Therapy involves you and your clients working collaboratively to describe and understand patterns of feeling, thinking, and behaving. This is the first step to helping your clients strategically and systematically hold on to their existing positive coping responses while also targeting and developing new effective habits that fit their specific cultural, social, and physical environments. Work in one area (e.g., behaviors or thoughts) is expected to help shift your clients' experiences in other domains (e.g., feelings). Because the focus is on person–environment fit, sometimes therapy focuses on helping clients adapt their actions and thoughts to their environment. Other times, the emphasis is on helping clients change some facet(s) of their environment to better fit their abilities and needs. The case conceptualization is often changed during therapy as more relevant information becomes available, and this guides your treatment planning and implementation.

Middle Phase of Therapy

At this point, your clients should be acquainted with the general structure and procedures used in this CBT for depression in later life. You and your clients, working together, should have converted several target complaints into initial treatment goals and prioritized them by their importance and likelihood of achieving improvement in a reasonable, brief period of time. Once that is done, the middle phase of therapy begins, during which you help your clients develop key skills to address these goals. This phase is typically the longest: It can range from four to 20 additional sessions, depending on the client needs, resources, and organizational policy, as well as progress in attaining therapy goals. Closed structured groups most commonly last six to eight sessions. We provide several different suggested group treatment approaches in Appendix B.

This middle phase comprises the modules on emotion regulation (*Skills for Feeling*), behavioral activation and problem solving (*Skills for Doing*), self-compassion and cognitive reappraisal (*Skills for Thinking*), and any of the selected personalized modules. The middle phase of closed groups will vary depending upon the focus of that specific group, and these are likely to include a focus on behavioral activation and problem solving.

Before the conclusion of therapy, your clients should be familiar with behavioral activation and have experience tracking and increasing rewarding and valued daily activities. You also want your clients to have some experience applying the DEEDS problem-solving approach, described in Chapter 8 of this guide.

Across the various personalized modules, the amount of time spent on each section and the order in which they are covered will vary depending on the nature of your clients' problems and their characteristic ways of dealing with internal and interpersonal stress in their lives, as well as institutional policies and reimbursement patterns. If your clients can only have a small number of sessions at this point (i.e., four to six sessions), we recommend focusing on behavioral activation, as this component of CBT is extremely helpful in itself to reduce depressive symptoms. For many individuals with depression, behavioral activation is a sufficient standalone treatment.

Ending Phase of Therapy

Whether in structured, time-limited groups or within individual psychotherapy, your attention to termination issues is as important as the other phases of therapy. As described in Chapter 10 of this guide, *Skills for Wrapping Up* is considered a core required module. We provide within-session Learn pages and between-session Practice forms to maximize the likelihood that therapy gains can be maintained over time. The longer a specific client has been working with you in therapy, typically the more sessions are devoted to this process.

Clinical Skill Domains

You will be working with most (if not all) of your clients on the core skills of emotion regulation and managing arousal within session (*Skills for Feeling*), behavioral activation and problem solving (*Skills for Doing*), and cognitive reappraisal (*Skills for Thinking*). At the same time, the conceptualization shared by you and your clients is the hub that connects these core change strategies. The Revised Cognitive Rating Scale (CTS-R) was developed jointly by clinicians and researchers in the United Kingdom to help therapists develop and assess CBT competencies (Blackburn et al., 2001; James et al., 2001). Figure 4.3 shows that conceptualization is at the heart of the CTS-R, just as in therapy. This collaborative conceptualization focuses on how depression is manifested in the daily life of each of your clients and is developed and revised through guided discovery. The Learn pages and Practice forms facilitate an emphasis on guided discovery both within and between sessions.

What is also evident from this model is the pivotal role for your use of therapeutic skills that facilitate movement around the circle. As shown in the list of "Items facilitating movement around circle" in Figure 4.3, CBT clinicians are aware of and manage several processes throughout each therapy session and across the course of therapy (i.e., agenda setting, feedback, collaboration, pacing and efficient use of time, and interpersonal effectiveness).

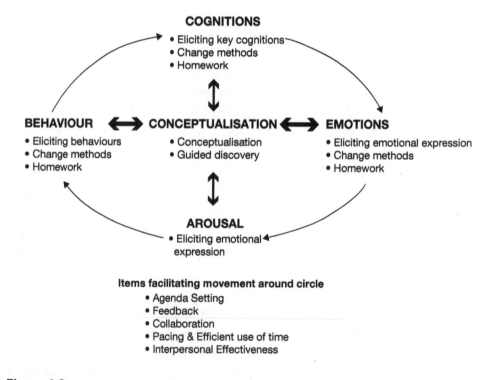

Figure 4.3

Processes and Skills in CBT

Adapted with permission from James et al. (2001)

Session Structure and Pacing Challenges with Clients Across the Lifespan

When first learning CBT, clinicians tend to struggle more with agenda setting, agenda adherence, and session pacing than with other core CBT skills. This is true with clients of all ages, whether within individual psychotherapy or with groups. For that reason, we find it helpful to spend some time here on the importance of session structure. Box 4.1 provides a typical recommended structure for CBT therapy sessions.

Use warmth and encouraging statements to support skill development and implementation. As we note throughout this guide, one of your important roles as a clinician is to remind your clients of their personal strengths, which have been demonstrated through past successful coping efforts. These reminders, combined with tangible

---

Box 4.1 Recommended Structure of Therapy Sessions

Prior to session, have clients complete:

- Preparing for Session form (Start 4 Practice: Preparing for My Next Session) to assist with agenda setting

- Brief assessment to track progress (e.g., mood, activities)

At the start of session:

- Review GDS-SF/PHQ-9 scores and any other assessments.

- Set the agenda collaboratively for the session.

- First on the agenda is always *Review home practice* (before any other "updates").

- Identify a treatment goal to be the focus of the session (e.g., increasing my daily involvement in everyday positive activities or questioning my negative thinking).

- Select an appropriate cognitive or behavioral strategy to address the goal and work on the steps of learning to apply the skill (e.g., reviewing daily activity logs or reviewing thought records). Get into the details of troubleshooting and problem solving.

- Periodically stop to review and summarize; also ask client to summarize to determine level of understanding.

- Review rationale for the strategy, and develop next home practice assignment; problem solve barriers.

- Summarize and assist client in completing Start 3 Practice: My Session Summary.

- Obtain and share feedback on the session.

signs of skill use in daily life, are effective means of building clients' self-efficacy beliefs. Keep in mind that expert opinion ranks low in sources of information that impact self-efficacy. This means that your simply telling a client that you see progress in their use of specific skills is helpful but not sufficient. Highest on the list of influences on improving self-efficacy is personal mastery experiences, usually achieved in a gradual, one-step-at-a-time fashion. Your ability to collaboratively implement session structure and set up "do-able" home practice assignments makes personal mastery experiences in daily life possible for your clients.

When training clinicians, our observations are that therapeutic skills in managing those five therapy processes (i.e., agenda setting and adherence, feedback, collaboration, pacing and efficient use of time, and interpersonal effectiveness) are commonly experienced by trainees as in competition with each other. The first four are especially seen by beginning CBT clinicians as potentially undermining the therapeutic relationship instead of being viewed as a means of developing and enhancing alliance. Rather than asking which should be sacrificed in the service of others, we find it more helpful to focus on the order of skill acquisition and effective implementation. Skillful and interpersonally effective agenda setting (and following the agenda), managing session pacing, and efficient use of time become the means by which time is available for working collaboratively and routinely asking for feedback (both of which foster the working alliance). Interpersonal effectiveness is not a stand-alone skill but becomes maximally therapeutic when used in the service of the other elements, which are all essential to supporting your clients' progress toward their therapy goals.

If this feels like a lot, it is! We understand that your development and use of these CBT skills takes time, practice, and feedback via supervision and consultation. Just as your clients have to develop and repeatedly practice new habits for healthy living in daily life, the process of developing and implementing these CBT skills involves focused effort and repetition. In addition to the professional development resources we list in Appendix A, the manual for the Cognitive Therapy Rating Scale—Revised (James et al., 2001) has become a valuable way for trainees and clinicians to develop and refine core CBT skills.

Describe, Demonstrate, Do, and Discuss (the 4 "Ds")

These four steps help your clients develop new skills and transfer established skills to more challenging situations. Your within-session role play of stressful situations with a client is an example of a strategy that easily incorporates the 4 Ds. You and your client together develop a *description* of the situation/feelings/thoughts/behaviors, then *demonstrate* and practice responses to the situation, and then *discuss* in detail what happened during the role-play exercise. This process segues nicely into a negotiation for an out-of-session practice to *do* the work.

An array of assignments and practice strategies can incorporate the 4 Ds; these include behaviorally based experiments such as relaxation exercises (*Skills for Feeling*) or positive activity logs (*Skills for Doing*) and written exercises like Thought Diaries (*Skills for Thinking*). Doing a portion of any assignment in session is essential for increasing compliance.

Overcoming Common Barriers to Home Practice Assignments

Home practice matters and is an essential component of CBT. The research literature is quite clear that engaging clients in developing and completing meaningful between-session assignments is linked to better outcomes for both individual (Kazantzis et al., 2010) and group CBT interventions (Neimeyer et al., 2008). If you are not routinely working with clients to set up and review between-session assignments, you are not engaging in CBT. When clients fail to either begin or finish home practice assignments, your first step as a clinician is to examine what actions or inactions on your part may be responsible. Often, the session time to initially set up the assignment was rushed, and the rationale and instructions were unclear to your client or were not developed collaboratively with the client. It is also common for clinicians to either rush or completely omit review of home practice assignments in the next session.

When there are concerns about compliance with home practice, the first steps for correcting the situation involve you as the clinician, not your client. Only after you are confident that (1) you have selected and developed the home practice assignment collaboratively with input from your client, (2) your client understands and agrees with the rationale and instructions for the home practice, (3) your client has explicitly indicated that this home practice feels "do-able," (4) you have together worked on a personally relevant example for the client that is written down on the home practice sheet, and (5) you have provided sufficient time to review home practice for several consecutive sessions, then you can direct attention to client factors that may be influencing compliance with home practice. Talk with your clients directly, and work together to find strategies to enhance completion. Again, a process of Socratic questioning can be particularly useful in addressing home practice problems (Wright et al., 2017). The classic book on homework in CBT by Tompkins (2004) remains an especially helpful resource for clinicians who are relatively new to implementing CBT.

Validation Strategies in CBT

Clients of all ages with depression benefit from skillful application of validation strategies. Validation is far more complex than simply agreeing with the perspective of your clients (which is not always possible or therapeutic). We find the detailed consideration of levels of validation within Dialectical Behavior Therapy (DBT) to be very useful and relevant for CBT (Koerner, 2012; Koerner & Linehan, 2004; Linehan, 1997) within both individual and group therapy settings. From this perspective, there are a range of ways to validate the experiences of your clients. Choice of strategy depends upon the therapy context and the needs of a particular client. The detailed recommendations provided by Koerner (2012) are particularly helpful for clinicians. At the very core of all validation strategies is a foundational premise of CBT: that all behavior makes sense in light of a specific learning history and current environment. We can use this clinically to help our clients feel heard, supported, and then ready to continue the challenging work of change.

Metaphors in CBT

There is a long history of the use of metaphor within psychotherapy, including in CBT. Metaphors provide cognitively efficient means of communicating complex material in a visually rich manner and can be important tools within CBT (Stott et al., 2010). Your skillful use of metaphors that are relevant to your clients can help them understand, remember, and apply therapeutic material. In the workbook, we utilize several metaphors that most of our aging patients have found understandable and useful. One example in *Skill for Feeling* is in Feel 5 Learn: Feelings Are Just the Tip of the Iceberg, which uses an iceberg metaphor for the concept of emotions being the most noticeable part of a complex array of positive and negative behaviors and thoughts. For clients who find that metaphor less useful, a similar one that conveys the same idea can be used as a culturally appropriate replacement (e.g., a branch sticking out of a river is usually a sign that an entire tree is submerged underneath the water; a stone that just breaks the surface is likely to be mostly buried underneath the earth). In the same module, Feel 7 Learn: Nurturing Positive Emotions provides the metaphor of cultivating a large plant from an initial small seed; this conveys how positive emotions can develop in daily life with attention and care. Within *Skills for Doing*, the interactive cycle of depressed mood and inactivity is compared in Do 8 Learn: The Importance of Doing to the downward tailspin of an airplane (i.e., each phase triggers things getting worse and worse). In *Skill for Thinking*, we use two different metaphors for unhelpful thinking habits (i.e., cooking without a recipe, lenses in a pair of glasses). We encourage you to know enough about the personal interests and leisure activities of your clients to be able to craft metaphors that resonate with their personal experience. Fortunately, there are several excellent resources available to help clinicians understand when and how to apply metaphors in psychotherapy. We especially recommend the works by Stott and colleagues (2010) and by Törneke (2017).

CBT in Groups: Procedures, Skills, and Processes

There is a long and successful history of CBT applications within groups. We realize that clinicians who may be new to working with groups, or new to group interventions within CBT, often have a large number of questions and concerns. Groups are attractive in many health care settings due to efficiencies of using staff time, combined with the many benefits that clients have from working alongside others experiencing similar problems. In addition to the knowledge and skills already discussed in this chapter, there is an additional layer of knowledge and skills specific to implementing CBT within groups. That could be a book in itself—wait, that book already exists! We direct readers with specific interest and professional development needs in group CBT to the excellent work by Bieling and colleagues (2009).

CHAPTER 5

Psychotherapy Modifications with Aging Clients

This chapter walks you through some very practical tips and strategies for therapy sessions with your aging clients. As we described in Chapter 4, our treatment approach retains core elements of CBT for individual and group psychotherapy sessions (and for behavioral health sessions integrated within primary care settings). Age-related adaptations to individual (Thompson et al., 2005) and group therapy (Thompson et al., 2000) are generally in the area of contextual modifications (Stirman et al., 2019); that is, the "how" of implementing specific change strategies within sessions. In the second edition of our workbook, we have revised therapy materials to make these adaptations clearer and easier to implement.

Because of the tremendous variability associated with aging that was discussed in Chapter 2, not every client of a specific age with depression requires significant, if any, modifications to central CBT processes. Our aim is to support your work with clients with depression across the second half of life (i.e., individuals in their 50s, 60s, 70s, 80s, and 90s). It is also the case that sometimes best practices for clinical work with aging clients are in fact best practices for working with clients of all ages. (Thus, some of the "modifications" described in this chapter may also improve your effectiveness in CBT with younger clients!)

This chapter is organized by specific challenges that arise in working with some aging clients, followed by potential remedies. There are many excellent resources available to advance knowledge and skill development in applying CBT to aging individuals. We've provided suggestions throughout this chapter, and especially recommend the work by Laidlaw and colleagues (Laidlaw, 2015; Laidlaw et al., 2003; Laidlaw & Thompson, 2014). Reviews of the principles and practices and the strong evidence base for using CBT with older adults are available (Braun et al.,

2016; Conti et al., 2017; Scogin & Shaw, 2012; Sorocco & Lauderdale, 2011). Beyond this chapter, expanded discussions and case studies are also available (Bilbrey et al., 2020b; Gallagher-Thompson et al., 2020b; Gallagher-Thompson & Thompson, 2010; Steffen et al., 2021; Steffen & Schmidt, in press; Zeiss & Steffen, 1996).

Successful Home Practice with Older Adults: Points for Consideration

We begin this discussion with a focus on home practice for several essential reasons. A fundamental premise of CBT is that insight alone is an insufficient means of achieving lasting change in psychotherapy. Discussing your clients' patterns of life problems and generating possible solutions is not nearly as helpful as developing specific plans that are then actually tried out between sessions (and then revised based on the results of that behavioral experiment). Asking your clients to recall details of their mood and daily events without the use of memory aids is unlikely to provide the level of accurate details needed to make meaningful changes.

Home practice is therefore an important component of CBT for clients across the lifespan. We encourage you to use your own creativity to help tailor home practice to meet the needs of your diverse aging clients and to employ a variety of strategies to address challenges to home practice. We outline a number of strategies here, with more details provided by Coon et al. (2003, 2007). Successful home practice rests on a number of "points for success." Note that many critical points that are common for individuals at all ages have not been covered. This section focuses on specific strategies to use with aging clients.

Point 1: Recognizing Beliefs About "Home Practice"

Home practice suffers when ageist assumptions and clinician pessimism lead to poorly articulated assignments. The following are some common clinician beliefs:

I am being disrespectful when I assign home practice to older clients; they have done it this way for over 60 years, so how can I question that habit now?

Consistent assignments aren't as important as my relationship with my clients, are they? I do not want to do anything that would weaken our therapeutic alliance.

Clinicians may need to ask themselves:

What evidence exists that my clients cannot complete home practice appropriately tailored to meet their needs?

What evidence is there that my clients cannot collaborate in developing home practice, taking into account their situations (including the sociocultural context in which they live)?

Older clients also have views about home practice, and clinicians need to be sensitive about this from the outset. Some older clients find the term "homework" to be amusing or engaging, yet "homework" can hold unpleasant connotations or may be considered demeaning, especially for those who did poorly in school or for those who completed little formal education. In this treatment, we have replaced standard CBT "homework" language with "home practice" language; additional phrases can be used, including "learning new habits," and assignments can be referred to as "experiments," "practice sheets," or "action steps."

Point 2: Tailoring Home Practice for Individual Differences

Diversity increases rather than decreases with age when we consider the wide range of personal histories and individual sociocultural contexts of aging individuals (Llorente, 2018). Seek out ways to acknowledge these histories and cultural contexts to foster collaborative development of suitable assignments and to maximize out-of-session practice (Lau & Kinoshita, 2019). It can be helpful for you to gain a clear understanding of the important role of significant others (e.g., family, community leaders, and cultural institutions) with regard to home practice. Increase your understanding of and respect for the use of religion and other spiritual practices in tandem with CBT. Do not make automatic assumptions about what will or will not work as home practice. Take it slowly: Gather the necessary information from the client (and from other reliable sources as needed), consistently check in about home practice assignments along the way, and be mindful to work within the client's sociocultural context.

Point 3: Recognize Later-Life Physical Challenges

Successful home practice completion with physically ill, disabled, or frail clients often requires you to develop new approaches, including (a) increased knowledge of common illnesses and functional impairments, (b) more frequent contact with various health care providers, (c) greater flexibility in treatment appointment times and locations (e.g., nursing homes, hospitals, clinics, and family residences), (d) more emphasis on teamwork with your older clients' support systems, and (e) an even closer collaboration with clients in the development of assignments.

Begin with modest steps to support success, and recalibrate the pace to fit client progress. Break assignments into several steps or components and celebrate accomplishments. Design assignments that minimize fatigue and discomfort. Consider securing permission to contact formal and informal network support members to facilitate home practice compliance, such as helping with writing tasks, setting up audiovisual equipment, or joining positive activities. Work with your clients and their support systems to resolve practical barriers to home practice completion. Avoid, however, the development of coercive systems or tactics to promote home practice compliance, and take the appropriate steps to protect confidentiality and respect privacy. Finally, remain mindful of "excess disability" and educate your clients and their support systems that depression is a reversible problem that can be distinguished from the older adult's physical challenges.

Point 4: Modify Home Practice for Clients with Mild Cognitive Impairment (MCI)

Several modifications can be used to enhance home practice for aging clients with MCI (e.g., record sessions for home review; use the Learn pages and Practice forms that provide structured and simple activity schedules for routine use). Simplify and reduce the number of concepts used, and then reuse and reliably reinforce them. For example, for some clients with MCI, the thought record can be effectively reduced to three columns of "Thought," "Feeling," and "New Thought" or "Thought," "New Thought," and "New Feeling/New Action." Design and use a simple notebook or calendar to schedule sessions and to hold intervention and home practice materials. Brainstorm with the client (and, as appropriate, a family member of the client) to pick one place at home to consistently keep the notebook or calendar.

Common Psychotherapy Challenges (and Remedies)

Excessive Details and "Staying on Track"

The Challenge

You have thoughtfully and collaboratively set an agenda at the beginning of session, but it falls apart within the first 15 minutes of session! Following the agenda can be very difficult to do with older adults who appear to need to "tell their story" at length. Often, this leads to wandering off track when talking, along with taking up valuable session time with details that are not directly important or relevant to the task at hand. Rather than viewing this as (1) a sign of loneliness, (2) just part of the client's "personality," or (3) essential to relationship building, you can remind yourself that there are age-related cognitive changes in attentional processes and executive functioning, including the ability to inhibit irrelevant information. These cognitive processes are additionally impaired in some individuals with depression, exacerbating this problem. It is very possible to develop strong, warm, and effective working relationships AND to maintain focus on session content that is most relevant for clinical improvement. This is true for clinical work both with individuals and with groups.

Your Main Remedy

You will need to learn the *art of gently redirecting the conversation*. Many clinicians, who are often one to three generations *younger* than these clients, find it difficult to interrupt an older person who is speaking. Begin in the first treatment session (once assessment is complete) to structure the time, and discuss the following points:

- Therapy time is very valuable and quite short, given that it is 45 minutes once a week (or shorter/less frequent in primary care), and so it is necessary to use the time well so that the client can feel better as soon as possible.
- To use the time well, you (the clinician) will have to interrupt the conversation at times and redirect it back to the topic at hand. To interrupt effectively, it is a good idea to have an agreed-upon signal such as raising a finger, holding your hand out palm forward, or using the "time-out" sign (i.e., crossed "T" with both hands). You want to interrupt in a respectful way, and it is important that you both agree on this course of action early in the therapy relationship.

Essentially, you are asking permission to interrupt, which will make you more comfortable doing it as the need arises. Within the very first or second session, you can say something like:

At some point during our time together, you will be saying something important that I want to be sure I understand. I might need you to pause, so that I can stop and make sure that I am getting the key points before you say much more. How would you like me to stop or interrupt you? I can raise my finger (demonstrate), or use a "time-out" sign (demonstrate), or put my hand up and say your name, like this (demonstrate). What feels good for you?

For clinicians implementing this treatment in groups, we recommend a group consensus on one gesture to be used for everyone, rather than attempting to remember which gesture is preferred by individual clients in the group.

You will also need to periodically (for some clients) or frequently (for others) reassure your clients that you really do have sufficient information to understand the nature of a specific problem. Often clients think that all of the specific details must be disclosed before the clinician can really, really, really understand the problem and the dilemma. When you decide it is time to curtail the deliverance of unnecessary details, you need to convey to the client in some way that you really, really, really understand and "we need to move on."

Other Remedies

Start 4 Practice: Preparing for My Next Session is an important tool to help your individual and group clients write down—ahead of session time—the information and points that seem most important to them. We see this as an essential form for all clients, because this helps you collaboratively set the session agenda together AND helps clients stay focused within session. You will write the agenda on a whiteboard or on a flipchart or at least on a piece of paper. Point out to clients that there is only so much time in therapy and the focus is on steps to help them feel better as soon as possible. Placing time estimates next to each agenda item is also helpful. It is very common for updates that are intended to last no more than 5 to 10 minutes to end up expanding to take over the majority of session. At the very minimum, review the home practice first. Many times, we place both home practice review and core skill building items ahead of the types of updates on daily life that clients "just think you should know about." Many times, these updates can get moved toward the end of session because you will have had the chance to glance over the Preparing for My Next Session form to determine if any of those updates do seem truly relevant to the therapy work at hand. There are natural limitations on time allotted for individual sharing in group sessions. We refer you to the discussion of within-session skills for managing CBT groups provided by Bieling et al. (2009).

A related issue is that quite possibly clients DO have a lot to share with you; perhaps several important things happened since the last session. You can then take the opportunity to rearrange the agenda and add items that directly impact treatment or therapy progress. A key question for you and your clients to consider together is, "How does this information impact the specific goals for therapy or the specific strategies we are using to work on those goals?" Asking clients to prioritize possible agenda items in light of those two questions at the beginning of session is helpful, because it is unlikely that all can be covered in the time available. Our experience is that most 45-minute individual psychotherapy sessions with older adults allow for two main agenda items, including the focused area of skill development, rather than three or more.

Pacing of How Rapidly New Material Is Presented

The Challenge

Mild cognitive impairments in memory and executive functions are commonly comorbid with later-life depression (see Chapter 2). If material is presented at the same pace as if the client were in their 20s or 30s, there is likely to be confusion and misunderstanding. In the typical course of CBT, there is a lot of material to cover, there are many skills to teach, and there are not that many sessions to work with. There are ways to help your aging clients who are experiencing changes to their memory and executive functioning (Harvey et al., 2014).

Slow Down the Pace

In general, it is recommended to start out by slowing the pace in which material is presented in session. You can begin by talking more slowly than may be typical for you, check that what you are saying is being heard clearly (as discussed earlier), and check for comprehension by asking clients to give frequent summaries of what they are learning throughout the session. In this way, you can check for how much is really being absorbed and adjust accordingly. Do not be discouraged if the pace is slower than you would like; it is better for some key material to be processed well than for a lot of material to be processed poorly.

Present Material Multimodally

Say it, show it, and do it. Dual processing (both hearing and reading information) is an important component to learning for all of us; this becomes increasingly important with age. Conducting therapy via conversation and discussion without written materials is like paddling from only one side of a canoe; you are working hard and feel like something is happening, but you are likely to move in circles! Each concept within this treatment approach has at least one or two didactic Learn pages that have been developed for this purpose. By having printed material in front of clients *during* session, and provided for review *between* sessions, both understanding and retention are enhanced. This kind of multimodal involvement reinforces learning.

Use Memory Aids

Our entire treatment approach has been developed to maximize the use of memory aids. The session summary form (Start 3 Practice: My Session Summary) is used in each session; clients write down key points, home practice assignments (which will be forgotten very quickly if they are NOT written down), and the date/time of the next scheduled appointment. This enhances memory. For this reason, plan to provide each of your clients with multiple copies of this form. It is also possible for clients with smartphones to use a voice-recording app to record key parts of session for review between sessions. This helps with memory problems for details. When indicated and possible, brief 5- to 10-minute reminder calls between sessions can greatly increase home practice compliance. Clients frequently say that they forgot to do their home practice, and with older adults that may be very accurate. The Practice forms in this treatment are also designed to maximize application and retention.

Therapeutic Relationship Concerns Due to Generational Differences

The Challenge

The client is typically at least one generation (often two or three) older than the clinician. What else can the clinician do (besides the norm) to enhance the working relationship?

Main Remedies

Clarify how your clients wish to be addressed, and how they wish to address you, and remember to follow those wishes from session to session, on the phone, and so on—even if it is not initially that comfortable for you. Remember important details of the individual's life history (keep specific notes; know the names of children and grandchildren; pay attention!). Learn to be nondefensive when the client asks about personal details of your life (which almost all do). Common questions include:

- "How old are you?"
- "Are you married?"
- "Do you have children or grandchildren?"
- "Have you worked with many older adults?"

Such questions are also common among clients of all ages from some racial and ethnic minority groups, so this is a good opportunity to practice skills in cultural sensitivity. Spend some time reflecting in advance and have answers ready to give that you are comfortable with. Dodging the issue by refusing to give any personal information (e.g., "Why are you interested? What difference would it make if I said _____?") makes the client suspicious of you and seems to damage the therapeutic relationship. Of course, you should disclose the minimum that seems to satisfy the client and that you are comfortable with. If you are uncertain about where the line of appropriate boundaries is for you, this is a great topic for peer consultation.

Other Remedies

For clients who raise generational concerns (e.g., "I'm not sure you really understand me. How could you? You haven't been married 50 years" or "You don't have to watch your adult children bringing up your grandchildren with no self-discipline or responsibilities"), it is important not to be defensive about your younger age or lack of certain life experiences. You can underscore that you have special training in the problems of later life, and believe that your knowledge and skills will be helpful to the person. Often, it is helpful to point out that you both can learn from each other.

Negative Reactions to Some Aging Clients

The Challenge

As we discussed in Chapter 2, we all live with the consequences of being immersed in an ageist society. Clinicians may sense that they are developing a bit of a negative attitude toward specific clients, hoping clients start canceling appointments, and/or stop expecting them to reach appropriate therapy goals. Many of the issues and triggers for you are likely similar for clients across the lifespan, but there can be some that are more common when working with aging clients. Compared to your younger clients, you may have some older individuals who are more likely to trigger your own feelings of frustration and pessimism, with thoughts such as "I don't feel I am helping them; they are so slow to change; they are very difficult to work with."

Remedies

Because of the historical baggage associated with countertransference language, we prefer to simply label these as emotional reactions to clients. The recommendations provided by Kimerling et al. (2000) for understanding and processing these emotional reactions using learning-based language can be quite useful. Use your own feelings as a chance to refocus on what this particular client is doing to create them. Avoid overly general labels for such clients such as "resistant" or "manipulative"; instead describe the difficult pattern in behavioral "if/then" terms. Maintain a problem-solving attitude and consider how you can present CBT differently and/or renegotiate therapy goals, which will help you remain appropriately optimistic about the client's ability to learn and to improve mood management skills. As with clients of any age, consult with a colleague if these negative feelings are strong.

Acknowledge that therapy can be difficult and requires hard work and commitment; indicate that you, too, for example, do "home practice" between sessions in order to make the best use of the time together. Give clients credit for specific accomplishments, but avoid generic compliments such as "You are doing a great job in therapy!" Specific and directed compliments can be much more useful; for example,

"Monique, you did a great job on the thought record this week. I can see that you are learning how to use it effectively. Good for you." Some clients do not get direct praise or compliments in daily life; a little goes a long way!

Need for Interprofessional Collaboration

The Challenge

Most clinicians in private practice settings tend to operate "solo" and tend not to make contact with other professionals who are also treating the client. It is far easier to work as a member of a multidisciplinary team in institutional settings than when you are working solo in private practice. Even though it requires more effort, it is important to set up communications with professionals who are treating other problems your client might have. Some clients may have health conditions that are being treated by a multidisciplinary or interdisciplinary team (Decaporale-Ryan et al., in press; Steffen et al., 2015; Steffen & Zeiss, 2017). In most instances you'll find that working together will result in more positive outcomes for your clients.

Remedies

With older adults, given their medical complexities, we recommend that you obtain written permission to communicate with the primary care physician, at least, to understand their medical problems and their functional limitations (as discussed earlier). If a physical therapist, occupational therapist, social worker, or case manager is involved, these professionals are also good to get to know as they are coordinating other aspects of the client's life that can have an impact on therapy.

Developing collegial relationships with other providers in the area who serve older adults is also helpful so that referrals can be made more readily, if necessary, when the course of CBT is over. For example, you should know about senior centers in the region (where they are and how to contact them). Such centers can be an excellent resource for increasing pleasant activities. It's surprising how few seniors know about the centers in their area and have ever actually visited one. It is helpful to become knowledgeable about self-help groups in the area that deal with common problems of later life, such as a support group for people living with a specific chronic illness. Expecting the *client* to seek out this kind of information is unrealistic. It generally saves time and frustration for the clinician to make the initial contact, obtain the basic information, make the referral, and so on, to lay the groundwork before passing it along to the client. Suggested national resources to help you get started are included in Appendix A.

Telemental Health: Video Conference and Telephone-Only Sessions

The research evidence is clear: Telemental health services provided via video conference or telephone sessions can be an effective means of providing treatment to clients of all ages (Varker et al., 2019) and to your aging clients who are experiencing depression in later life (Barrera et al., 2017; Gentry et al., 2019; Harerimana et al., 2019). There are now a variety of resources available for behavioral health practitioners who are interested in developing their professional competencies in telemental health (Luxton et al., 2016; Myers & Turvey, 2012; Riper & Cuijpers, 2016) and specifically their use of CBT within telemental health sessions (Nelson & Duncan, 2015).

Although some providers may have concerns about generational differences in client comfort using technology, the technical literacy of older adults and their interest in telehealth is higher than clinicians assume (Glueck et al., 2013; Greenwald et al., 2018). In addition to the common recommendations for telemental health to facilitate comfort with procedures for signing on, maintaining privacy, and risk management, there are also specific things for clinicians to do to establish and maintain therapeutic rapport in telemental health (Glueck et al., 2013). Our placement of emotional literacy and work with anxiety early within the treatment (*Skills for Feeling*) is consistent with this, given the key role of focus on emotional communication in enhancing therapy alliance early in treatment.

We had the opportunity to beta-test materials in the workbook during the spring and summer of 2020. This was when the COVID-19 global pandemic began causing so many clinicians to provide telemental health services for the first time in their professional careers. Our gratitude goes out to those clinicians who helped us identify the materials within the workbook that seemed to work best in telemental health sessions. One of us (AMS) also has years of experience working with individuals with depression, who were dementia family caregivers, via telephone sessions that were supported by use of weekly written materials (i.e., bibliotherapy) and, in some cases, videos. In addition to these caregivers showing a reduction in depression scores (Steffen & Gant, 2016), our team learned quite a bit about enhancing the effectiveness of these interventions. A key function that use of workbook materials can have in telemental health sessions is to enable dual processing of material (verbal and visual) and facilitate more elaborate encoding and memory. When clients do not yet have a copy of the workbook at home to refer to and use during session, we scan or copy relevant pages and send them either via email or in regular mail. This strategy can do much to help with a client's ability to focus and benefit from treatment.

In the beginning of this clinician guide, we provide a master list of all Learn pages and Practice forms that are in the workbook. The pages that are a particularly good fit for telehealth sessions have been identified there with a ^{T}; these are also identified in each chapter of this guide devoted to a specific workbook module. These pages and forms reflect a balance between simplicity and allowing for some elaboration and re-flection. We also aim to include Learn pages and Practice forms that recognize and reinforce existing personal strengths of your clients.

PART II

Core Modules
(For Most Clients)

CHAPTER 6

Module 1: Skills for Getting Started: Planning Your Treatment

Therapy Orientation and Goal Setting

This core module of the workbook is focused on the skills of:

1. Developing positive expectations for treatment
2. Understanding depression
3. Respecting values, identities, and life experiences
4. Personalizing the CBT model
5. Developing therapy goals
6. Shifting expectations for how change happens
7. Setting agendas for treatment sessions
8. Engaging in home practice

This chapter is provided to help you use workbook Module 1: *Skills for Getting Started* with your clients. We start with a brief overview, followed by some practical tips based on the most common questions we hear from clinicians during professional trainings. The bulk of this chapter is devoted to reviewing skills involved in the early phase of treatment, with a description of the specific Learn pages and Practice forms available for your use in sessions. We provide recommendations for a standard progression of material (i.e., Learn pages and Practice forms that typically go with each other in the same session, estimates of how much can be accomplished in a given session), with the understanding that this may vary quite a bit depending upon your practice setting and specific client needs. We end the chapter with some comments about related topics that are not included in this treatment approach.

As you read this chapter, we encourage you to have the workbook open so that you can refer to the specific Learn pages and Practice forms as they are described and explained. You will use these Learn pages and Practice forms during sessions, encouraging your clients to review the Learn pages between sessions and try out/record between sessions using the Practice forms. Your reviewing these items as you read through this chapter will prepare you to make the most of the treatment materials. Using these pages and forms means more than having them available to look at or read over with your clients during sessions. Instead, you'll be engaging your clients in exploring the meaning this has to them, through discussion and careful application. Your goal each session is to help your clients apply specific Learn and Practice material to their recent experiences in daily life, and to the problems that bring them into treatment.

Overview

The research literature on preventing premature dropout from psychotherapy is clear. There is much that we can do in these first sessions that has a powerful impact on whether clients remain in treatment long enough to benefit (Fernandez et al., 2015; Swift et al., 2017). These steps include explaining the therapy approach, setting expectations for treatment length, directly linking the treatment approach to the client's presenting problems, instilling hope, and asking for and responding to feedback. This *Skills for Getting Starting* module is designed to help you begin to develop a strong therapeutic alliance with your clients, engage them actively in treatment, and create a climate of hope (Spencer et al., 2019).

When to Use This Module

When you use our approach for individual and group psychotherapy with middle-aged and older adults with depression, this module is recommended for *all clients* because there is very strong empirical support for the importance of orientation to treatment in preventing premature termination. Clinicians using this program in groups will likely make some decisions regarding which materials are the best fit, depending upon the setting of the group (i.e., inpatient, partial hospitalization, outpatient). Those clinicians who are doing very brief behavioral health interventions integrated into primary care settings may use some but not all of the materials in this module in their work with clients. For all clinicians, the first step in preparing to use this module is a thorough review of all Learn pages and Practice forms. When this module is used to begin psychotherapy, we expect that (a) you have already completed a separate intake interview and assessment process as described in Chapter 3 and (b) a decision for beginning treatment has been made.

Tips for Clinicians

Directly Address Expected Length of Treatment

Many older adults without previous psychotherapy experience initially expect that just a few sessions will be enough to help them feel better, and they are often surprised at hearing anything else. The analogy of a cycle of physical therapy is often useful at this point, because after a fall or surgery, many older adults have engaged in several months of physical therapy. For middle-aged and older clients with a diagnosis of major depressive disorder (MDD), the core treatment should be expected to last at least 4 to 5 months. It is important to reassure your clients that the two of you will be focusing on specific and concrete goals that are important to them, and that you will be routinely tracking how therapy is helping them reach those goals.

Emphasize That Treatment Has Started and Will Build over Time

Active treatment strategies begin with Session 1, in addition to the process of orienting your clients to therapy. Your clients will track times of the day in which their mood is lighter (Start 2 Practice: One Daily Exception), reflect on their personal values and strengths (Start

5 Practice: My Values and Strengths), articulate therapy goals (Start 10 Practice: My SMART Therapy Goals), and develop skills for self-encouragement (Start 12 Practice: Ways to Encourage Myself)—all active interventions that we have intentionally woven into this module. Beginning use of the My Session Summary form (Start 3 Practice) and Preparing for My Next Session (Start 4 Practice) actively promotes engagement early in treatment.

Manage "Story Telling"

Many older adults may begin to "tell stories" about themselves and can use up most of the session time talking about problem areas in a longwinded manner. As we described in Chapter 2, some of this may well be due to changes in the frontal lobe of the brain that impact executive functioning involved in abstract thinking and organizing; these changes create difficulties inhibiting irrelevant information. Some older clients also tend to be very concerned that the clinician get the maximum amount of information about their physical condition and possible bases for their problems. You can reassure your clients that you understand their issues and will ask for more information when it is needed. (You will also resist the urge to ask questions just out of habit or as a way of communicating that you care about your clients.) It is necessary to gently but firmly bring clients back to focus on the agenda and the topic at hand. Over time, older clients learn to curb their desire to just talk, but initially this can be a struggle.

We recommend that in the very first treatment session you establish some sort of signal for interrupting and redirecting the discussion (e.g., a raised finger, making the "time-out" [T] sign with both hands, or touching your watch). You will need to explain *why* you are doing this (because therapy time is precious and relatively short, and there is a lot to be done), and establish that making the signal is going to be acceptable to the client. Contrary to what you might expect, older adults are generally appreciative of your efforts in this regard. This issue is also discussed in Chapter 5.

We have designed this module to emphasize important steps for you to take early on. Before each psychotherapy session, at home or in the waiting room your clients will complete the PHQ-9, the GDS-SF, or another appropriate self-report measure for depressive symptoms. This routine assessment should be described as an ongoing part of treatment and an important way to track reactions to therapy, in the same way that blood pressure readings are taken at the beginning of each primary care medical appointment.

Developing Positive Expectations for Treatment

When using this *Skills for Getting Started* module within individual psychotherapy, you will provide an orientation to treatment, using Start 1–4 Learn. Those using this approach in group psychotherapy will most likely use Start 3–5 Learn. One of the first things you will do is describe CBT, using Start 4 Learn: What to Expect from Cognitive-Behavioral Therapy (CBT) to help set expectations. Explanations of the client role, the clinician role, the collaborative relationship, and the importance of home practice are often necessary. The heart and soul of CBT is the formation of a collaborative relationship between the client and the clinician. You begin to develop this by listening carefully to the client and validating the difficulties of their situation. It is helpful to discuss past therapy experiences by comparing and contrasting those experiences with CBT. Explain that the collaborative relationship means that *both* the client and the clinician take an active role in understanding the problems that brought the client to therapy, defining goals, and working to achieve goals through the end of therapy. When using this approach within individual psychotherapy for MDD, we suggest that, if possible, you set up the full 16- to 20-session schedule with the client so that times and days of the week become regular for you both. Laying out all the planned sessions can be also helpful in reassuring your client that therapy will continue, even if the client is not responding yet or doesn't know how helpful it will be. This discussion of future termination at the very beginning of treatment is also a way of expressing your firm belief that this treatment will help the client feel better and they will not be in therapy forever.

Using both Start 3 Learn: Making This Workbook Work for You and Start 4 Learn: What to Expect from Cognitive-Behavioral Therapy (CBT), emphasize the importance of practicing new skills in between sessions. Practice is how healthy new habits are formed, and it is one of the best ways we know to make the therapy skills a routine part of daily life. Assignments for home practice should be made collaboratively during session and reviewed at the end of every session. We also realize that many life circumstances make it difficult for clients to complete home practice. For example, time constraints, a difficult assignment, or fears of doing it "wrong" commonly interfere with completing home practice. Some clients may feel resentful of a clinician "telling them what to do," or sometimes clients think that the home practice is silly or useless. Avoiding home practice can seriously interfere with a client's progress, so it is important to routinely check on the feasibility of a specific home practice task and find strategies to enhance compliance. See Chapter 5 for suggestions for common problems. Start 3 Practice: My Session Summary is a key form that will be used throughout treatment at the end of each session to help the client review and remember important ideas and plans for moving forward. Be gentle about correcting erroneous ideas and also use this as an opportunity to reinforce what the client did correctly understand. You and your client should get into the habit of completing Start 3 Practice together at the end of each session. Just a few phrases are needed for each section. Be sure that the client writes down the time and date of the next appointment on this form.

After completing the Start 3 Practice form, allow about 5 minutes for mutual feedback at the end of each session:

- Feedback in session is designed to encourage clients to discuss what was helpful about the session and what was not.
- You also want to be able to give selective praise and positive reinforcement for the client's compliance with the session's focus. Ask the client for both negative and positive feedback. Encourage honesty, and explain that this is important information to help you adjust the pacing, tone, and content of future sessions. Some specific questions we recommend asking are *"What did you like about today's*

session?" "Were there things I said or did that didn't sit well with you or that you thought were off base?"

- Also, problems in the relationship can be discussed (e.g., *"I don't think we are understanding each other as well as I'd like us to; let's talk about what seems to be the problem in communication between us"*). Psychotherapy process research has demonstrated that this common practice within CBT is very successful at early identification and resolution of potential ruptures of the therapeutic relationship. Routinely engaging in mutual feedback at the end of each session leads to a strong working alliance.

Understanding Depression

Typically, the pre-therapy assessment sessions have provided a chance to engage in some psychoeducation about depression and treatment options (Start 6–9 Learn). There are times when Start 6 Learn: Overview of Clinical Depression is particularly useful to use as treatment begins, because it helps set up the first between-session assignment in which the client writes down some details of their experiences of depression (using Start 1 Practice: My Depressive Symptoms) and begins to monitor occasions of lighter mood (on Start 2 Practice: One Daily Exception).

Respecting Values, Identities, and Life Experiences

One important goal of these initial sessions is to begin to develop a therapeutic alliance and collaborative stance (i.e., *"I care about your well-being, and we are working on this together"*). In this early phase of therapy, you and your client are beginning to talk about parts of their life that are most important and central to them. This process helps clients trust that "you really know them" and helps you individualize therapy with each client. At the same time, you are helping each client begin to make their connections between personal values and strengths (Start 10 Learn: Your Life Values and Personal Strengths, Start 5 Practice: My Values and Strengths), the parts of identity that are most important to them (Start 11 Learn: Celebrating Diversity), and any adverse childhood experiences (ACEs) and other traumatic life events (Start 12

Learn: Childhood Experiences). This sets the background for the following discussion of their individualized CBT model of depression (Start 6 Practice: The Cognitive-Behavioral Model of My Depression).

We see these initial brief conversations of values and strengths, the role of cultural diversity, and trauma history as "planting seeds." Rather than considering this as the only time you will discuss any of these, use these tools (Start 10–12 Learn) to introduce topics that will continue to be a part of the rest of treatment in some way. Our strengths-based approach is developed for you to adapt to the preferences and needs of your client's individual racial, ethnic, sexual, and gender identities (among others). In keeping with the multicultural guidelines for psychological practice (Clauss-Ehlers et al., 2019), we see age as just one of many different facets of cultural diversity that intersects with others (Lau & Kinoshita, 2019). Start 10 Learn: Your Life Values and Personal Strengths helps you have an important early discussion of values and strengths that are most important to each client. Start 11 Learn: Celebrating Diversity helps you and your clients have an initial conversation about the identities that are most important to them, and this is one of the first steps to your adapting this treatment to the values, beliefs, and preferences of individual clients. Behavioral health professionals are especially unlikely to solicit information and discussion about their clients' spiritual and religious beliefs and practices, despite their importance for so many older adults (Krause et al., 2019). There are a number of ways that clinicians can link this initial discussion of spirituality and religion to work with clients (Vieten et al., 2016; Wilt et al., 2019).

The question at the bottom of Start 11 Learn about chosen family is especially relevant to many diverse middle-aged and older adults and communicates your sensitivity to important relationships in their lives. For all of your clients, you would ideally like to know which family member or members are key and most likely to be sources of support for medical issues and for this treatment.

We also encourage you to have an early conversation about traumatic life experiences, as many clients do not bring these up during the intake assessment process unless directly asked (Kaiser et al., 2019). By the time individuals have reached midlife, the vast majority have experienced at least one traumatic event (Rapsey et al., 2019). This means that any traumatic life event does not necessarily signal current traumatic stress or posttraumatic stress disorder, and it may not need specific attention during treatment. We focus on ACEs because of the strong relationship between the number of such experiences and mental health problems in early adulthood that may persist in some form into later life (https://www.cdc.gov/violenceprevention/acestudy/index.html). When a client discloses a trauma history, you want to thank them for sharing, ask how it felt to share that information, and ask if they see any connections between that history and their current depression. While validating the difficulty of a trauma history, our focus will be on posttraumatic growth and resiliency. You can emphasize that you see your client as someone who has developed a number of internal strengths that will help in this treatment. Thus, your intent is to tie this brief discussion of traumatic life experiences back to the earlier focus on values and strengths, and link this to the concept of bravery (drawing upon internal strengths during challenging times) and resilience. For this reason, we have Start 5 Practice: My Values and Strengths as a suggested between-session assignment after all of these conversations; completing this exercise emphasizes the positives as clients continue to reflect on their values and strengths.

Personalizing the CBT Model

As shown in Start 13 Learn: What Is the Cognitive-Behavioral Model?, these four components of the CBT model include the client's current physical symptoms, thoughts, behaviors, and emotions. Point out that each connection has an arrow in two directions. Although the client may well be concentrating on how to change negative emotions, note that the relationships within this model also work for positive emotions. Also emphasize the word "environment" surrounding the model. Explain that environment refers to the events and people around the client that affect what the client does and thinks, as well as how the client feels physically and emotionally. Inform them that in the course of therapy, they are going to be looking at many different situations in their environment to see how they affect these four components. You can say something like:

People usually come to therapy because they do not feel good emotionally for one reason or another. (Circle emotions on the diagram.) *Unfortunately, it is not possible for me to reach in and change how you feel. This program also does not try to change your physiology directly through drugs or other means. That leaves us with two factors, behaviors (actions) and thoughts. CBT can help you change what you do and what you think. You can make changes by learning to build more positive activities into your schedule and becoming more aware of the things you tell yourself, among other changes.*

You will teach each client about the CBT model using Start 13 Learn and can help them understand the model by presenting the example of Winnie. You can say something like:

For example, Winnie is 79 years old and has lived alone since the death of her husband 3 years ago. She doesn't have any children but has a god-daughter, Emily, who says Winnie is her "second mom," and they talk a few times a week. Winnie describes herself as feeling "blah" most days and sometimes feels downright sad (emotions = "blah," sad). Winnie finds herself thinking of some things to do and then talks herself out of them (thoughts = "Why bother; nothing will help"). This often leads her to spend much of her day in her chair watching TV (behaviors = watch TV most of day, low activity). The long periods of sitting have led to un-planned naps and made her arthritis worse (health/physical = stiff knees, sleep problems). Winnie's environment includes both physical (living alone in an older house) and social (her relationship with Emily) features.

You can point to the different parts of the model and talk with your clients about which details from Winnie's story would fit the various parts of the model. Then, transition to talking with your clients about their own experiences of depression. With your help, your clients will use Start 6 Practice: The Cognitive-Behavioral Model of My Depression during the session to begin to write in how their experiences fit into the CBT model, and then take Start 6 Practice home to review and write in additional ideas.

Developing Therapy Goals

A fundamental assumption of CBT is that people improve their mental health and well-being by making specific and concrete changes to behaviors, thoughts, and emotional patterns. At least one session of this phase of therapy is devoted to the collaborative efforts of the client and clinician to turn target problems (Start 14 Learn, Start 7 and 8 Practice) into specific therapy goals. This helps define ways of routinely monitoring progress to-ward meeting those goals (Start 15 and 16 Learn, Start 9 and 10 Practice).

"Target complaints" refer to the client's description of which situations or symptoms are troublesome. We ask about these so that specific and measurable behavioral goals for change can be set. We recommend the identification of two (maximum of three) target complaints for the course of therapy. Use Start 14 Learn: Identifying and Prioritizing Target Problems, Start 7 Practice: Problems to Target in Treatment, and Start 8 Practice: My Target Problems within session to identify both the "chief complaint" (i.e., what is bringing the person into treatment at this time) and other complaints so that you and your client can work collaboratively to select one where improvement is likely to be seen in a reasonable period of time. For home practice, ask the client to review, add to, and be prepared to discuss in the next session both Start 7 Practice and Start 8 Practice.

The difference between a target complaint and a goal is that a goal helps establish a well-defined plan of change (whether focusing on behaviors or beliefs) that is important, time-limited, specific, realistic, positive, and measurable. Each of these properties of SMART goals is defined in Start 15 Learn: Translating Problems into SMART Goals. You will discuss these together in session, and then you will work with the client to complete both Start 9 Practice: My Goals for this Program and then Start 10 Practice: My SMART Therapy Goals for each of their goals. Be sure to ask key questions that may not have occurred to the client. For larger goals, help the client break them into smaller separate ones. Also address any limitations of time, money, material, or skills that may interfere with these goals. It will not be possible to complete all of this during one session. At least some of the remaining work can be assigned as home practice, to be brought to the next session, where it will be completed by the two of you together.

Shifting Expectations for How Change Happens

The *Skills for Getting Started* module ends with an important discussion of expectations for how change happens over time (Start 17 Learn: Ways to Think About Progress Toward Your Goals) and ways that clients can make the most of their time in treatment (Start 11 Practice: My Plan for Fully Participating). This is followed by how clients can encourage themselves (Start 12 Practice: Ways to Encourage Myself) and remember key points from this initial module (Start 13 Practice: My Review of Skills for Getting Started). It is important to use Start 17 Learn to explain that progress toward goals is not linear; rather, there are ups and downs with the overall progress showing improvement. It is important to discuss the process of change and help clients avoid thinking in extremes. This work takes time. It is accomplished via small steps and not suddenly in a single week. Notice and reinforce any small incremental improvement or action that is in the positive direction. Clarify for your clients that if goals are not reached quickly, this does not mean that nothing was accomplished. In addition, emphasize that progress on set goals rarely occurs at a steady pace, or in a continuous direction, like climbing steps. Explain that it is difficult to learn a new way of thinking and new behaviors. Furthermore, making the effort and showing progress is easier some days than others. Most change happens with setbacks in between and looks more like a "sawtooth" curve (i.e., jagged, with various ups and downs, but over time going up). When reviewing the progress of goals over the course of treatment, make sure clients evaluate the overall process, not just compare the results of one week against those of the previous week. Just as importantly, encourage your clients to recognize and then reward themselves for each step made toward achieving the goal.

Setting Agendas for Treatment Sessions

Rather than starting sessions with "*How are you?*" or "*What would you like to discuss today?*," instead start by saying something to the effect of "*It is good to see you; I'm glad you are here. Let's set the agenda together to find out how we will spend our time together today.*" It is very important to begin setting an agenda quite early on in treatment so that bad habits of rambling and unstructured use of time do not get established—it is harder to break them than it is to prevent them from occurring. Tell the client that setting an agenda will help you both make the best use of the available time. After a brief check-in that involves reviewing their depression scores, the first item on the agenda should always be home practice review (from Session 2 onward). If this is not done, the client will soon assume that home practice is not that important, despite what you might say, and so compliance will be minimal. A sizable body of research says that clients with depression who do at-home assignments regularly obtain greater benefit from therapy and have less difficulty generalizing what is learned in therapy to the rest of their lives. Also, doing home practice is a skill that the client can use after therapy is over.

It is wise in the early sessions to take most of the responsibility for setting what you think will be a useful, productive agenda. Besides home practice review, you will add in the one or two key areas/skills to be worked on in that session. You will ask the client to add to the agenda by having them refer to what they wrote down in Start 4 Practice: Preparing for My Next Session, and then work together to prioritize the top two agenda items. (Also later on, we recommend that you add time estimates for each item so that the session moves along and everything gets at least some time.) Table 6.1 presents a sample agenda for a 45-minute Session 3.

Your client will use Start 4 Practice: Preparing for My Next Session to prepare for all therapy sessions beginning with Session 2. Middle-aged and older clients are used to developing a list of topics to discuss ahead of medical appointments, so this will be a familiar idea. Explain that they can work on this the day before the next therapy session or the morning of the therapy session. When clients arrive for their check-in, which should be at least 15 minutes prior to the start of each session, have available a blank copy of Start 4 Practice along with whatever symptom measure you are using (e.g., PHQ-9, GDS-SF) in case they need to complete these items ahead of session time. Ensure that telehealth clients have multiple copies of that form that they can complete at home ahead of video- or telephone-only sessions.

Table 6.1 Sample Agenda for a 45-Minute Session 3

3 p.m.	Mood check/discuss scores
3:05 p.m.	Review values and strengths (Start 5 Practice)
3:10 p.m.	Review personal CBT model (Start 6 Practice)
3:25 p.m.	Begin to turn problems into goals
3:35 p.m.	Summarize and next steps (Start 3 Practice)
3:40 p.m.	Feedback

A significant percentage of problems related to home practice completion are due to clinician error, not client motivation. Before attributing compliance problems to the client, you must ensure that you are doing all that you can to promote compliance. It is on you as the clinician to make sure that sufficient time was spent discussing the reason for a specific home practice task and exactly what is expected, including doing an example together on the same form that the client will continue to work on at home. Try to set the specific time that the client will do the home practice, since increased structure and collaboration will improve the probability of the client completing the task. It is your job to help clients anticipate what might get in the way of completing home practice (e.g., specific daily events, thoughts, low mood). Identify these in advance, talk about them, and make plans ahead of time for a proactive response. Be sure the client writes down the assignment on their <u>Start 3 Practice</u> form (<u>My Session Summary</u>). Encourage questions if it's unclear what is to be done.

If the client does not do the home practice, work on your end to shore up your roles as just described. Then, you can also discuss what the problem might be: lack of clarity about the assignment, lack of time on the client's part, inability to articulate how it can help, no real belief in the model, and so on. You need to elicit reasons why the assignment was not done and respond within a CBT framework (e.g., *"Treat this as an experiment; it would be good for you to collect data about whether or not doing home practice is helpful rather than to just assume it isn't"*). See the home practice section in Chapter 5 for information on how to troubleshoot and suggestions for gaining cooperation.

Suggested Progression of Content

This important orientation to individual psychotherapy and goal setting takes approximately four sessions, depending on the client. Little progress will be made in addressing treatment goals until these initial steps have been accomplished. Sometimes, if the client is cognitively impaired or has other complications, the early phase may continue into an additional session. Table 6.2 presents the suggested sequence for this module.

Table 6.2 Session Outline

Each Session: Depression Measure + Start 3 & 4 Practice

GDS-SF or PHQ-9

Start 3 Practice	My Session Summary (begins Session 1)^T
Start 4 Practice	Preparing for My Next Session (begins Session 2)^T

Skills for Getting Started Session 1: Orientation to CBT

In Session 1: Start 1–4 Learn, Start 6 Learn, Start 1 Practice
Between Sessions 1 and 2: Start 1 and 2 Practice

Start 1 Learn	Introduction to Skills for Getting Started
Start 2 Learn	How Can This Workbook Help You?
Start 3 Learn	Making This Workbook Work for You^T
Start 4 Learn	What to Expect from Cognitive-Behavioral Therapy^T
Start 6 Learn	Overview of Clinical Depression^T
Start 1 Practice	My Depressive Symptoms
Start 2 Practice	One Daily Exception^T

Skills for Getting Started Session 2: Individualizing the CBT Conceptualization

In Session 2: Start 10–13 Learn, Start 6 Practice
Between Sessions 2 and 3: Start 5 and 6 Practice

Start 10 Learn	Your Life Values and Personal Strengths^T
Start 11 Learn	Celebrating Diversity^T
Start 12 Learn	Childhood Experiences
Start 13 Learn	What Is the Cognitive-Behavioral Model?^{T}
Start 5 Practice	My Values and Strengths^T
Start 6 Practice	The Cognitive-Behavioral Model of My Depression^T

Skills for Getting Started Session 3: Developing Therapy Goals

In Session 3: Start 14 and 15 Learn, Start 7–10 Practice
Between Sessions 3 and 4: Start 7–10 Practice

Start 14 Learn	Identifying and Prioritizing Target Problems
Start 15 Learn	Translating Problems into SMART Goals
Start 7 Practice	Problems to Target in Treatment

(continued)

Table 6.2 Continued

Start 8 Practice	My Target Problems
Start 9 Practice	My Goals for This Program
Start 10 Practice	My SMART Therapy Goals[T]

Skills for Getting Started Session 4: Expectations for Progress

In Session 4: Start 16 and 17 Learn, Start 10–13 Practice
After Session 4: Start 10–13 Practice

Start 16 Learn	Measuring Changes Using a Rating Scale
Start 17 Learn	Ways to Think About Progress Toward Your Goals[T]
Start 10 Practice	My SMART Therapy Goals[T]
Start 11 Practice	My Plan for Fully Participating
Start 12 Practice	Ways to Encourage Myself[T]
Start 13 Practice	My Review of Skills for Getting Started[T]

[T] Identified as particularly appropriate for telehealth sessions.

Not Included in This Treatment

Therapy Orientation for Family Members

Not all of your clients will wish to involve a family member in their therapy process, and some of your clients may not have someone available. For that reason, we have not provided specific Learn pages and Practice forms to facilitate discussions between your client and members of their social network whom they wish to involve in their treatment in some way. We have, however, noted on a number of Learn pages that clients may wish to share information they are learning in therapy with someone who is important to them.

Treatment Recommendations for Bipolar Depression

As described in Chapter 1 of this clinician manual, this treatment approach is appropriate for middle-aged and older adults who experience depressive symptoms due to subsyndromal unipolar depression or MDD. Treatment of depression that is a part of bipolar disorder is not addressed in this approach, but we would like to refer clinicians to Reiser et al. (2017).

Additional Resources for Clinicians

Hook, J. N., Davis, D., Owen, J., & DeBlaere, C. (2017). *Cultural humility: Engaging diverse identities in therapy.* American Psychological Association.

Scogin, F. R. (2000). *The first session with seniors: A step-by-step guide.* Jossey-Bass.

Swift, J. K., & Greenberg, R. P. (2015). *Premature termination in psychotherapy: Strategies for engaging clients and improving outcomes.* American Psychological Association.

Resources and Measures in Appendix D Related to This Module

(Recommendations for use are provided in Chapter 3 of this clinician guide.)

ADDRESSING Model Worksheet for Case Conceptualization

Geriatric Depression Scale—Short Form (GDS-SF)

GAD-7

Agnew Relationship Measure-5 (ARM-5)

CHAPTER 7

Module 2: Skills for Feeling: Recognizing and Managing Strong Emotions

This core module of the workbook is focused on the skills of:

1. Monitoring therapy progress and fine-tuning treatment goals
2. Understanding and describing emotional reactions
3. Nurturing positive emotions
4. Applying relaxation skills
5. Visualizing successful coping
6. Defusing anger or frustration
7. Revising therapy goals, staying encouraged and engaged in treatment

This chapter is provided to help you use the *Skills for Feeling* module of the workbook with your clients. We start with a brief overview, followed by some practical tips based on the most common questions we hear from clinicians during professional trainings. The bulk of this chapter is devoted to reviewing skills involved in this module, with a description of the specific Learn pages and Practice forms available for your use in sessions. We provide recommendations for a standard progression of material (i.e., Learn pages and Practice forms that typically go with each other in the same session, estimates of how much can be accomplished in a given session), with the understanding that this may vary quite a bit depending upon your practice setting and specific client needs. We end the chapter with some comments about related topics that are not included in this treatment approach, and point readers to resources for additional professional development related to this module's focus on emotional literacy and regulation.

Overview

CBT requires careful attention to your clients' emotional experiences, both within and outside of therapy. Some clinicians new to CBT have a misperception that emotional processes are relatively ignored in this treatment (sometimes merely because "emotion" does not appear alongside "cognitive" and "behavioral" in "CBT"). Attention to emotional experiences is viewed as validating by many clients, who may see clinicians as warm and caring especially in the context of processing emotions during session. There are also specific interventions in CBT that are impossible without a focus on emotions. Decisions about activity scheduling, for example, can only be made when you and your clients can identify changes in emotions following specific daily activities. Cognitive reappraisal strategies are only effective when the most current *and* emotionally loaded thoughts are identified, targeted, and modified.

We have placed both emotional literacy and interventions to foster positive emotions at the very beginning of this treatment. You will discuss the role of emotions, what emotions are, and how they work (e.g., de-bunk overly strong beliefs in catharsis as a primary change strategy). You will also be assessing your clients' abilities to label and describe emotional experiences.

When to Use This Module

We strongly recommend that you plan to use the first half of this module for all individual psychotherapy clients, early in treatment. That is why we have labeled this as a core module and placed it right after the *Skills for Getting Started* orientation to treatment. Clinicians using this module in groups will likely make some decisions regarding which materials are the best fit, depending upon the setting of the group (i.e., inpatient, partial hospitalization, outpatient) and whether it is a closed or open group. Clinicians who are doing very brief behavioral health interventions integrated into primary care settings may use some but not all of the materials in this module. For all clinicians, the first step in preparing to use this module is a thorough review of all Learn pages and Practice forms.

The core of the *Skills for Feeling* module includes basic psychoeducation about emotions (Feel 1 and 2 Learn), emotional literacy skills (Feel 3–6 Learn, Feel 2–4 Practice), a focus on cultivation of positive emotions (Feel 7–10 Learn, Feel 5–10 Practice), and an introduction to relaxation skills (Feel 11–14 Learn, Feel 11 and 12 Practice). Why did we select these skills? There are several good reasons. Distress over negative emotions can be a primary reason for seeking psychotherapy; this early focus on developing a shared understanding of emotions is used as a building block for the rest of therapy. Clients develop skills in labeling and describing the intensity of their feelings, which is a foundational CBT skill that will be applied in other modules. Importantly, individuals with depression and anxiety tend to ignore or minimize their positive emotional experiences. Spending time early in therapy to attend to and culti-vate positive emotions increases tolerance and savoring of positive emotions. We also suggest one or two sessions focused on relaxation

(<u>Feel 11–14 Learn</u>, <u>Feel 11</u> and <u>12 Practice</u>) to facilitate use of relaxation strategies within sessions.

We also provide materials to help you work with clients with anxiety and irritability, using more detailed relaxation training skills (<u>Feel 11–15 Learn</u>, <u>Feel 11</u> and <u>12 Practice</u>) and skills for managing frustration and anger (<u>Feel 15–18 Learn</u>, <u>Feel 13 Practice</u>). Particularly with highly anxious or irritable clients, using a relaxation exercise at the beginning or end of each session can improve focus and/or help them leave the session feeling better. Including relaxation exercises for home practice can increase the rate of compliance with other, more technical home practice assignments.

Tips for Clinicians

Discuss Limitations of Emotional Expression as a Treatment for Depression

One concrete benefit of this module's inclusion of psychoeducation about emotion is to debunk overly strong beliefs in emotional expression (i.e., catharsis) as a primary change strategy. As a clinician using this treatment approach, part of your job is to be a warm, trustworthy source of support as your client learns new skills. At the same time, it is important to find ways to repeat throughout therapy that simply talking about upsetting situations and feelings is not likely to be enough to reduce clinical depression.

Stay Aware of Generational Differences in Labeling Emotional Experiences

It can be helpful for clinicians new to working with older adults to be aware of cultural and generational differences in the labeling of emotions. Older women, for example, are less likely to endorse feeling "angry" than younger clients, instead preferring other labels such as "irritated" and "frustrated." The current cohorts of older adults are more likely to use words such as "nervous" or "tense" or describe that their "nerves are shot," more than feeling "anxious" (Wuthrich et al., 2015).

Respond to "I Relax By" (e.g., Reading the Newspaper, Dozing in My Chair)

Some of your older clients will respond to the material on relaxation by saying something to the effect of, "*Oh, I don't really need that because I relax by putting my feet up and reading the newspaper*" (or napping, etc.). Rather than contradicting this, we suggest you reply with,

> *I'm glad to hear that* _____ *is something you find relaxing. I would like to also suggest that you experiment with adding some other options. These might help during times when you are especially tense and need to relax on the spot. You may not always be able to relax in that way if you are in the middle of a difficult situation such as* _____ (insert example from the client's life). *Are you willing to try and see if this helps?*

Keep Relaxation Training as Simple as Possible

There are many effective methods of relaxation, but you should be somewhat cautious in selecting exercises for older adults. This module includes a few relaxation techniques that we have found helpful and that seem to be acceptable to most older adults. We suggest a trial-and-error method of selecting exercises for clients. Remember that some methods are more appropriate for some situations than others. A simple deep-breathing exercise can be done almost anywhere, whereas listening to music or going for a walk can be very relaxing but requires time and access. It is good to review with clients what they are already doing and whether or not it's working for them. Many are already practicing some form of relaxation that may not work so well anymore or that may consume too much time or energy to be effective at this point in their lives.

Some clients will be turned off by complexity. Learn what they are doing now, if anything, and see if it can be fine-tuned. Teach simple deep breathing, since it is so portable and, for most people, very easy to learn. Work with the client's lifestyle to suggest other relaxation methods, so that by the conclusion of therapy, the client has a repertoire of several relaxation techniques that are manageable and can be used as needed to reduce anxiety and improve quality of life.

Monitoring Therapy Progress and Fine-Tuning Treatment Goals

This module begins with the orientation provided in Feel 1 Learn: Introduction to Skills for Feeling and the important reminder to have a "state of therapy" discussion about therapy goals and progress. This is a good time to review the overall pattern of depression scores, using whichever weekly measure of depression is a part of this feedback-informed treatment. This is the first opportunity that your client has to review the two or three treatment goals developed in *Skills for Getting Started*, to see whether each goal is still a good fit. Allow for a third (15 to 20 minutes) of the first session in this module to discuss Feel 1 Practice: Review of My Treatment Goals, determine whether these goals need to be refined to be useful in treatment, and evaluate them.

Understanding and Describing Emotional Reactions

CBT involves careful attention to emotions and emotional experiences of clients. Within both inpatient and outpatient CBT, emotional regulation skills begin with the ability to label and describe emotional experiences (Berking et al., 2013). Begin with Feel 2 Learn: Understanding Emotions to discuss together what emotions are and how they work.

Across all of the following modules, you will ask clients to label and describe their emotional experiences and identify triggering situations. Feel 3–6 Learn and Feel 2 and 3 Practice and/or Feel 4 Practice are to be used in session, and reviewed between sessions, to help clients develop and use their emotional literacy skills. You will want to stick with the emotional vocabulary that is natural to your client. Feel 2 Practice: My Mood Scale helps you work together to develop that list of key words to describe emotions. All older clients can benefit from printed lists of feeling terms available to look at during the therapy session. Recognition memory is far easier than recall for all of us, and this increases with age. Use Feel 5 and 6 Learn and Feel 4 Practice to continue the education about the CBT model, and help clients begin to see the connections between situations, thoughts, emotions, and behaviors. Hofmann (2016) provides additional suggestions related to working with emotions in CBT. You will see the optional Feel 4 Learn: Recognizing Mixed Emotions (linked to Feel 3 Practice: A Pie Chart of Mixed Emotions) specific to processing mixed emotions. This is a more advanced skill and is particularly helpful when clients describe finding themselves confused about their reactions to specific situations.

Using first Feel 5 Learn: Feelings Are Just the Tip of the Iceberg and then Feel 6 Learn: The ABC Model, you will introduce the ABC model. You can give an example in session, such as the following:

Assume that you are going up on an elevator when suddenly you receive a sharp poke in the ribs. What goes through your mind? (The client will usually give a mixture of thoughts and feelings. Try to elicit both, while differentiating between the two.)

Good! So you think to yourself, "This person is going to rob me" (write this under the "Beliefs" column) *and you feel "scared,"* (write this under the "Consequences" column) *or you might think, "What an inconsiderate person!"* (write this under the "Beliefs" column) *and you feel "irritated"* (write this under the "Consequences" column). *Now assume that you turn around and you notice the person who poked you has a white-tipped cane and is blind. How do you feel now?* (Elicit responses separating "Beliefs" and "Consequences" column information.)

What is different in these two situations? (Try to get the client to explain some variation of "I learned something new about the situation.") *Right! You turned around and gained information that you didn't have before in order to have a more positive reaction.*

This is a small example of how CBT works. You will learn various ways to "turn around" your thoughts, assumptions, and perceptions in order to gain new insights and more helpful beliefs that will lead to more positive emotions.

Apply the ABC "chain" using Feel 6 Learn: The ABC Model, and discuss a specific example from the client's life to facilitate learning. Feel 4 Practice: ABC Form can be assigned between sessions; in Situation 1, help the client to write in an example that you discussed in session.

Nurturing Positive Emotions

In addition to the ongoing scientific advances in positive psychology and positive psychotherapy, there are accumulating data on the ways that individuals with depression and anxiety may actively avoid positive emotions. Feel 7 Learn: Nurturing Positive Emotions is an informational sheet to discuss together in session, followed by Feel 5 Practice: Recognizing Positive Emotions or Feel 6 Practice: Growing Positive Emotions to be used between sessions. Depending upon the preferences of your clients, the following session can focus on Feel 8 Learn: Highlighting the Positive (e.g., gratitude, kind acts, positive experiences), with Feel 7 and 8 Practice as a between-session assignment. Or, clients who prefer a focus on humor can choose to focus in session on Feel 9 Learn: Using Humor and Feel 10 Learn: One Funny Thing, and then use Feel 9 and 10 Practice as the between-session assignment.

Applying Relaxation Skills

We have provided Feel 11 Learn: Awareness of Tension as a way to begin the work on relaxation with a discussion of the client's specific experiences of tension or nervousness (i.e., anxiety). The more situations that the person is anxious about, the more important it is to address the anxiety as a problem in its own right. Spend a few moments discussing their physical symptoms that are signals of tension. Most clients judge their level of anxiety according to the severity of these symptoms, so it is important for you to know the full range of symptoms involved. Feel 11 Practice: Relaxation Diary can be used as a way for clients to become aware of both tension and relaxation each day across the week and to identify triggering situations.

Feel 12 Learn: Relaxation Is Important emphasizes the importance of relaxation in treating depression. Strong feelings of anxiety often accompany depression. Many people report that increased anxiety worsens their negative thinking, creates significant physical tension, and intensifies physical pain. Relaxation can be an effective tool to break this vicious cycle. We often hear clients describe themselves as feeling overwhelmed by these emotions, unable to find a way to reduce their impact. It is also common for these feelings to be so intense that people find it hard to imagine a time when these feelings were absent. Relaxation skills help clients gain at least some control.

Guided Relaxation Practice Within Session

You can't just talk about relaxation; you must actively help your clients practice within session. We recommend starting with a brief, guided relaxation exercise that is quite effective with middle-aged and older people who are experiencing significant anxiety along with depression. In addition to the <u>Relaxation Diary</u> provided in <u>Feel 11 Practice</u>, we provide <u>Feel 12 Practice: My Relaxation Practice Log</u>, which you will introduce and use during the following within-session exercise; this log will also help clients learn to practice between sessions.

In session, ask clients to first rate their tension before you start the exercise, and then have them rate it again after the exercise is completed. At that time, if the tension level has not dropped, ask for feedback (What interfered? Were there intrusive thoughts? Did the client have difficulty focusing attention on the breath?). Try to find out what the problem is, and then problem solve for a remedy. If there is time, repeat the exercise in session so that the client has an opportunity to experience the value of this technique.

Instructions for In-Session Controlled Breathing Exercise

Read the following exercise to your clients to allow them to experience a breathing exercise during session.

1. *Sit in a comfortable position, keeping arms and legs uncrossed.*
2. *Keep your eyes closed and try to block out all external sounds.*
3. *This deep-breathing exercise is very simple: I will ask you to breathe very slowly, inhaling through the nose and exhaling through the mouth. Focus on your breathing, and breathe with a steady pace. To help you breathe in slowly, I will count to five (IN—2, 3, 4, 5). Please inhale to that count, then exhale to the same count, if you can (OUT—2, 3, 4, 5). If that bothers you in any way, let me know, and we will shorten the intervals. If not, let's continue.*

Visual Imagery

You can ask the client to use visual imagery as well and to incorporate that with the deep breathing. We suggest you do not begin that until the client masters the slow, deep breathing; adding visual imagery helps them relax more deeply. Before starting, ask the client to select a safe and relaxing place and to picture it in their "mind's eye." If clients have a problem coming up with something, suggest scenes, such as the beach, a lake, a location in the mountains, or in the warm desert sun. Once the client has an image in mind, you can begin. The following are useful phrases for guiding the relaxation:

- *Imagine a (this) safe and relaxing place where there are no worries or cares or concerns.*
- *Now imagine yourself in that place.*
- *Gently keep that image in your mind's eye while breathing, all the while inhaling and exhaling slowly and deeply.*
- *Let all thoughts that float into awareness, float out again. This is not a time to think about things, but to just relax.*

Additional Relaxation Options

In <u>Feel 14 Learn: Options for Relaxing</u>, we provide additional options for relaxation, depending upon clients' preferences (i.e., music, mild exercise, religious/spiritual activities). Most people agree that music affects their moods, although they may not have consciously chosen to use music to *improve* their mood or to relax. Walking (or any other mild exercise that the person enjoys) can also be a reliable form of relaxation. For those who do not care or are unable to walk, recommend other forms of gentle exercise for stress reduction, such as stretching exercises (often done to music), gentle yoga, tai chi, qi gong, or chair exercise programs. Classes can often be found in community settings such as a senior center (which would add a socialization component that can also be extremely important for the isolated and lonely older client).

We start our list of religious and spiritual activities with nature to emphasize that you may have clients with a strong spirituality but who are not affiliated with a specific religious tradition. Connecting to nature and a variety of meditation practices can be a powerful means of relaxation. For older adults who have a religious orientation or background, significant stress reduction can be found in some forms of prayer, listening to or singing along with religious-affiliated music, reading religious or spiritual material, and/or attending a religious or spiritual gathering or service. Again, this is not for everyone, and prayer forms vary significantly in terms of whether they are meditative or energizing. The purpose and intent of prayer is not to relax, but relaxation may be one of many positive outcomes for some clients. If prayer is part of your client's life experience, some forms are options for potentially deep relaxation and should not be overlooked.

Ask clients to practice relaxation daily (at least once a day) to reduce their levels of tension and/or anxiety. Instruct them to do the exercise when they are tense if at all possible, so that they feel some immediate benefit. Clients should complete <u>Feel 12 Practice: My Relaxation Log</u> before and after doing each relaxation exercise. This is a crucial step so that even small decreases in perceived tension will be noted, and the client will be encouraged to continue to practice. For those clients who are not initially able to use a relaxation technique when they are actually tense, have them start out by setting aside specific times of day to practice, and frame it as *"relaxation is a treat you can give yourself."* Keep reminding them that practice is needed to enhance the effects and that different methods will likely have different results at different times.

Sometimes, the only effective remedy to deal with anxiety/tension is to rest (to lie down or take a nap) or to distract oneself (escape into reading a book or watching TV). We want, however, to reduce the number of times that clients use these avoidant coping strategies and instead encourage active coping by conscious use of a relaxation strategy that works for them. Relaxation can also be used to prepare clients for an upcoming stressful event. For example, if visits to a particular family member are stressful, encourage the client to spend a few moments in their "relaxation spot" prior to the visit. In addition, clients may want to try relaxation exercises as a nice way to start the day, even if they are not in a high-stress moment. Relaxation can also create a calm break to refocus throughout the day. Often, clients expect their tension to decrease more than it does after their first few practices. Remind them that the more they practice relaxation, the more relaxed they will feel immediately following the exercise. Also, with increased practice, there will be a decrease in the time it takes to reach a relaxed state. Encourage the use of Feel 12 Practice: My Relaxation Practice Log to note progress and identify problems.

Visualizing Successful Coping

Feel 15 Learn: Preparing for Stressful Events with Imagery provides information about how to use imagery as another tool to manage intense feelings. Clients create in their mind a "picture" of the stressful situation and its possible solutions. Visualization skills can help challenge clients' perceptions of the outcomes of stressful situations and manage intense emotions. Clients picture a stressful event and the feelings, thoughts, and outcomes they associate with it. Then, they are instructed to return to imagining the situation, this time picturing the outcome using a different perspective. Elicit a description of this outcome. Is the original negative outcome as likely as it seemed before considering other possible outcomes? This exercise is aimed at helping clients re-imagine the situation as less emotionally charged and with more confidence in their ability to manage it effectively.

Defusing Anger or Frustration

Simple, brief relaxation exercises can also be done in session to help clients learn that negative feelings such as irritation, frustration, and anger can be reduced with practice. You can use Feel 16 Learn: Managing Irritation, Frustration, and Anger and Feel 17 Learn: "Stop Signs" to Manage Irritation, Frustration, and Anger in session to help the client recognize that the anger is getting out of hand and learn about "danger signals" and "stop signs." Danger signals are the particular changes in the body that occur when feelings of anger are rising. Stop signs are strong visual images that can be used to interrupt the negative feelings and the train of thoughts long enough to enable the client to gain cognitive control. When used correctly, individualized stop signs enable the client to take a short breather when feeling overwhelmed by negative emotions or the physical sensations associated with them. Stop signs are mental images that make the client "stop and think." To be effective, they need to be powerful, meaningful to the individual, and effective in interrupting negative feelings and thoughts. The point is that clients should be encouraged to use whatever is both dramatic and meaningful to them. Between sessions clients can use <u>Feel 13 Practice: What to Do After Danger Signals and Stop Signs</u> to help them recognize danger signals, use stop signs, and then apply coping strategies that involve new thoughts or new actions. We find that by linking this model to action at the end, we increase the likelihood that the client will use it.

Revising Therapy Goals, Staying Encouraged and Engaged in Treatment

<u>Feel 19 Learn: Setting Personal Goals Related to Your Feelings</u> provides the option for you and your client to collaboratively decide whether you should change or revise therapy goals. Again, it is important to emphasize that therapy can focus on addressing no more than two or three overall goals. Sometimes as work in a specific module is wrapping up, it becomes clear that focused work on change in one area is likely to be an important part of ending the depression. Either <u>Feel 1 Practice</u> or <u>Do 1 Practice</u> (both are <u>Review of My Treatment Goals</u>) could be used as a form to write down and rate those revised goals. <u>Feel 20 Learn: Ways to Think About Progress Toward Your Goals</u> reminds clients of the most common pattern of change with therapy (sawtooth curve, not a straight line or stair steps). We recommend using <u>Feel 14 Practice: As I Continue with Treatment: My Plan for Fully Participating</u> for times when you already have some concerns about a client's engagement in treatment, either within session or in compliance with between-session practice.

<u>Feel 15 Practice: My Review of Skills for Feeling</u> can be used with all clients to review and consolidate key points and skills that were worked on in this module.

First, you need to thoroughly review all related Learn pages and Practice forms, so you are familiar with their content and can think about the fit between different skills and the needs of your specific clients. We realize that behavioral health providers working within primary care may use materials from this module in very brief sessions and will select individual Learn pages and Practice forms that fit the concerns and needs of their clients. Similarly, there may be occasions within individual or group psychotherapy when clinicians choose specific Learn and/or Practice materials.

This module will generally require four to six sessions to complete the recommended core components (i.e., psychoeducation, emotional literacy, enhancing positive emotions, basic relaxation). The additional segments can be used as needed and can be interwoven into the other modules. In almost all therapy cases, this module will be initiated after clinicians have worked on goal setting and therapy orientation in the *Skills for Getting Started* module. Sessions will use the same basic structure: (a) set an agenda, (b) review home practice, (c) select at least one topic to work on in depth, (d) summarize, (e) set up new home practice assignment, and (f) do mutual feedback. Start work on all Practice forms within session, or wait for the next session to introduce them. Don't send a client home with a Practice form without a personal example already inserted. Be sure to allow time to review any Practice forms in the next session.

For most of your clients, you will move directly from finishing with this module into behavioral activation in *Skills for Doing*. There will also be times when you have finished *Skills for Feeling*, have started work with clients in another module, and will find yourself coming back to key Learn pages and Practice forms in this module. This is especially true for skills in cultivating positive emotions and relaxation.

Table 7.1 presents the suggested sequence for this module.

Table 7.1 Session Outline

Each Session: Depression Measure + Start 3 and 4 Practice

GDS-SF or PHQ-9

Start 4 Practice	Preparing for My Next Session[T]
Start 3 Practice	My Session Summary[T]

Skills for Feeling Session 1: Assess Progress and Psychoeducation

In Session 1: Feel 1 and 2 Learn, Feel 1 Practice (+ prior session review)

Between Sessions 1 and 2: Feel 1 Practice

Feel 1 Learn	Introduction to Skills for Feeling
Feel 2 Learn	Understanding Emotions[T]
Feel 1 Practice	Review of My Treatment Goals[T]

Skills for Feeling Session 2: Emotional Literacy

In Session 2: Feel 3 Learn, Feel 5 and 6 Learn

Between Sessions 2 and 3: Feel 2 Practice, Feel 4 Practice

Feel 3 Learn	Emotional Literacy[T]
Feel 5 Learn	Feelings Are Just the Tip of the Iceberg[T]
Feel 6 Learn	The ABC Model[T]
Feel 2 Practice	My Mood Scale[T]
Feel 4 Practice	ABC Form[T]

Skills for Feeling Session 3: Nurturing Positive Emotions

In Session 3: Feel 7 Learn

Between Sessions 3 and 4: Feel 5 Practice or Feel 6 Practice

Feel 7 Learn	Nurturing Positive Emotions[T]
Feel 5 Practice	Recognizing Positive Emotions[T]
Feel 6 Practice	Growing Positive Emotions

(You may skip Session 4 for some clients.)

(continued)

Table 7.2 Continued

Skills for Feeling Session 4: Highlighting the Positive / Humor

In Session 4: Feel 8 Learn or Feel 9 and 10 Learn

Between Sessions 4 and 5: Feel 7 and 8 Practice or Feel 9 and 10 Practice

Feel 8 Learn	Highlighting the Positive[T]
Feel 9 Learn	Using Humor
Feel 10 Learn	One Funny Thing
Feel 7 Practice	Highlighting the Positive I[T]
Feel 8 Practice	Highlighting the Positive II[T]
Feel 9 Practice	One Funny Thing I
Feel 10 Practice	One Funny Thing II

Skills for Feeling Session 5: Relaxation

In Session 5: Feel 11–14 Learn

Between Session 5 and 6: Feel 11 and 12 Practice

Feel 11 Learn	Awareness of Tension[T]
Feel 12 Learn	Relaxation Is Important[T]
Feel 13 Learn	How to Relax[T]
Feel 14 Learn	Options for Relaxing[T]
Feel 11 Practice	Relaxation Diary[T]
Feel 12 Practice	My Relaxation Practice Log[T]

(You may skip Session 6 for some clients.)

Skills for Feeling Session 6: More Relaxation

In Session 6: Feel 11–14 Learn, Feel 15 Practice

After Session 6: Feel 12 Practice

Feel 11 Learn	Awareness of Tension
Feel 12 Learn	Relaxation Is Important[T]
Feel 13 Learn	How to Relax[T]
Feel 14 Learn	Options for Relaxing[T]
Feel 12 Practice	My Relaxation Practice Log[T]
Feel 15 Practice	My Review of Skills for Feeling[T]

[T] Identified as particularly appropriate for telehealth sessions.

A Variety of Relaxation Exercises

It can be quite difficult for older adults with joint or muscular difficulties to engage in exercises requiring the physical tensing and releasing of their muscles, as is commonly found in the technique called progressive muscle relaxation. Therefore, that particular method, although very effective, is not generally recommended for use with older adults. Our experience with older adults has led us to emphasize very simple cued controlled breathing and imagery/visual-based relaxation methods.

Mindfulness Training

The past two decades have seen an explosion of interest in mindfulness meditation training. Some of this has been incorporated into mindfulness-based CBT, as well into other treatment approaches. There may be clients who already have a history of using and enjoying mindfulness meditations or other practices to be mindful throughout the day. Such clients can certainly continue to use those as they go through this treatment. It is also the case that mindfulness practices are intended to increase acceptance of strong emotions rather than to generate feelings of being relaxed. More focused development of mindfulness skills is beyond the scope of our approach.

Strategies to Target Generalized Anxiety Disorder

The attention that we give to anxiety in this module is in recognition of the high rates of comorbidity between depression and anxiety. Many older adults who are in treatment for depression experience significant anxiety symptoms. Clinicians should keep in mind that there are evidence-based treatment approaches for generalized anxiety disorder (GAD) in older adults. When a clinical interview early in treatment suggests GAD, in addition to high GAD-7 scores, it is possible that the depression is secondary to (a result of) a lifetime of GAD. In those circumstances, treatment should likely move away from this program and involve one of the evidence-based treatments specific to GAD (Ayers et al., 2015; Bower et al., 2015).

Additional Resources for Clinicians

Hofmann, S. G. (2016). *Emotion in therapy: From science to practice.* Guilford Press.
Thoma, N. C., & McKay, D. (Eds.). (2014). *Working with emotion in cognitive-behavioral therapy: Techniques for clinical practice.* Guilford Press.

Measure in Appendix D Related to This Module

GAD-7

CHAPTER 8

Module 3: Skills for Doing: Values-Based Living and Solving Problems

This core module of the workbook is focused on the skills of:

1. Monitoring therapy progress and fine-tuning treatment goals
2. Understanding the role of activities in depression
3. Recording daily activities
4. Developing a written list of positive activities
5. Scheduling and engaging in positive activities
6. Applying the steps of problem solving
7. Revising therapy goals, staying encouraged and engaged in treatment

This chapter is provided to help you use the *Skills for Doing* module of the workbook with your clients. We start with a brief overview, followed by some practical tips based on the most common questions we hear from clinicians during professional trainings. The bulk of this chapter is devoted to reviewing behavioral activation and problem-solving skills, with a description of the specific Learn pages and Practice forms available for your use in sessions. We provide recommendations for a standard progression of material (i.e., Learn pages and Practice forms that typically go with each other in the same session, estimates of how much can be accomplished in a given session), with the understanding that this may vary quite a bit depending upon your practice setting and specific client needs. We end the chapter with some comments about related topics that are not included in this treatment approach, and point readers to resources for additional professional development in behavioral activation.

Overview

Considerable research done over the past 50 years has shown that as individuals become more active, depressive symptoms decrease. Clients are able to view stressful events from a different perspective in light of experiencing positive activities. Our clinical observations have led us to coin the phrase "*Four* positive activities a day keeps the blues away." These activities are to be consciously chosen and deliberately done. It is not enough for positive events to "happen"; rather, they must be planned into the client's day and implemented in order to be effective, becoming a new lifestyle habit so that clients can gain some control over their mood.

Refer back to Figure 2.1: Model of Depression in Older Adults, shown on page 21 of this guide, where we see that the specific function of daily activities is key. On the left side of this figure, we can see many of the life circumstances that may have created the context for depression (e.g., medical conditions, physical limitations, bereavement, residential moves, other losses). These losses are possible contributors, but they affect depression indirectly—largely through decreases in daily meaningful and rewarding activities. The right side of the figure shows how these decreases in daily activities play an especially strong role in perpetuating the cycle of depression in middle-aged and older adults. For that reason, working to increase daily rewarding, meaningful, and valued activities is a priority in this treatment.

When to Use This Module

Behavioral activation (BA) is recommended for use early in treatment with all middle-aged and older adults with depression because there is strong empirical support for BA as an effective strategy on its own to treat depression across the lifespan (Richards et al., 2016). The conceptual development of BA was given impetus by the research and subsequent theoretical model developed by Peter Lewinsohn and colleagues confirming that increasing pleasant events and/or decreasing unpleasant events results in improved mood states in individuals with depression (Dimidjian et al., 2011; Fishman, 2016). Dismantling research studies, which investigate whether specific components of a treatment package are needed for change, have led to the conclusion that BA (*Skills for Doing*) is a powerful and effective change strategy on its own (Kanter et al., 2010; Moshier & Otto, 2017). Importantly, BA has been shown to be effective for a diverse range of adults (Aguilera et al., 2010) and older individuals, including African American older adults in the United States (Szanton et al., 2014).

The first step in preparing to use this module is a thorough review of all Learn pages and Practice forms so you are familiar with the content and can begin to think about the fit between different skills and specific clients. Because BA is a practical, individually tailored treatment that emphasizes clients' values and preferences, it is inherently culturally sensitive (Kanter & Puspitasar, 2016). Your job is to help your clients identify simple activities that can be done most (if not all) days of the week and that are culturally friendly for each individual (e.g., family and/or faith based, connection with nature).

Our aim in the *Skills for Doing* module is for you to work collaboratively with your clients to develop and use these skills in daily life. We recommend that following therapy orientation (*Skills for Getting Started*) and emotional literacy (*Skills for Feeling*), you start with BA (not cognitive skill building) with middle-aged and older adults with depression.

An exception to this treatment order is when the onset of therapy is dominated by a major stressor (e.g., caregiving, pain, bereavement) that leads the client to dismiss any interventions not explicitly focused on that stressor. For example, we have found that the circumstances of caregiving can lead clients to discount the focus on their own BA at the very start of treatment. In those cases, after completing *Skills for Getting Started*, begin with the assessment and intervention strategies in *Skills for Caregiving*, and then circle back to portions of the *Skills for Feeling* and *Skills for Doing* that appear to be a good fit with the client's needs. There may also be some clients with chronic pain or recent major losses for whom the same strategy is helpful (e.g., transition from *Skills for Getting Started* directly to the specific personalized module in *Skills for Managing Chronic Pain* or *Skills for Living with Loss*, and then circle back to *Skills for Feeling* and *Skills for Doing* when such clients believe that you are taking their life circumstances seriously and they better understand the applicability of those skills).

Tips for Clinicians

Stay Specific

It can be easy to fall into a common pitfall of discussing daily activities in a general and abstract way (e.g., "Whenever I try X, it doesn't work because of Y or because Z happens"). Those abstract discussions create difficulties in helping your clients develop new healthy lifestyle habits that include rewarding activities. For BA to be an effective treatment strategy, you need to work with specifics and details (e.g., experiences on a specific day, future plans for a specific time and day).

Focus on Increasing Activities That Are Already Considered Positive

Our values- and strengths-based approach encourages you and your clients to look for daily activities that they already experience as rewarding, positive, and/or meaningful (currently or in the past) but in which they do not frequently engage. Resist the urge to target activities and experiences that are so-so or negative in terms of positivity in the hopes that therapy can increase enjoyability (e.g., attempting to increase pleasure of contact with a family member when there is a history of conflict). Especially in this early phase of BA, we are looking for the "low-hanging fruit" of activities that are enjoyable or valued when they occur but are just not happening often enough. The next level is to identify things that the client has valued or enjoyed in the past but that need some modification to fit the client's current circumstances and abilities.

Prioritize Physical and Social Activities

Because of the vital role of exercise for physical, cognitive, and emotional health, physical activities are especially important. Virtually any movement is beneficial, so help your clients get moving however possible. Break this down into as many steps/phases as needed to get started. We provide additional resources in Do 13 Learn: Your Plan for Physical Activity. A very useful website sponsored by the National Institute on Aging on how to incorporate physical activity into one's life is https://www.nia.nih.gov/health/exercise-physical-activity. Similarly, any activities that are experienced as positive and that increase a sense of connection with others are especially useful in combating depression and reducing loneliness in older adults. This can include any activities actually done with others (e.g., going to lunch with a friend) as well as activities that encourage the client to feel more connected to others (e.g., looking at pictures or videos of past good times).

Return to Material in Skills for Feeling

Some clients report a solid level of daily positive activities and do not appear to be socially isolated but still struggle with depression. Often, this anhedonia (i.e., absence of enjoyment) is accompanied by a reluctance to savor positive emotions. Beliefs such as "this is good now but won't last" and "I don't want to be disappointed in the future" may lead some individuals to avoid or abruptly discontinue activities that are pleasurable. The *Skills for Feeling* module, which includes material on cultivation of positive emotions, is intentionally provided ahead of

BA for this reason. In therapy where you have used only the emotional literacy material from *Skills for Feeling*, you may need to cycle back to that module to spend more time on cultivating and savoring positive emotions through the positive psychology interventions provided there.

Re-emphasize Problem-Solving Skills—DEEDs!

Middle-aged and older adults can experience a number of life stressors that pose true difficulties in daily life. Some of these stressors tax their existing coping abilities, especially in depressed individuals with poor concentration and/or cognitive limitations. In *Skills for Doing* (<u>Do 16–18 Learn</u>, <u>Do 6 Practice</u>), we have provided a DEEDS clinical tool to help your clients learn problem-solving skills. This is different than merely having session time filled with solving the problem of the week (which can take up entire sessions and the bulk of psychotherapy if you and your client fall into that pattern). The DEEDS tool is designed to be used repeatedly, across different problems that interfere with BA, to reinforce client learning and then using problem-solving skills on their own. Learning to use this tool will take multiple repetitions.

Embrace Collaborative Empiricism

At its heart, CBT for later-life depression is deeply humanistic in its focus on each client as an individual. In addition to the strong emphasis on grounding BA in each client's values and personal strengths, we encourage an open "let's see what is true for you" experimental approach. Collaborative empiricism refers to clinicians and clients working together, often side by side in the therapy room, finding the patterns and behavioral solutions that fit for that individual.

Remember That Behavioral Changes Can Lead to Cognitive Changes

We recognize that starting with BA may be counter to many clinicians' (and some clients') tendencies, for whom upsetting situations and thoughts are more salient and feel more pressing. Just keep in mind that changing daily experiences is a powerful way to impact thoughts and feelings. Behavioral work gradually leads to changes in negative expectations and other unhelpful thought patterns. After working on behavioral changes and development of new habits, it becomes more apparent where the "stuck" points are regarding thoughts, and then it may be appropriate to work on development of cognitive reappraisal skills in *Skills for Thinking*. While doing any cognitive reappraisal work, however, keep in mind that this is usually in the service of leading toward additional behavioral changes, which then influence both thoughts and feelings. Thus, the CBT model of reciprocal relationships and interactions is very much at work here.

Adapt Positive Activities for Clients with Physical or Cognitive Disabilities

Older clients often have physical disabilities that make it difficult to participate in cherished activities. Due to their depression, they don't see real alternatives; some don't even see the point in trying. These issues usually become apparent during the assessment. Your job is to help clients figure out what they still can do and what physical resources are needed to make this happen. Problem solving helps to find substitute activities that clients *can* do and to modify activities they previously enjoyed so that they can engage in them now. There are also some depressed individuals with multiple comorbidities (e.g., severe osteoporosis with fear of falling) and no family nearby; they may be cared for by paid assistants who also provide companionship. With such clients, we recommend discussing how these paid caregivers can help.

Older adults with mild cognitive impairment (MCI) are also very likely to benefit from increasing everyday positive activities. The presence of mild (or greater) cognitive impairment (regardless of cause) can be determined through use of the measures described in Chapter 3 of this clinician guide. We recommend including an involved family member when working with clients with cognitive impairments.

Monitoring Therapy Progress and Fine-Tuning Treatment Goals

This module begins with the orientation provided in <u>Do 1 Learn: Introduction to Skills for Doing</u> and the important reminder to have a "state of therapy" discussion about therapy goals and progress. This is a good time to review the overall pattern of depression scores, using whichever weekly measure of depression is a part of this feedback-informed treatment. Complete and review <u>Do 1 Practice: Review of My Treatment Goals</u> during session so that the overall therapy goals stay in the forefront while working on this module. The first session of this module will likely include some time following up with practice related to the previous *Skills for Feeling* module.

Understanding the Role of Activities in Depression

You will help your clients explore the role of activity in their depression through activity monitoring. Clients then identify, list, schedule, and engage in rewarding and meaningful activities, modifying activities as they learn what really does impact their mood. You will help them develop problem-solving skills, which can also be applied in later personalized modules that are focused on specific life domains (e.g., sleep, pain management). Encourage your clients to continue integrating daily activities as part of a healthy lifestyle (i.e., both important in treating their current depression and in preventing future occurrences of depression). You will frame all of this work within the context of clients' personal life values and strengths to ensure that they are engaging in culturally congruent daily activities that are consistent with their values and strengths.

You will use <u>Do 1–4 Learn</u> to introduce this module and discuss the relationships between activities and mood. Clients with depression are usually engaging in very few activities. On the other hand, as negative filtering is a characteristic way for them to misperceive events, they also may underestimate the number of activities they are doing and how positive such activities might be.

Recording Daily Activities

It is important to obtain an objective assessment of what the client is doing during the week and how enjoyable various things are. Do 2 Practice: First Steps (along with Do 3 Practice: First Steps Instructions) is designed to assist with this assessment. Once the form has been filled out for the previous week, collaboratively review it with the client, using the questions provided in Do 5 Learn: Using the First Steps. This will help your client recognize the link between activities and mood and begin to identify positive behaviors or thematic areas to expand upon in the activity scheduling process. Do 6 and 7 Learn provide an example for any clients who struggle with seeing this in their own lives.

Do 8 Learn: The Importance of Doing uses the concept of a downward spiral of depressed mood and low activities. This concept illustrates that "giving in" to the "slowed down" feeling that often comes with depression leads to a downward spiral (do less → feel worse → do even less, and so on). Clients will learn ways of stopping this tailspin and also reversing it. This therapy aims to also prevent future recurrences of depression; clients learn to stop a tailspin before it gets started by changing behaviors and thoughts that could lead to a downward spiral. Clients will also learn techniques to reverse the tailspin and move themselves in an upward spiral.

Developing a Written List of Positive Activities

The initial focus is on activities that the client has already been engaging in or has the immediate opportunity to do so. As the client understands more at the experiential level about the relationship between activities and mood, it is helpful to identify and write down other positive activities that they might plan to try in the future. *The development of a written list is key!* The Do 9–13 Learn pages and Do 4 Practice: List of Positive Activities are designed to assist with this. Aim for clients to list at least 10 (preferably 15 to 20) activities they *may* enjoy. They will then experiment to find out which they actually *do* enjoy.

You can also assign the California Older Person's Positive Experiences Schedule-Revised (COPPES-R; client workbook) as a between-sessions home practice; be sure to help your clients begin completing this within session. If clients are unable to complete this material on their own, do it with the client during session and use it as a springboard for discussion. Scoring information and detailed instructions for using the COPPES-R are provided in Appendix C of this clinician guide. Additional resources for the COPPES-R, including an online administration and scoring tool, are provided at the Optimal Aging Center's website (www.optimalagingcenter.com).

Scheduling and Engaging in Positive Activities

Using Do 5 Practice: PAL: Positive Activities Log in collaboration with your client, take the information obtained from the past week to revise the list of activities and update it for the coming week so that the activities become more likely to happen. Remember to keep activities simple and achievable. Do 14 Learn: Schedule Your Activities provides tips and reminds clients to keep it simple, and Do 15 Learn provides an example. You can also ask some questions to help guide your client, such as "*How likely is it that you actually will do these activities?*" "*Can you think of things that might get in your way of following the schedule? How do you think you might prevent that from happening?*"

It is vital for treatment success to continue the use of Do 5 Practice: PAL: Positive Activities Log (which helps clients with mood monitoring and recording of daily positive events) for a minimum of 2 consecutive weeks. Using it for 4 weeks is preferred so that this practice becomes incorporated into daily life. Increased positive activities will assist clients greatly in maintaining a positive mood. Do 5 Practice is one of the most important skill-development tools in this entire treatment approach.

When reviewing home practice at subsequent sessions, be sure to discuss what did *not* work, as well as what did, and revise accordingly. You want clients to understand that their activities are likely to change over time (e.g., in winter, they may not want to walk outside, so where else could they walk? Or, if walking isn't likely to happen in the winter months, what other activity can be substituted?). The point is that PAL is a dynamic tool, not a static "one and done"; it changes as clients' health and life circumstances change. It is vital that the client understands this.

Applying the Steps of Problem Solving

Problem solving is a skill that can be helpful throughout this treatment. We include it here to help your clients deal with concrete issues in activity scheduling and in keeping up their practice, but it can help in other modules as well. You will use <u>Do 16–18 Learn</u> in session to help your clients learn a five-step technique for developing alternatives and options for managing a situation or solving a problem. This technique is referred to as DEEDS:

- Define the problem.
- Explore possible solutions.
- Evaluate solutions.
- Decide on one alternative.
- Select another alternative.

Step 1: Define the Problem

The first task is to define the problem as specifically as possible. This step can often be the most challenging, as sometimes several different problems can be embedded into one. Clients need to sort out each problem and pick the one that appears to cause the greatest distress. If not immediately apparent, monitoring between sessions may be necessary to identify the antecedents and consequences of the problem behavior or event.

Step 2: Explore Possible Solutions

This is a brainstorming step in which potential solutions to a problem are proposed. The key to brainstorming is not to evaluate each potential solution, but just allow suggestions to be presented.

Step 3: Evaluate Solutions

This step allows possible solutions to be evaluated based on any criteria desired. For example, clients may evaluate whether they have time to devote to one solution or another, or they may evaluate each solution based on money, energy, or how much help they would need from other people, and so on. As each item is examined, some of the alternatives proposed may seem unrealistic and therefore will get a higher rank order than others. In ranking the options, the client may assign numbers to them or may choose to just use plus (+) or minus (–) signs.

Step 4: Decide on One Alternative

In this step, clients should select the first alternative solution and see what develops.

Step 5: Select Another Alternative

Step 5 instructs clients to go back to the list of options and select another alternative or, if necessary, get more information about contingent events that precede or follow the problem.

Ask clients to complete an example DEEDS form on their own. Do 6 Practice: DEEDS is a worksheet that instructs clients on how to problem solve. Again, although you are introducing DEEDS during this module, we encourage this approach to development of problem-solving skills throughout treatment and across other modules.

Revising Therapy Goals, Staying Encouraged and Engaged in Treatment

Do 19 Learn: Setting Personal Activity Goals provides the option for you and your client to decide together on whether you should change or revise therapy goals. Again, it is important that therapy focus on addressing no more than two or three overall goals. Sometimes as work in a specific module is wrapping up, it becomes clear that focused work on one area is likely to be an important part of ending the depression.

Do 1 Practice: Review of My Treatment Goals can be used to write down and rate those revised goals. Do 20 Learn: Ways to Think About Progress Toward Your Goals reminds clients of the most common pattern of change with therapy (sawtooth curve, not a straight line or stair steps). Do 7 Practice: As I Continue with Treatment: My Plan for Fully Participating is recommended for times when you have concerns about a client's engagement in treatment, either within session or in compliance with between-session practice. We suggest using Do 8 Practice: My Review of Skills for Doing as a way to review and consolidate key points and skills that were worked on in this module.

Suggested Progression of Content

The first step in preparing to use this module is a thorough review of all Learn pages and Practice forms so you are familiar with the content and can begin to think about the fit between different skills and specific clients. We realize that behavioral health providers working within primary care may use materials from this module in very brief sessions and will select individual Learn pages and Practice forms that fit the concerns and needs of their clients. Similarly, there may be occasions within individual or group psychotherapy when clinicians choose specific Learn and/or Practice materials.

In our experience, it will take six to eight sessions to do BA effectively and for the requisite skills to be learned. Four sessions is the minimum needed to see results. Almost always, this module will be used after clinicians have worked on goal setting and therapy orientation in the Skills for Getting Started module and after facilitating emotional literacy skills in Skills for Feeling. Sessions will use the same basic structure: (a) set an agenda, (b) review home practice, (c) select at least one topic to work on in depth, (d) summarize, (e) set up new home practice assignment, and (f) do mutual feedback. Start work on all Practice forms within session, or wait for the next session to introduce them. Don't send a client home with a Practice form without a personal example already inserted. Be sure to allow time to review any Practice form in the next session.

Table 8.1 presents the suggested sequence for this module.

Table 8.1 Session Outline

Each Session: Depression Measure + Start 3 and 4 Practice

GDS-SF or PHQ-9

Start 4 Practice	Preparing for My Next Session[T]
Start 3 Practice	My Session Summary[T]

Skills for Doing Session 1: Assess Progress and Psychoeducation

In Session 1: Do 1–3 Learn, Do 1 Practice (+ prior session review)

Between Sessions 1 and 2: Do 1 Practice and Do 4 Practice

Do 1 Learn	Introduction to Skills for Doing
Do 2 Learn	Activities Affect Your Mood[T]
Do 3 Learn	What Are Positive Activities?[T]
Do 1 Practice	Review of My Treatment Goals[T]
Do 4 Practice	List of Positive Activities[T]

Skills for Doing Session 2: Activity Monitoring

In Session 2: Do 4–7 Learn

Between Sessions 2 and 3: Do 2 and 3 Practice

Do 4 Learn	Snapshot of Where You Are Right Now[T]
Do 5 Learn	Using the First Steps[T]
Do 6 Learn	Example of First Steps: Days 1–4
Do 7 Learn	Example of First Steps: Days 5–7
Do 2 Practice	First Steps[T]
Do 3 Practice	First Steps Instructions[T]

Skills for Doing Session 3: Finding and Listing Valued Activities

In Session 3: Do 8–11 Learn

Between Sessions 3 and 4: Do 4 Practice

Do 8 Learn	The Importance of Doing[T]
Do 9 Learn	Making Your List[T]
Do 10 Learn	Using Past Activities[T]
Do 11 Learn	Using Values and Purpose[T]
Do 4 Practice	List of Positive Activities[T]

Table 8.1 Continued

Skills for Doing Session 4: Finding and Listing Physical Activities

In Session 4: Do 12 and 13 Learn

Between Sessions 4 and 5: Do 4 and 5 Practice

Do 12 Learn	Physical Activity Is Important[T]
Do 13 Learn	Your Plan for Physical Activity[T]
Do 4 Practice	List of Positive Activities[T]
Do 5 Practice	PAL: Positive Activities Log[T]

Skills for Doing Session 5: Scheduling Activities

In Session 5: Do 14 and 15 Learn

Between Sessions 5 and 6: Do 5 Practice

Do 14 Learn	Schedule Your Activities[T]
Do 15 Learn	Example of Positive Activities Log
Do 5 Practice	PAL: Positive Activities Log[T]

Skills for Doing Session 6: DEEDS for Problem Solving

In Session 6: Do 16–18 Learn

Between Sessions 6 and 7: Do 5 and 6 Practice

Do 16 Learn	Problem Solving with DEEDS—Step 1
Do 17 Learn	Problem Solving with DEEDS—Steps 2 & 3
Do 18 Learn	Problem Solving with DEEDS—Steps 4 & 5
Do 5 Practice	PAL: Positive Activities Log[T]
Do 6 Practice	DEEDS

Skills for Doing Session 7: Putting It All Together

In Session 7: Review Do 5 and 6 Practice

Between Sessions 7 and 8: Do 5 and 6 Practice (maybe Do 7 Practice)

Do 5 Practice	PAL: Positive Activities Log[T]
Do 6 Practice	DEEDS
Do 7 Practice	As I Continue with Treatment: My Plan for Fully Participating

(continued)

Table 8.1 Continued

Skills for Doing Session 8: Personal Goals and Expectations

In Session 8: Do 19 and 20 Learn, Do 1 Practice

After Session 8: Do 5 and Do 8 Practice

Do 19 Learn	Setting Personal Activity Goals[T]
Do 20 Learn	Ways to Think About Progress Toward Your Goals[T]
Do 1 Practice	Review of My Treatment Goals[T]
Do 5 Practice	PAL: Positive Activities Log[T]
Do 8 Practice	My Review of Skills for Doing[T]

[T] Identified as particularly appropriate for telehealth sessions.

With some clients, especially those with MDD, you will move on to *Skills for Thinking*. With others, you can move directly into preparation for therapy termination using the *Skills for Wrapping Up* module. There will also be times when you have finished this module with a client, start work in another module, and come back to key Learn pages and Practice forms in this module to continue to reinforce the use of rewarding and valued daily activities.

Not Included in This Treatment

Values Clarification Tools

Successful BA requires a collaborative focus on your client's unique values, strengths, and most salient cultural identities. In younger adults, it would be common to integrate values clarification exercises to assist with this process of identifying valued and meaningful activities. We have found that by midlife, most adults are able to articulate these with just a little prompting, using the resources we have provided for this (Start 10 and 11 Learn, Start 5 Practice). There are a range of clinical tools for values clarification that may also help but that are beyond the scope of this workbook.

Specific Physical Exercise Routines

Aging clients will vary dramatically in their physical condition and tolerance for exercise. Many will have neuromuscular conditions that impact range of motion, pain following specific physical activities, and explicitly proscribed activities. In the same way that you would not provide specific advice or suggestions regarding medications, we caution against your suggesting specific forms of exercise that have not been volunteered as options by your clients. Start with what the individual suggests as possibilities, and then encourage communication with their primary care provider (and nurse), physical therapist, or local senior centers to identify physical exercise that fits their abilities and limitations.

Additional Resources for Clinicians

Hershenberg, R. (2017). *Activating happiness: A jump-start guide to overcoming low motivation, depression, or just feeling stuck.* New Harbinger Publications.

Martell, C. R., Dimidjian, S., & Herman-Dunn, R. (2010). *Behavioral activation for depression: A clinician's guide.* Guilford Press.

Mazzucchelli, T. G., Kanter, J. W., & Martell, C. R. (2016). A clinician's quick guide of evidence-based approaches: Behavioural activation. *Clinical Psychologist,* 20(1), 54–55. https://doi.org/10.1111/cp.12086

Measure Instructions in Appendix C Related to This Module

Scoring information and instructions for the California Older Person's Positive Experiences Schedule-Revised (COPPES-R)

CHAPTER 9

Module 4: Skills for Thinking: Self-Compassion and Helpful Thoughts

This core module of the workbook is focused on the skills of:

1. Monitoring therapy progress and fine-tuning treatment goals
2. Replacing self-criticism with self-compassionate thoughts and actions
3. Building cognitive reappraisal skills
4. Rating the strength of unhelpful thoughts and upsetting feelings
5. Identifying unhelpful thought patterns
6. Modifying thoughts and using the 6-Column Thought Diary
7. Revising therapy goals, staying encouraged and engaged in treatment

This chapter is provided to help you use the *Skills for Thinking* module of the workbook with your clients. We start with a brief overview, followed by some practical tips based on the most common questions we hear from clinicians during professional trainings. The bulk of this chapter is devoted to reviewing self-compassion and cognitive reappraisal skills, with a description of the specific Learn pages and Practice forms available for your use in sessions. We provide recommendations for a standard progression of material (i.e., Learn pages and Practice forms that typically go with each other in the same session, estimates of how much can be accomplished in a given session), with the understanding that this may vary quite a bit depending upon your practice setting and specific client needs. We end the chapter with some comments about related topics that are not included in this treatment approach, and point readers to resources for additional professional development in cognitive therapy.

Overview

This module can take from three to eight sessions to complete, depending on whether therapy is targeting self-compassion strategies alone or both self-compassion and cognitive reappraisal. First, we reorient clients to the CBT model and discuss the role of thoughts in maintaining depression. Clients then learn to recognize and respond to their most common self-criticisms, and use self-compassionate thoughts and actions during difficult times. The second and larger part of this module involves clients learning to identify their own common unhelpful thoughts, typically using a thought diary and/or some of the other Practice forms. Clients then practice examining and modifying unhelpful thoughts, across multiple recent daily experiences, to enhance the ability to use this skill on their own during challenging life circumstances. All of this work is framed within the context of their personal life values and strengths to ensure that specific cognitive strategies are consistent with those values and strengths. This continued emphasis on values-consistent therapeutic strategies is vitally important for building and maintaining a therapeutic alliance with all clients, including middle-aged and older adults from cultural minority groups.

How do you know if a specific client needs some of the skills emphasized in this module? A key consideration is how well the client has been able to engage with and benefit from the behavioral activation strategies provided in *Skills for Doing*. If a client's difficulties in benefiting from the behavioral activation strategies in the *Skills for Doing* module appear strongly related to self-criticism or perfectionism, then we suggest a few sessions devoted to applying self-compassionate behaviors and thoughts in daily life. That may be sufficient, and sessions devoted to cognitive reappraisal strategies may not be needed. On the other hand, for clients who consistently have negative views about themselves, their experience, and the future, cognitive reappraisal work is needed. This is also indicated for clients whose depression has not responded well to behavioral activation as well as for clients who come into therapy already doing a number of positive activities but who still have depression.

There are other clients who respond reasonably well to behavioral activation but need attention to *specific* cognitions related to sleep, pain, grief, or caregiving. In those cases, we suggest that you transition from *Skills for Doing* into one of those personalized sections. Then, add material from this *Skills for Thinking* module if it becomes apparent that patterns of negative thinking are interfering with that work. Cognitive reappraisal may be especially appropriate for clients who find themselves in life circumstances that allow for little control and that do not fit well with a problem-solving approach.

Tips for Clinicians

Consider Whether Problem Solving Is a More Appropriate Strategy

Not all upsetting thoughts about situations are distorted. Middle-aged and older adults can experience a number of life stressors that pose true difficulties in daily life. Some of these stressors may tax existing coping abilities, especially in depressed clients with poor concentration and/or cognitive limitations. In *Skills for Doing* (Do 16–18 Learn, Do 6 Practice), we have provided a DEEDS clinical tool to use as you help clients learn problem-solving skills. This is different than merely having session time filled with solving the problem of the week (which can take up entire sessions and the bulk of psychotherapy if you and your client fall into that pattern). Instead, the DEEDS tool is intended for use when you and your client collaboratively decide that it is important to spend time in session to problem solve a particularly challenging situation. More information about strategies to help clients develop and use problem-solving skills is provided in Chapter 8 of this clinician guide. Our reminder here is that, when the most upsetting thought about a situation appears realistic and related to something that is amenable to problem solving, use of DEEDS is the better clinical choice. In such circumstances, some application of self-compassion strategies may help your clients lower their emotional arousal enough to be able to engage in applying the problem-solving skills that they first learned in *Skills for Doing*.

Help Your Clients Focus on Specific Situations

It can be easy to fall into a common pitfall of discussing general thoughts and beliefs about relationships and situations in life. Those abstract discussions are not cognitive therapy, and they create difficulties in helping clients develop self-compassion and cognitive reappraisal skills. For example, a client may report having a conflictual relationship with an adult child and want to discuss a common pattern of negative interactions. To work on unhelpful thoughts that are involved in this, the clinician should invite the client to apply the skills in this module to a recent example that was upsetting. Remind your clients that therapy is most helpful when the two of you focus on a fairly recent situation that can be given a date and time (e.g., last Monday night after dinner). If therapy sessions focused on cognitive reappraisal don't seem to be particularly helpful, check that you and the client are spending the majority of time focusing on specific recent examples when distressing emotions and upsetting thoughts were elicited. When clients have a hard time identifying the exact situation, remind them that a situation can occur when they are alone, as in, "Last Wednesday morning, sitting in my chair with nothing much to do, I felt very apathetic and bored, and had the thought that nothing I do matters or helps."

Listen for Extreme Language

Clinicians can miss hearing the extreme nature of some unhelpful thoughts. Many older adults have chronic health conditions and may also be recovering from surgery or an acute medical problem. Thoughts such as "I was in too much pain to do anything at all today" can sometimes sound reasonable to clinicians who wish to support their clients. Listening carefully for extreme language (e.g., "always," "never," "anything") is a good way to find places to look for baby steps or some wiggle room to make small changes that over time can make a big difference.

Focus First on Evaluating the Helpfulness of Thoughts, Not the Evidence

Cognitive therapy has received an undeserved reputation in the past for being cold, overly logical, and thus perhaps inappropriate for culturally diverse clients from non-European American backgrounds. This is an unfortunate misunderstanding because in the history of cognitive therapy, examining the evidence has always been just one among a number of different questions used to facilitate a new perspective on emotionally distressing or behaviorally paralyzing thoughts. The reappraisal strategies developed by the internationally recognized Beck Institute, for example, have always included several other questions to help shift perspective, such as considering what one would tell a friend in the same situation; asking whether the thought is helpful; and asking what the worst, best, and most likely outcome would be if the thought was true. Thus, examining the evidence for a thought can be a part of clients learning how to reappraise their thoughts, but it is certainly not the only technique. It can be important for clients to grasp that just because they think something doesn't make it true, and that beliefs are not facts. Beliefs can change over time with new facts (just the way scientists used to believe that the world was flat but changed this belief with new information). Sometimes, examining the evidence has been overused by clinicians who consider this to be the primary tool in cognitive therapy. Working with culturally diverse individuals requires clinicians to be especially aware of how an overfocus on evaluating evidence can be experienced by clients as invalidating (Hays, 2016). For that reason, we encourage you to start by helping clients ask, "Is this thought helpful?" Then, additional reappraisal questions can be added in as needed.

Teach Clients to Ask Themselves Reappraisal Questions

When teaching reappraisal skills, your aim is to help your clients learn to ask themselves questions to shift their perspective. You might say something like:

> *As you develop new ways of seeing upsetting situations, you will ask yourself some questions about your most upsetting thoughts. For example, as we look at your* Think 5 Practice *form from this past week, let's look together at what you wrote about last Tuesday afternoon after your doctor's appointment. I see that you wrote down* _____ [insert specific thought]. *When you ask yourself the question, "Is this thought helping me?", what is your answer to that?*

Your role as the clinician is to help clients learn to ask reappraisal questions. Early on in working on *Skills for Thinking*, you may pose reappraisal questions and strategies, but your intent is to move clients toward having in-session practice with asking themselves those questions. This may sound something like:

> *Let's look at* Think 13 Learn. *Read a few of these aloud. What ideas do you have about how you can reconsider this perspective as you apply some of those lenses to your situation?*

If you find yourself as the clinician being the one who is directly challenging unhelpful thoughts, work toward shifting to helping clients ask themselves those questions. Anytime you find yourself and the client debating the accuracy of a thought, this is a sign that you as the clinician need to step back and shift to the role of collaboratively facilitating the client selecting a reappraisal strategy that fits them (or, moving into a problem-solving mode instead, using the DEEDS tool in *Skills for Doing*). One occasion in which a clinician should directly jump in and be the one to challenge an unhelpful thought is when working with an acutely suicidal client who is very stuck in suicidal ideation; a direct approach to challenging thoughts is appropriate in those circumstances.

Focus on "Hot Thoughts"

All of us, including our clients, have situations that create strong feelings and unhelpful thoughts at the time of the situation but in retrospect aren't as bothersome or upsetting. We call these unhelpful thoughts "cold cognitions" or "cold thoughts" because when reconsidered in a therapy session, they do not retrigger that negative emotional experience. Leave those thoughts alone, and praise your client for coping successfully on their own (or with the help of a friend, which is a form of coping). Therapy time is precious, and cognitive reappraisal efforts should be reserved for those "hot thoughts" that, when discussed in therapy, still elicit a strong emotional response. If you attempt to work with cold cognitions during therapy sessions, clients will have the sense of therapy being academic and not really relevant to daily life or their problems. Therapy time spent on cold thoughts instead of hot thoughts is part of what leads clients to have the "I know this (new perspective) in my head but don't really feel it in my gut."

Remember the Importance of Experiences (Behavior) in Daily Life

Self-efficacy, which is the confidence to engage in behaviors (including thoughts) that are important to an individual in specific life domains, is best influenced by personal experiences of mastery in daily life (Bandura, 1997). Rather than expecting a series of cognitive therapy sessions to immediately result in thoughts that lead to lasting improvement in emotional functioning, clinicians should always be asking themselves and their clients the question, *"So what does this mean for the next time you find yourself in a similar situation? What might you do differently?"*

We are looking for cognitive reappraisal strategies to nudge clients toward more flexible ways of thinking, with the aim of influencing behavioral responses (which then will lead onward to additional changes in thoughts and feelings). Thus, the CBT model that we first discuss with clients in Start 13 Learn: What Is the Cognitive-Behavioral Model?, with those arrows pointing in multiple directions, needs to stay a living and breathing conceptual model throughout your work with clients.

Work hard at keeping that model in the front of your mind as you work with clients.

Key Skills in This Module

Monitoring Therapy Progress and Fine-Tuning Treatment Goals

This module begins with the orientation provided in <u>Think 1 Learn: Introduction to Skills for Thinking</u> and the important reminder to have a "state of therapy" discussion about therapy goals and progress. Copy the current two or three therapy goals into <u>Think 1 Practice: Review of My Treatment Goals,</u> and have your client rate before or in session. Be sure to *discuss these in session.* This is a good time to review the overall pattern of depression scores, using whichever weekly measure of depression is a part of this feedback-informed treatment. The first session devoted to this module will likely include some time following up with ongoing behavioral activation efforts and/ or work related to whichever module comes ahead of this one. <u>Think 2 Learn: Preventing a Downward Spiral</u> should then be used to reinforce the concept that was first applied in *Skills for Doing.*

Replacing Self-Criticism with Self-Compassionate Thoughts and Actions

In the past decade, there has been increasing interest in compassion-focused therapy for depression (Gilbert, 2010) and other approaches to foster self-compassion (Neff & Germer, 2018). As we re-examine the Model of Depression in Older Adults (Fiske et al., 2009) that is shown in Figure 2.1 (on page 21 of this guide), the specific function of self-critical thoughts comes to the fore. On the left side of this figure, we can see that negative and pessimistic thinking may have created the context for depression across an individual's lifetime. These "depressogenic cognitive styles" are possible contributors to a lifetime of vulnerability to depression. Clinically, however, we do not start with a focus on those. The right side of the figure shows that self-critical thoughts play an especially strong role in perpetuating the cycle of depression in middle-aged and older adults. For that reason, softening self-criticism and strengthening self-compassion have precedence in this treatment.

We recommend that you listen for self-critical thoughts while working with clients in other modules of the workbook. Begin any focus on unhelpful thoughts with psychoeducation on self-criticism and opportunities to practice self-compassion (Diedrich et al., 2016). Many middle-aged and older adults grew up in households and communities where harsh criticism was used as a way to "motivate." Think 3 Learn: Self-Criticism vs. Self-Compassion is especially important to help counter that view; have your clients describe how they would encourage a very young child who is taking on something that is quite difficult for them. We all do our best in managing hard situations when others are patient and encouraging; it is now time for your clients to apply that to themselves. Think 3–6 Learn help your client move from a pattern of self-critical thoughts to more compassionate thoughts and actions. Think 2–4 Practice are possible between-session assignments to build use of self-compassionate thoughts and actions in daily life. With its focus on specific self-encouraging thoughts, Think 11 Practice: Ways to Encourage Myself can also be used as a part of this work on self-compassion. We want to emphasize that a client agreeing that self-compassion is a good thing (i.e., having insight) is not at all the same as being able to apply specific self-compassionate strategies during particularly difficult times. Practicing during daily events is key to using self-compassion amid life's struggles.

Building Cognitive Reappraisal Skills

Think 7–17 Learn and Think 5–10 Practice are all devoted to developing, practicing, and using cognitive reappraisal skills. One premise of CBT is that our unhelpful thoughts (sometimes experienced as images or pictures in our head) contribute to negative emotions. This process happens so quickly that we are often unaware that thoughts occur between a stressful situation and uncomfortable emotions. It thus becomes important to teach clients to slow down their thought processes in order to identify the thoughts and/or internal images associated with stressful situations that lead to intense negative feelings (DiGiuseppe et al., 2016). We break this part of therapy into more steps than are typically used in cognitive therapy with younger adults.

Use <u>Think 7 Learn: Unhelpful Thinking Habits</u> and <u>Think 8 Learn: Introduction to the 3-Part Thought Diary</u> as you teach clients to use a 3-Part Thought Diary to slow down their thoughts and to keep track of what they are thinking/imagining once they have noticed a strong emotional reaction. You will use <u>Think 5 Practice: 3-Part Thought Diary</u> when introducing clients to a simple 3-Part Thought Diary (brief description of the stressful situation, a list of automatic thoughts and/or images connected with this situation, and a list of the emotions experienced as a result). Recording these three pieces of information will help clients begin to notice and monitor the thoughts that are associated with situations that arouse negative emotions. Emphasize to clients that they cannot make any changes in their thoughts unless they know *what* to change. <u>Think 5 Practice</u> is a very important part of developing cognitive reappraisal skills, so don't skip this. It is very useful to complete a few thought diaries in session to get started. You and your client will use this together within session, and then your client will continue to use <u>Think 5 Practice</u> as a between-session assignment for at least 1 or 2 weeks. Be sure to provide written examples from the client's recent experiences to help with between-session assignments.

Because the module on behavioral activation preceded this one, your clients should be familiar with the concept of monitoring mood and identifying possible contingencies of mood change. Having spent at least several sessions on emotional literacy skills in the *Skills for Feeling* core module will also pay off during work on cognitive reappraisal. Understanding that feelings/emotions are best described using a single word becomes key when working on reappraisal strategies. You will find, for example, that many older clients initially have difficulty in distinguishing between a feeling and a thought (e.g., "I felt that he really didn't care about me" instead of "I thought, 'He really doesn't care about me.' I felt hurt and lonely"). With practice, most clients are able to complete this task, and many can eventually do thought diaries effectively in their mind without using the form.

Rating the Strength of Unhelpful Thoughts and Upsetting Feelings

Help your clients learn to assign a value to their thoughts and feelings by rating how strongly they believe in each one right at the moment of rating (not merely when the situation or event happened or immediately after). Encourage clients to use the scale 0% (not strong at all) to 100% (strongest possible) shown in the 3-Part Thought Diary (Think 5 Practice). Likewise, it is important that clients measure the strength of their emotional reactions as they record the situation. The range of the rating scale is the same: 0% means that the emotion is not at all present and 100% means that the emotion is completely present, or as strong as it could possibly be. Rating thoughts and emotions is important because you will focus cognitive reappraisal efforts on only the strongest thoughts and feelings (i.e., rated 60% or higher). You do not want to spend session time on thoughts that may have been upsetting at the time of the situation or event but that no longer trigger a strong reaction. When in-session and between-session efforts focus on thoughts and resulting emotional reactions that are weaker than 60%, it is hard to see the benefits of reappraisal efforts. This clinical mistake of focusing in-session reappraisal efforts on relatively weak thoughts and feelings is what has given cognitive therapy a sometimes bad reputation of being "cold" or overly rational. So, take time to help your clients get in touch with the intensity of their thoughts and feelings at the time the situation occurred (e.g., *"Try to think back to the time when this happened. Give me as many details as you can. This will help you experience now just how strong your feelings were at that time"*). Ask questions if needed to facilitate this. If the client continues to report that the thought is no longer upsetting, then it is better to move on rather than spend session time on that thought.

Rating the strength of thoughts and feelings also helps your client understand the impact that unhelpful thoughts can have on mood. The rating exercise guides the two of you toward a focus on key thoughts that will benefit from reappraisal. These ratings are also useful later in comparing how the strength of these thoughts has changed over time. Explain that we can gain similar information regarding which emotions are present and the strongest, and we can also compare initial ratings to the later type and intensity of emotions as the client's thoughts change.

Identifying Unhelpful Thought Patterns

As your clients begin to identify and examine their unhelpful thoughts more regularly, they will begin to notice specific patterns in both the types of thoughts and the situations that are difficult. Many clients recognize a particular manner or style to the way they interpret stressful situations. In Think 9 Learn: Unhelpful Ways of Seeing Situations, we use the common metaphor of different eyeglass lenses to explain this concept to the client. These negative lenses can be exhibited through different patterns or styles of thinking, and a person can be employing several different styles at any one time. Think 10 Learn: Unhelpful Thought Patterns or "Cognitive Lenses" can be used in session; have clients hold this list in their hands, read it aloud (rather than you reading it to them), and talk through which patterns feel most familiar. People often find that some of these thought patterns fit them better than others. The identification of the more common thought patterns can be very helpful in later exercises of examining and modifying unhelpful thoughts. Think 6 Practice: Unhelpful Thought Patterns and Think 7 Practice: Situations and Unhelpful Thought Patterns are two options for clients to start to recognize these across the week. This step of recognizing unhelpful patterns is important and happens *before* teaching the steps of questioning and changing/replacing unhelpful thoughts. At this point, the focus is on recognizing that stressful situations are fueled by negative thoughts, identifying the most upsetting and unhelpful thoughts as soon as they occur, and labeling the patterns that these thoughts reflect. Think 11 Learn: Finding Your Patterns and Think 12 Learn: Identifying Negative Beliefs Through Imagery are provided as optional pages that may be helpful for some clients who need extra work in this area. Think 12 Learn is especially suited for clients who may think in images.

Modifying Thoughts and Using the 6-Column Thought Diary

You will use Think 13 Learn: Put on New Lenses: Changing Your Thoughts as a way to learn how to change and/or soften unhelpful thoughts. As you work with your clients on understanding and using Think 13 Learn, you will help them experiment with a variety of ways of holding unhelpful thoughts more lightly and developing more helpful and flexible ways of thinking about specific situations. This is done by listening for extreme language and replacing that with less extreme words and phrases. You are looking to soften the focus on absolutes and help your clients shift their perspective. What would someone who is a caring friend or a very wise person say about the situation?

As you and your client begin to challenge the unhelpful thoughts, the expanded version of the thought diary is needed. Think 10 Practice: 6-Part Thought Diary contains six sections for the following information:

1. Antecedents: a brief description of the stressful situation
2. Beliefs: a list and rating of the negative thoughts that occurred in conjunction with this situation and which patterns are present
3. Consequences: a list and rating of the emotions that were experienced as a result
4. Develop Responses: a list of more realistic adaptive thoughts that can replace the unhelpful thoughts, followed by rating strength of the old thoughts
5. Effect: rating strength of new thoughts, along with a list and rating of the emotions experienced now
6. Function: a brief description of behavior that will follow

For many older clients, this process goes very slowly. It's a new way of thinking for many of them. With time, most begin to understand how to use the form. It's a good idea to help them with this in session until they really get the concept. This will take more than one session; generally two to three sessions are needed at this point. This work should continue until clients express confidence that they know how to recognize negative thinking patterns and how to modify them to be more adaptive and helpful.

It is quite common for people to have difficulty with the first 6-Part Thought Diary (Think 10 Practice) they complete. We provide Think 16 Learn as an example to look at and discuss together in session. Even when clients are able to come up with helpful responses to their negative thoughts, they may not have a great deal of confidence in these new thoughts. It takes time for the newer, more helpful thoughts to "sink in." It is helpful to remind clients that they are challenging thoughts they have had for a very long time. Emphasize that the way that changes can be made is through practice, practice, practice! Encourage your clients to get into the habit of completing thought diaries.

As you help your client develop cognitive reappraisal skills, include reminders and refreshers of the earlier work that you've done in self-compassion. The actual content of an unhelpful thought can be accompanied by a harsh tone of voice within one's head. In the same way, merely developing an alternative thought is insufficient if the tone of one's inner voice remains harsh.

Revising Therapy Goals, Staying Encouraged and Engaged in Treatment

Think 21 Learn: Setting Personal Goals Related to Your Thinking provides the option for you and your client to collaboratively decide whether you should change or revise therapy goals. Again, it is important that therapy focus on addressing no more than two or three overall goals. Sometimes when a specific module is moving toward completion, it becomes clear that focused work in another area is needed to reduce depression and prepare clients for termination. Think 1 Practice: Review of My Treatment Goals can be used as a form to write down and rate those revised goals. Think 22 Learn: Ways to Think About Progress Toward Your Goals reminds clients of the most common pattern of change with therapy (sawtooth curve, not a straight line or stair steps). Think 12 Practice: As I Continue with Treatment: My Plan for Fully Participating is recommended for times when you already have some concerns about a client's engagement in treatment, either within session or in compliance with between-session practice. Use Think 13 Practice: My Review of Skills for Thinking at the end of this module to review and consolidate key points and skills.

Throughout the remainder of the therapy, you should continue to use Think 10 Practice: 6-Part Thought Diary (or Think 8 Practice: Putting on New Lenses or Think 9 Practice: Putting on New Glasses: Changing Unhelpful Thoughts) to help the client identify and challenge unhelpful thoughts when they occur in response to other stressful situations and in other modules (e.g., pain, caregiving). The more the client practices with this tool, the more likely the application of this tool will occur, nearly as automatically as the occurrence of unhelpful negative thoughts.

If goals are now sufficiently met and the level of depressive symptoms is significantly less than at the start of therapy, then move on to *Skills for Wrapping Up* to prepare for termination.

The first step in preparing to use this module is a thorough review of all Learn pages and Practice forms so you are familiar with the content and can begin to think about the fit between different skills and specific clients. We realize that behavioral health providers working within primary care settings may be using materials from this module in very brief sessions and will select individual Learn pages and Practice forms that fit the concerns and needs of their clients. Similarly, there may be occasions within individual or group psychotherapy when clinicians choose specific Learn pages and/or Practice forms. You will ideally be sitting next to clients in individual psychotherapy (instead of across from them) during most sessions in this module. Working side by side while looking at the same information on a table in front of the client helps focus attention and facilitates the collaboration process between clinician and client. For telehealth sessions, we recommend selecting a platform that allows you to screen share in order to accomplish the same thing.

When this module is being used in its entirety to help clients develop and use self-compassion *and* cognitive reappraisal skills to reduce depression, we suggest an eight-session approach. In many cases, this will be after you have started work with your clients in other modules and have found that a specific set of unhelpful cognitions is interfering with a client's ability to benefit from those other strategies (i.e., a client's thoughts are getting in the way of being able to learn, practice, and apply other change strategies). Sessions will use the same basic structure: (a) set an agenda, (b) review home practice, (c) select at least one topic to work on in depth, (d) summarize, (e) set up new home practice assignment, and (f) do mutual feedback. Start work on all Practice forms within session or wait for the next session to introduce them. Don't send a client home with a Practice form without a personal example already inserted. Be sure to allow time to review any Practice form in the next session.

Session Outline—Self-Compassion

Table 9.1 presents the suggested sequence for the self-compassion section of this module.

Table 9.1 Self-Compassion Session Outline

Each Session: Depression Measure + Start 3 and 4 Practice

GDS-SF or PHQ-9

Start 4 Practice	Preparing for My Next Session[T]
Start 3 Practice	My Session Summary[T]

Skills for Thinking Session 1: Progress Assessment and Psychoeducation

In Session 1: Think 1 and 2 Learn, Think 1 Practice, Start 5 Practice (+ prior session review)

Between Session 1 and 2: Think 1 Practice and Start 5 Practice

Think 1 Learn	Introduction to Skills for Thinking
Think 2 Learn	Preventing a Downward Spiral[T]
Think 1 Practice	Review of My Treatment Goals[T]
Start 5 Practice	My Values and Strengths[T]

Skills for Thinking Session 2: Self-Criticism vs. Self-Compassion

In Session 2: Think 3–6 Learn

Between Sessions 2 and 3: Choice of Think 2, 3, or 4 Practice

Think 3 Learn	Self-Criticism vs. Self-Compassion
Think 4 Learn	Self-Compassion[T]
Think 5 Learn	Self-Compassion Strategies[T]
Think 6 Learn	Building Self-Compassion
Think 2 Practice	Strategies for Building Self-Compassion
Think 3 Practice	Building Self-Compassion in Situations[T]
Think 4 Practice	Responding to My Inner Critic

Skills for Thinking Session 3: Self-Compassion Continued

In Session 3: Think 3–6 Learn

After Session 3: Choice of Think 2, 3, or 4 Practice

Think 3 Learn	Self-Criticism vs. Self-Compassion
Think 4 Learn	Self-Compassion[T]
Think 5 Learn	Self-Compassion Strategies[T]
Think 6 Learn	Building Self-Compassion

Table 9.1 Continued

Think 2 Practice	Strategies for Building Self-Compassion
Think 3 Practice	Building Self-Compassion in Situations[T]
Think 4 Practice	Responding to My Inner Critic

[T] Identified as particularly appropriate for telehealth sessions.

Clinician Note

For some clients, you will stop this module after completing practice on self-compassion strategies.

Session Outline—Cognitive Reappraisal

Table 9.2 presents the suggested sequence for the cognitive reappraisal section of this module.

Not Included in This Treatment

Treatment for Moderate to Severe Suicide Risk

If your client expresses suicidal thoughts during therapy, we recommend a focused assessment using the SAFE-T Protocol with C-SSRS (Columbia Risk and Protective Factors) Lifetime/Recent, available at the Columbia Lighthouse project site (http://cssrs.columbia.edu/). This provides you with clinically rich information that helps you evaluate the extent of risk and develop a targeted treatment plan. Depending on the outcome of that evaluation, you can decide on the next steps. If the client is assessed as being at low risk, one option is to focus therapy time on the skills described in this chapter—that is, identify specific thoughts (and triggers) that are related to suicidal ideation, identify unhelpful thinking patterns associated with suicidal ideation, and work with the client to re-evaluate their persistent negative thoughts—while also continuing behavioral activation. This may require modification of the therapy schedule so additional sessions can be arranged in a timely manner.

Table 9.2 Cognitive Reappraisal Session Outline

Each Session: Depression Measure + Start 3 and 4 Practice

GDS-SF or PHQ-9

Start 4 Practice	Preparing for My Next Session[T]
Start 3 Practice	My Session Summary[T]

Skills for Thinking Session 4: Unhelpful Thinking Habits

In Session 4: Think 7 and 8 Learn (+ prior session review)

Between Sessions 4 and 5: Think 5 Practice

Think 7 Learn	Unhelpful Thinking Habits[T]
Think 8 Learn	Introduction to the 3-Part Thought Diary[T]
Think 5 Practice	3-Part Thought Diary[T]

Skills for Thinking Session 5: Recognizing Unhelpful Thinking Habits

In Session 5: Think 9 and 10 Learn

Between Sessions 5 and 6: Think 5, 6, or 7 Practice

Think 9 Learn	Unhelpful Ways of Seeing Situations[T]
Think 10 Learn	Unhelpful Thought Patterns or "Cognitive Lenses"[T]
Think 5 Practice	3-Part Thought Diary[T]
Think 6 Practice	Unhelpful Thought Patterns[T]
Think 7 Practice	Situations and Unhelpful Thought Patterns

Skills for Thinking Session 6: Replacing Unhelpful Thoughts with Adaptive Ones

In Session 6: Think 13–16 Learn

Between Sessions 6 and 7: Think 8, 9, or 10 Practice

Think 13 Learn	Put on New Lenses: Changing Your Thoughts[T]
Think 14 Learn	New Ways of Seeing Things[T]
Think 15 Learn	6-Part Thought Diary[T]
Think 16 Learn	Maria's 6-Part Thought Diary
Think 8 Practice	Putting on New Lenses[T]
Think 9 Practice	Putting on New Glasses: Changing Unhelpful Thoughts
Think 10 Practice	6-Part Thought Diary[T]

Table 9.2 Continued

Skills for Thinking Session 7: Replacing Unhelpful Thoughts with Adaptive Ones

In Session 7: Think 17–20 Learn

Between Sessions 7 and 8: Think 8, 9, or 10 Practice

Think 17 Learn	Completing a Thought Diary
Think 18 Learn	Encouraging Yourself[T]
Think 19 Learn	Other Skills for Thinking[T]
Think 20 Learn	Consider Other Perspectives
Think 8 Practice	Putting on New Lenses[T]
Think 9 Practice	Putting on New Glasses: Changing Unhelpful Thoughts
Think 10 Practice	6-Part Thought Diary[T]

Skills for Thinking Session 8: Personal Goals and Expectations

In Session 8: Think 21 and 22 Learn

After Session 8: Think 11–13 Practice

Think 21 Learn	Setting Personal Goals Related to Your Thinking[T]
Think 22 Learn	Ways to Think About Progress Toward Your Goals[T]
Think 11 Practice	Ways to Encourage Myself[T]
Think 12 Practice	As I Continue with Treatment: My Plan for Fully Participating
Think 13 Practice	My Review of Skills for Thinking[T]

[T] Identified as particularly appropriate for telehealth sessions.

If, however, assessment with the SAFE-T Protocol with C-SSRS identifies your client as being at moderate or high suicide risk, then other options need to be considered and implemented. As noted in Chapter 3, it is important to target suicide risk factors directly in therapy using an evidence-based treatment for suicide risk reduction. Although considered appropriate in the past, treating depression and seeing a reduction in other depressive symptoms is no longer an evidence-based practice for treating suicidality.

Consult with your clinical supervisor, care manager, or psychiatrist on the team (common in mental health clinics) while also following whatever protocol is in place at your facility or agency for handling clients who are acutely suicidal. Risk management responses may include psychiatric referral (depending on availability), referral for voluntary inpatient psychiatric hospitalization, or enlisting services such as calling 911 to institute involuntary psychiatric hospitalization, depending on the circumstances and degree of lethality. Working with suicidal clients is not for everyone. If it is beyond your skill level as a clinician, you have an ethical obligation to refer the client to a more appropriate level of care and/or provider.

We specifically recommend obtaining additional training in this area to increase both your skill level and comfort in providing clinical services to at-risk clients. If you are already trained and functioning as a CBT clinician, then receiving training and consultation in using Cognitive Behavioral Therapy for Suicide Prevention (CBT-SP: Bryan & Rudd, 2018; Wenzel et al., 2009) is appropriate. For all other clinicians, we suggest training in use of the Collaborative Assessment Method for Suicidality (CAMS) in light of the detailed guidance available through the CAMS workbook (Jobes, 2016) and the CAMS-care professional training site (https://cams-care.com).

Schema Therapy and Focus on Core Beliefs

On the basis of data from other research teams suggesting that working at the level of core beliefs can activate and increase depressive symptoms in some clients (Hawley et al., 2017), we have made the decision not to include a focus on core negative schemas in this edition. Thus, we would suggest that clinicians using our approach with middle-aged and older adults with depression first work at the level of automatic thoughts (i.e., those that are activated in clients during specific current situations). We encourage cognitive therapists who are already trained and certified in schema-related work to listen for and consider how core beliefs are manifested in specific situations in daily life. That will allow clinicians to decide when and how to address negative longstanding beliefs using the cognitive reappraisal strategies emphasized in this treatment approach. For clients who may meet criteria for a personality disorder, we refer readers to the works of Videler and colleagues (2018) and Lynch and colleagues (2007) for further suggestions.

Additional Resources for Clinicians

Beck, J. S. (2020). *Cognitive behavior therapy: Basics and beyond* (3rd ed.). Guilford Press.

Laidlaw, K. (2015). *CBT for older people: An introduction.* Sage Publications. https://doi.org/10.4135/9781473910799

Module 11: Skills for Wrapping Up: Finishing Treatment

Although *Module 11: Skills for Wrapping* up is placed at the end of the *Treating Later-Life Depression Workbook*, this chapter of the clinician guide is located in Part II, along with the other core components of treatment. We want to emphasize that termination processes involve a distinct and essential phase of treatment. Careful application of this module will help you prepare your older clients for termination with the same individualized planning and intentionality that have been present throughout therapy.

This core module of the workbook is focused on the skills of:

1. Processing termination issues
2. Developing a Maintenance Guide
3. Reviewing skills learned
4. Planning for future stressful situations
5. Recognizing and planning for danger signals

This chapter is provided to help you use the *Skills for Wrapping Up* module of the workbook with your clients. We start with a brief overview, followed by some practical tips based on the most common questions we hear from clinicians during professional trainings. The bulk of this chapter is devoted to reviewing termination processes and relapse prevention, with a description of the specific Learn pages and Practice forms available for your use in sessions. We provide recommendations for a standard progression of material (i.e., Learn pages and Practice forms that typically go with each other in the same session, estimates of how much can be accomplished in a given session), with the understanding that this may vary quite a bit depending upon your practice setting and specific client needs. We end the chapter with some comments about related topics that are not included in this treatment approach, and point readers to additional resources.

Clinician Note

As you read this chapter, we encourage you to have the workbook open so that you can refer to the specific Learn pages and Practice forms as they are described and explained. You will use these Learn pages and Practice forms during sessions, encouraging your clients to review between sessions using the Learn pages and try out/record between sessions using the Practice forms. Your reviewing these items as you read through this chapter will prepare you to make the most of the treatment materials. Using these pages and forms means more than having them available to look at or read over with your clients during sessions. Instead, you'll be engaging your clients in exploring the meaning this has to them, through discussion and careful application. Your goal each session is to help your clients apply specific Learn and Practice material to their recent experiences in daily life, and to the problems that bring them into treatment.

Overview

Termination is anticipated and discussed from the beginning of treatment, but this can be a difficult aspect of treatment for some older patients. You will periodically talk about termination throughout the course of therapy, each time you review progress toward therapy goals (e.g., the first Practice form of most modules). The first session of each personalized module includes some discussion of current treatment goals and progress toward ending treatment. In our approach, the final three or four sessions are devoted to termination and maintenance issues.

The same components are incorporated into the basic structure of each session as throughout therapy: (a) set an agenda, (b) review home practice, (c) select at least one topic to work on in depth, (d) summarize, (e) set up new home practice assignment, and (f) do mutual feedback. The focus of these sessions, however, is on termination itself, and we have provided Learn pages and Practice forms for you to use with clients to support this work. As with other modules, termination preparation is framed within the context of the personal life values and strengths (Start 5 Practice: My Values and Strengths) of each client, to ensure that the termination process and Maintenance Guide are consistent with those values and strengths.

Termination of the relationship with the clinician can be stressful for any client. It may be particularly difficult for socially isolated older clients who have few friends and family members or who report that loneliness is one of their primary target complaints. The clinician often becomes an important person in the client's life who provides some companionship. We have provided Wrap 2 Learn: What Does Ending Treatment Mean to You? as a resource to use during the termination process to facilitate these discussions of the therapy relationship, including what was helpful, what will be missed, and what was challenging. Increasing time intervals between sessions at the very end of therapy can help the client adjust to this loss. Spacing out sessions also gives clients an opportunity to try the skills they have learned on their own. Clients can observe whether or not they are now able to deal effectively with stressful situations without immediate consultation. When a client returns for a spaced session, you and your client can then decide together what changes may be required, if any, to help the client maintain the gains made during therapy.

When to Use This Module

For individual psychotherapy clients, we recommend that therapy end in a gradual and systematic way whenever possible. The final few sessions are ideally spaced out (i.e., instead of held weekly, perhaps biweekly to monthly) to give clients time to disengage from the therapeutic relationship and to use the skills learned in therapy independently to deal with stressful events and negative moods. We have found that more gradual terminations are easier for clients to adjust to and are associated with increased long-term improvement. We also recommend, if needed, the possibility of scheduling booster sessions after the last formal session. Booster sessions are designed as a check-in to see how clients are using these skills on their own. We often schedule booster sessions to occur anywhere from 3 to 6 months after the official last session. Knowing that there is at least one booster session planned also makes it easier for clients to move forward with termination.

Tips for Clinicians

Manage Time Spent on New Stressors

The focus of these sessions is on termination itself. Clients may still wish to update or report on events in their lives, but these conversations should be focused on emphasizing how they have been using therapy skills on their own to manage these problem areas or stressful life events. Your aim is to continue to build clients' self-efficacy for coping on their own, and help them recognize examples of healthy and effective coping efforts (even when imperfect). During termination, do not introduce new topics/problem areas. To do so may interfere with planned termination. The best way of managing new issues is while setting the agenda. Let clients know that the focus of termination sessions includes highlighting what they are already doing to cope, while also developing a list of skills that they are finding most helpful. If a true major new problem arises at this time, it may be necessary to renegotiate for several additional sessions before getting into this final phase of the work.

Individualize Termination

It is useful to reflect back on earlier sessions and identify which additional strategies seemed to work best for the client. In this phase more than others, maintain the basic elements, but keep assignments as simple and concrete as possible, with an emphasis on tailoring them to the client's needs. It is critical to help clients appreciate and use their own abilities to cope with losses and negative changes. Themes such as "coming to terms with the meaning of one's life" may also emerge at this point, and helping clients develop highly specific and structured strategies for dealing with these issues can be helpful.

Support Disengagement from You

Another important issue to discuss is the loss of the relationship with the clinician. As noted earlier, termination is often stressful. Clients may become anxious and experience thoughts that they won't be able to make adjustments without your help. It then becomes important to clarify that clients are ultimately responsible for their mastery of the skills. Clients need to make attributions that they are the agents of behavioral and emotional change as opposed to you. The successful client will have the belief that "I can do this on my own." This facilitates the development of high self-esteem and self-efficacy, which are important contributors to a client's ability to use their new skills during times of distress.

Offer Reminders of Behavioral Activation as a Core Strategy for the Future

In this treatment approach, we were very intentional about the emphasis on activity scheduling and the focus on daily positive, rewarding, and meaningful activities. Research evidence is very strong for behavioral activation in both treating depression and preventing relapses. This means that as you work with clients in the termination phase, find opportunities to review and highlight key *Skills for Doing* strategies that work for the individual client.

Organize Learn Pages and Practice Forms as a Resource

Reminders of key skills and how they have been applied to a client's life can be found in the Learn pages and Practice forms that have been used during treatment. A good between-session assignment during the maintenance phase of treatment is for clients to spend time reviewing important forms in the workbook and/or organizing these materials in a folder or binder. Instruct clients to keep this in a place where it is easily found after therapy (e.g., on a bookshelf, underneath the bed near the nightstand). Encourage the use of these materials as a written record of the work done in therapy. Clients often find it helpful to review certain sections as needed.

Review Specific Thought Diaries

For clients who worked on cognitive reappraisal using the *Skills for Thinking* module, termination processing can be a good time to review copies of actual thought diaries completed during treatment. This review can be used to see what were some important issues and the progression over time in the client's understanding of the problems. You should provide your clients with at least a few blank thought diaries (Think 10 Practice: 6-Part Thought Diary) for future use.

Facilitate Referrals to Community Resources

In these final sessions, we recommend that consideration be given to referring clients to appropriate community resources, to help them continue to get needed support. For example, encouraging clients to find local support groups for coping with chronic illness can promote continued well-being long after formal therapy is over. In addition, a list of national resources is included in Appendix A of this clinician guide and may be of relevance to some clients at this point in the process.

Key Skills in This Module

Processing Termination Issues

During the final sessions, encourage discussions about what ending therapy means to clients, their ideas about what was more helpful and what was less helpful during treatment, and their feelings about their relationship with you (the clinician). We have specifically provided Wrap 2 Learn: What Does Ending Therapy Mean to You? as a resource for you to use. Rather than thinking of this as a page that is used in one termination session, it may be helpful to look at it together toward the beginning of several termination sessions. (Keep in mind that recognition is easier than recall, and your clients will be able to process more issues if they can have a list of topics to look at.)

Talking directly about these issues helps create a more positive ending and will give clients a sense of closure that is very important. Ask clients to come prepared to talk about these things; they may, perhaps, want to write out some notes on these topics. Other topics that may come up at this point in time are whether or not clients should continue with another professional clinician, start taking antidepressant medication, and/or join a self-help group or a support group.

Developing a Maintenance Guide

This phase begins with a review of the skills and techniques your clients have learned for dealing with stressful situations—and of these, which seemed to work best and what might be possible explanations for why this is the case. We recommend that at the start of this phase, you introduce the idea of developing a Maintenance Guide that clients will complete over the next couple of sessions with your help. The resources provided in Wrap 3–6 Learn will facilitate this work within session, and Wrap 3–7 Practice are provided for use within and between sessions.

Encourage your clients to continue to apply the skills they have learned. Research has documented that at a 2-year follow-up, clients who continue to use the skills they learned are much less likely to experience a high level of depressive symptoms (Powers et al., 2008). Furthermore, how helpful skills were rated upon use was more highly correlated with the level of symptoms than with the frequency of skill usage. This suggests that during the late phase of therapy, it is important to determine which skills are most helpful to the client and to set up explicit guidelines detailing when and how these should be applied. Wrap 5–7 Practice within the Maintenance Guide helps with this. During booster sessions, work with your clients to determine the helpfulness level of specific skills and encourage or dissuade their continued use accordingly.

The Maintenance Guide (Wrap 5–7 Practice) is a specific document created together by both you and your clients that consolidates their experience in therapy; it is used to review skills and prepare for possible problems in the future. We recommend creating this guide over three sessions before the final goodbye session. This guide can be started in session and clients can complete or add to it for home practice.

An example of a Maintenance Guide has been provided in <u>Wrap 3–6 Learn</u>, using the case example of John. Discuss this case in session to demonstrate how helpful the guide can be if a negative event or some crisis occurs that might trigger a depressive episode.

Reviewing Skills Learned

To begin preparation for creating the Maintenance Guide, ask clients to review the skills they have learned throughout therapy. <u>Wrap 4 Learn: The Maintenance Guide, Part 2</u> provides examples continuing with the case of John to help stimulate this discussion with clients. <u>Wrap 3 Practice: Planning for Future Stressful Situations</u> lists all the modules of this treatment and is a starting place to check off or circle the modules that were included in therapy. Then, <u>Wrap 5 and 6 Practice: My Maintenance Guide</u> include space to list specific emotional, behavioral, cognitive, and interpersonal skills that were a part of treatment.

Planning for Future Stressful Situations

Ask clients to think about the situations that are likely to arise in the future that may exacerbate symptoms and result in depression. <u>Wrap 5 Learn: Future Stressful Situations and Danger Signals</u> gives the case example of John to help generate ideas. Then, clients should use <u>Wrap 3 Practice: Planning for Future Stressful Situations</u> to list their top three ideas of future stressful situations. Have them think of specific cognitive, behavioral, and interpersonal skills (from their earlier list) that would help in each particular situation, and record these in the space provided on the form.

Recognizing and Planning for Danger Signals

Encourage clients to talk about "danger signals" that should serve as warning signs that low moods are again present and getting more severe. Let clients know that sometimes depressive reactions occur, despite our best efforts. For example, a person may become overwhelmed by one very big negative event (such as death of a loved one) or by a series of smaller but frequent negative events (several bad things happen at once and overtax one's ability to cope). Emphasize that this can happen to anyone. It is important that clients think back to their most recent bout of depression and try to remember what the main symptoms were. Wrap 5 Learn: Future Stressful Situations and Danger Signals provides an example using the case of John. In session, help clients use Wrap 4 Practice: My Danger Signals to make a list of the symptoms that they would consider to be their danger signals. This way they can notice them right away when they happen and make immediate plans for constructive action. Discussing clients' prior history will help a great deal here. Some clients may benefit from looking at the list of depression symptoms provided on Start 7 Learn: Recognizing Common Signs of Depression.

The final task is to develop a concrete plan for what to do if/when serious depressive symptoms resurface. Who can the client call? What is the best strategy if you are no longer in the area, or are not available, and the client needs therapy again? You should have specific answers to these questions so that you can terminate with your clients in confidence. A related issue is that of making referrals at this time to community resources (e.g., appropriate support groups) that are likely to be of benefit to clients to help them maintain their gains. This is, of course, an individual decision, but in our experience, helping clients to connect with community-based services is often very helpful as they transition out of formal therapy. A listing of a wide variety of national resources is included in Appendix A to give you direction and assistance in locating appropriate follow-up services. Because finances are often an issue for older clients, being able to provide them with specific information about free or low-cost services is usually very much appreciated. It also helps to ease the termination process and conveys the message that ongoing support is out there and may be worth considering to help with maintenance of gains.

The first step in preparing to use this module is a thorough review of all Learn pages and Practice forms so you are familiar with the content and can begin to think about the fit between different skills and specific clients. We realize that behavioral health providers working within primary care may use materials from this module in very brief sessions, and will select individual Learn pages and Practice forms that fit the concerns and needs of their clients. Similarly, there may be occasions within individual or group psychotherapy when clinicians choose specific Learn and/or Practice materials.

This module usually requires three or four sessions, and we recommend that you space out the last few sessions (e.g., biweekly rather than weekly). For clients who have been seen for a year or longer, it may help to have one or two sessions scheduled monthly. In the suggested outline in Table 10.1, this is noted by labeling specific sessions as "spaced." A booster session roughly 3 to 6 months after termination to evaluate progress and make any necessary adjustments in the skills being used can also be helpful to minimize relapse.

Not Included in This Treatment

Therapy Termination Resources for Family Members

Not all of your clients will wish to involve a family member in their therapy process. Some of your clients may not have someone available. For that reason, we have not provided specific Learn pages and Practice forms to facilitate discussions between your clients and members of their social network regarding therapy termination and development of the Maintenance Guide. We have, however, noted on a number of Learn pages that clients may wish to share their thoughts and plans for therapy termination with someone who is important to them.

Table 10.1 Session Outline

Each Session: Depression Measure + Start 3 and 4 Practice

GDS-SF or PHQ-9

Start 4 Practice	Preparing for My Next Session[T]
Start 3 Practice	My Session Summary[T]

Skills for Wrapping Up Session 1: Progress and Discussion of Termination

In Session 1: Wrap 1 and 2 Learn, Wrap 1 Practice (+ prior session review)

Between Sessions 1 and 2: Wrap 1 and 2 Practice, continued focus on key skills

Wrap 1 Learn	Introduction to Skills for Wrapping Up
Wrap 2 Learn	What Does Ending Treatment Mean to You?[T]
Wrap 1 Practice	Review of My Treatment Goals[T]
Wrap 2 Practice	My Values and Strengths That Help Me[T]

Skills for Wrapping Up Session 2 (Spaced): Discussion of John's Termination Preparation

In Session 2: Wrap 3–5 Learn

Between Sessions 2 and 3: Wrap 3 and 4 Practice

Wrap 3 Learn	The Maintenance Guide, Part 1[T]
Wrap 4 Learn	The Maintenance Guide, Part 2[T]
Wrap 5 Learn	Future Stressful Situations and Danger Signals[T]
Wrap 3 Practice	Planning for Future Stressful Situations[T]
Wrap 4 Practice	My Danger Signals[T]

Skills for Wrapping Up Session 3 (Spaced): Work Together on Maintenance Guide

In Session 3: Wrap 6 Learn

Between Sessions 3 and 4: Wrap 5–7 Practice

Wrap 6 Learn	Making a Plan[T]
Wrap 5 Practice	My Maintenance Guide, Page 1[T]
Wrap 6 Practice	My Maintenance Guide, Page 2[T]

(continued)

Table 10.1 Continued

Skills for Wrapping Up Session 4 (Spaced): Maintenance Guide, Say Goodbye

In Session 4: Wrap 6 and 7 Learn; Wrap 5–7 Practice

Wrap 6 Learn	Making a Plan[T]
Wrap 7 Learn	One Important Resource: Your Learn Pages and Practice Forms!
Wrap 5 Practice	My Maintenance Guide, Page 1[T]
Wrap 6 Practice	My Maintenance Guide, Page 2[T]
Wrap 7 Practice	My Maintenance Guide, Page 3[T]

Booster Session (3–6 months after termination): Review and Reinforce Skills

---

[T] Identified as particularly appropriate for telehealth sessions.

Specific Referrals for Support Groups

Some of your clients, especially those who are relatively socially isolated, will miss the emotional connection along with the structure of having someplace specific to go each week. We have not developed Learn pages or Practice forms specifically focused on how clients might find other structured ways of feeling socially engaged and emotionally connected with others once therapy has ended. AARP's Connect2Affect (https://connect2affect.org) and COVIA's Well Connected programs (https://covia.org/services/well-connected/) are two good resources for socially isolated clients who reside in the United States.

Additional Resource for Clinicians

O'Donohue, W. T., & Cucciare, M. (Eds.). (2010). *Terminating psychotherapy: A clinician's guide*. Routledge.

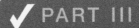

PART III

Personalized Modules (For Some Clients)

CHAPTER 11

Module 5: Skills for Brain Health: Healthy Cognitive Aging

This personalized module of the workbook is focused on the skills of:

1. Monitoring therapy progress and fine-tuning treatment goals
2. Understanding cognitive aging
3. Engaging in brain-healthy habits
4. Navigating health care and managing medications
5. Considering a cognitive evaluation
6. Revising therapy goals, staying encouraged and engaged in treatment

---

Clinician Note

As you read this chapter, we encourage you to have the workbook open so that you can refer to the specific Learn pages and Practice forms as they are described and explained. You will use these Learn pages and Practice forms during sessions, encouraging your clients to review between sessions using the Learn pages and try out/record between sessions using the Practice forms. Your reviewing these items as you read through this chapter will prepare you to make the most of the treatment materials. Using these pages and forms means more than having them available to look at or read over with your clients during sessions. Instead, you'll be engaging your clients in exploring the meaning this has to them, through discussion and careful application. Your goal each session is to help your clients apply specific Learn and Practice material to their recent experiences in daily life, and to the problems that bring them into treatment.

This chapter is provided to help you use the *Skills for Brain Health* module of the workbook with your clients. We start with a brief overview, followed by some practical tips based on the most common questions we hear from clinicians during professional trainings. The bulk of this chapter is devoted to reviewing skills to enhance cognitive health, with a description of the specific Learn pages and Practice forms available for your use in sessions. We provide recommendations for a standard progression of material (i.e., Learn pages and Practice forms that typically go with each other in the same session, estimates of how much can be accomplished in a given session), with the understanding that this may vary quite a bit depending upon your practice setting and specific client needs. We end the chapter with some comments about related topics that are not included in this treatment approach, and point readers to additional resources.

Overview

The science and practice of brain health is developing at a rapid pace. We now understand that there are many things that middle-aged and older adults can do to make a difference in their cognitive health and functioning. The Fingers Project, a breakthrough research study of older adults in Finland, showed that a multidomain lifestyle intervention can prevent cognitive decline (Ngandu et al., 2015); a replication in the United States called the Pointer Study is now under way (www. wwfingers.com). Across multiple studies, evidence is building to support physical activity, stimulating daily activities, social connections, heart-healthy dietary practices, and managing cardiovascular risk factors as interconnected ways to improve brain health and cognitive functioning. A review by the Lancet Commission (Livingston et al., 2017) and their updates (Livingston et al., 2020) clearly validate that what is good for the heart is truly good for the brain; behavioral changes can significantly impact brain structures and functions. In fact, as illustrated in Figure 11.1, they conclude that 40% of the risk factors for dementia are modifiable!

This means that, contrary to popular belief that dementias are entirely genetically determined, there are many daily health habits that can reduce risk for dementia and that are under our control. Many middle-aged and older clients are eager to learn about and apply this to their lives. The aging cohort of baby boomers are especially concerned about and interested in

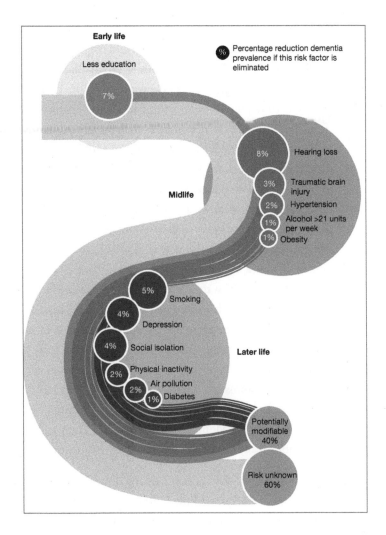

Early life

Less education

7%

% Percentage reduction dementia prevalence if this risk factor is eliminated

Midlife

8% Hearing loss

3% Traumatic brain injury

2% Hypertension

1% Alcohol >21 units per week

1% Obesity

5% Smoking

4% Depression

4% Social isolation

2% Physical inactivity

2% Air pollution

1% Diabetes

Later life

Potentially modifiable 40%

Risk unknown 60%

Figure 11.1

Life Course Model of Contributions of Modifiable Risk Factors for Dementia

Republished with permission of Elsevier Science & Technology Journals, from Livingston et al. (2020). Dementia prevention, intervention, and care: 2020 Report of the Lancet Commission. *Lancet, 396*(10248), p. 428; permission conveyed through Copyright Clearance Center, Inc.

maintaining their cognitive health. They are also comfortable with using mental health services and expect behavioral health clinicians to be prepared to work with them on brain health efforts. There is much that you can do to support the physical health and well-being of your clients (Haber, 2016). This module is designed for you to use with middle-aged and older adults who want to stay as healthy and functional as possible.

With depressed clients, it is also important to be aware of the complex relationships between depression and cognitive functioning (Blazer & Steffens, 2015; Blazer & Wallace, 2016; Blazer et al., 2015). For individuals of all ages, clinical depression impairs concentration. Some adults with depression who complain about memory concerns, when formally assessed, are determined to have no substantive changes in their memory. Instead, the poor attention and disruptions in concentration that are associated with depression lead to information not being processed and consolidated from short-term into long-term memories. Other research has shown a number of areas of cognitive functioning to be negatively impacted by depression in older adults, compared to those who are not depressed (Ranjan et al, 2017). Early-onset depression is linked to more cognitive decline than for older adults experiencing depression for the first time later in life. More severe forms of depression in older adults are also associated with a host of cognitive difficulties, including slower processing speed and impairments in executive function, working memory, episodic memory, reading, and understanding what others are saying (Ranjan et al., 2017; Sheline et al., 2006). These cognitive symptoms can improve as depression lifts, but these are generally slower to improve than other depressive symptoms (e.g., depressed mood, fatigue, anhedonia). You will need to emphasize to clients that daily habits really do make a difference in their recovery process.

Even with clients who are experiencing decreased functioning, there are things that can help. As shown in Figure 11.2, our treatment approach emphasizes those factors that are at the intersection of increasing cognitive reserve, reducing brain inflammation, and reducing brain damage (i.e., reducing depression, supporting a rich social network, exercise, and adherence to a Mediterranean diet).

The *Skills for Brain Health* module includes clinical tools for healthy cognitive functioning. The heart of this module is devoted to helping clients develop healthy lifestyle habits that support optimal cognitive functioning. This extensive module also provides resources for:

- Learning about cognitive aging
- Exploring evaluation of cognitive concerns
- Understanding key areas of differential diagnosis for cognitive problems (i.e., depression, delirium, dementia)

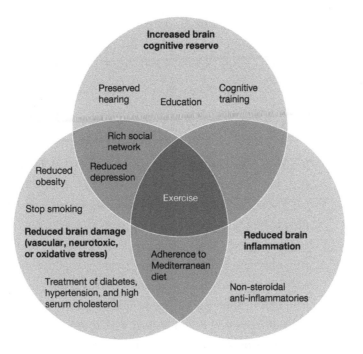

Figure 11.2

Potential Brain Mechanisms for Preventive Strategies in Dementia

Reprinted from Livingston et al. (2017). Dementia prevention, intervention, and care. *Lancet, 390*, p. 280, with permission from Elsevier.

- Maximizing helpfulness of medical appointments, including the annual Medicare Wellness Visit
- Managing medications

At the end of the module, there is an option for clients to develop personal goals related to their brain health. All of this work is framed within the context of their personal life values and strengths to ensure that treatment goals and strategies are consistent with these.

In the context of treating later-life depression, it is important to have first engaged clients in therapy orientation and treatment planning (*Skills for Getting Started*). The psychoeducation and skills developed within this *Skills for Brain Health* module are grounded in an understanding of the cognitive-behavioral model, which is presented and discussed in *Skills for Getting Started*. The values clarification work done at the beginning of treatment is especially key to promoting brain health. A focus on priorities in life can help clients do the hard work of developing and maintaining a brain-healthy lifestyle. Behavioral activation (*Skills for Doing*) continues to be critically important because of how central physical and social activities are to cognitive health and functioning.

When to Use This Module

The materials provided in this module will be helpful for some middle-aged and older clients who are interested in brain-healthy routines and practices. Many individuals with depression worry that their cognitive symptoms are not simply a part of depression and may signify lasting deficits. Middle-aged clients with family members diagnosed with Alzheimer's disease or another neurocognitive disorder are especially likely to have questions and concerns about protecting their own brain health. Some middle-aged and older adults will present in primary care and behavioral health settings with specific cognitive concerns and complaints that are currently undiagnosed.

> ### Clinician Note
>
> *We consider behavioral health clinicians who work with this optional module to be "brain health coaches" and would like to caution you not to go beyond your training and scope of practice in terms of assessment and evaluation of suspected neurocognitive disorders. In most cases, clinicians using this treatment approach will screen and then refer clients to other providers for formal evaluation of cognitive complaints. Screening and assessment of cognitive complaints are addressed in Chapter 3 of this guide, and we refer you to that section for details.*

Tips for Clinicians

Modify Sessions to Accommodate Cognitive Symptoms

There are important within-session strategies to manage cognitive symptoms of depression. For some of your clients, these symptoms will interact with age-related changes and become magnified. Other clients may already have mild cognitive impairment or be in early stages of a progressive neurocognitive disorder. There are specific things that you can do in session to help these individuals benefit from treatment (Gallagher-Thompson & Thompson, 2021). Because more time is needed to focus attention and process new information, session structure (e.g., setting and keeping agendas, periodic reviews and summaries) is important. With both depression and cognitive aging comes increased distractibility; it is easier for clients to lose their train of thought and move from topic to topic unintentionally. Reduce distractions within session and prioritize agenda items with the expectation that you will only get to two or three items in session. Help your clients get in the habit of writing things down during session, not just to help with memory but also as a way to think about and process information. Do not expect your clients to think about and solve complex problems "in their head." Clients should use written logs/records of clinically important material. We provide more detailed recommendations in Chapter 5 of this clinician guide.

Attend to Culture-Specific Beliefs About Cognitive Health

There are important culture-specific beliefs about cognitive health and the dementias, and these can shape your clients' understanding of cognitive aging, their expectations for their own brain health, and communication within families and with health care providers (Yeo et al., 2019). Because expectations about aging are embedded within culture, awareness of the facets of diversity most important to specific clients is very important. Throughout this entire module, you are implementing culturally sensitive ways for clients to share their interests and concerns about brain health with family members and health care providers.

Support Social Connections

Positive social interactions support brain health while also reducing depression; the cognitive stimulation that accompanies social activities is important. Individuals with longstanding difficulties in their interpersonal relationships may find it especially difficult to elicit and use support for developing brain-healthy habits. Relationships are also significantly impacted by cognitive impairments. The social withdrawal and/or irritability that sometimes accompany depression can also be early signs of frustration and passivity that are a part of a progressive neurocognitive disorder. For clients who already have a diagnosed condition such as mild cognitive impairment or a neurocognitive disorder such as Alzheimer's disease, communication with members of their social network can be challenging but important. These clients may improve their interpersonal effectiveness with use of the personalized *Skills for Relating* module; developing skills involved in asking for help may be particularly useful.

Key Skills in This Module

Monitoring Therapy Progress and Fine-Tuning Treatment Goals

Health 1 Learn: Introduction to Skills for Brain Health provides an important reminder to have a "state of therapy" discussion about therapy goals and progress. Now is the time to review the overall pattern of depression scores from whichever measure of depression is being used weekly as a part of this feedback-informed treatment. Complete and review Health 1 Practice: Review of My Treatment Goals during session so that overall therapy goals stay in the forefront, even while spending time addressing brain health. Clients should take that review of therapy goals home so they can re-read it between sessions. This may be a point in therapy where the client has made significant progress on one of their therapy goals and wishes to revise or replace it with another.

Understanding Cognitive Aging

A basic understanding of how the brain does, and doesn't, change with normal healthy aging is important. The psychoeducation provided in Health 1–6 Learn will be of interest to many of the clients who use this module. Because this is a rather complex module with a number of different subsections, devote a little session time to outlining the topics listed on Health 1 Learn: Introduction to Skills for Brain Health and discuss which ones are of primary interest to the specific client. There is a reminder to encourage clients to share information with a key family member or the family members who are most involved in their medical treatments, who may be special sources of support. If you are unsure who those family members are, including chosen family, now is the time to explore that within session. Across the entire module, you will encourage your clients to communicate with family care partners about their brain health concerns and what they are working on in treatment, while being sensitive to the ways in which cultural differences impact this process.

The information in Health 2–6 Learn conveys important core concepts. Different cognitive functions are listed in Health 2 Learn: Brain Health Is Important at Every Age, emphasizing that brain health involves a range of abilities that are used in daily life and that are linked to core personal values. Health 3 Learn: Key Points About Brain Health: Cognitive Aging explains intra- and inter-individual variability of cognitive functioning, leading to a focus on values-consistent lifestyle habits and practices that support brain health and daily activities. Health 4 Learn: How Our Brains Do and Don't Change as We Age outlines normative age-related changes in cognitive functioning, and Health 5 Learn: Brain Health and Depression reviews how depression and cognitive functioning are related to each other. Health 6 Learn: Some Brain Changes Are Not Due to Aging describes atypical changes that indicate a need for evaluation; repeat the point that the warning signs are problematic when they occur repeatedly and frequently, not just on rare occasions. Health 2 Practice: Maintain My Physical Health by Knowing My Numbers is a way for clients to begin work in this module by collecting details of their cardiovascular risk all in one place. This sometimes motivates clients to have an annual medical appointment with their primary care physician to have blood tests ordered and reviewed. In this initial psychoeducation section of the module, we introduce the planning sheet for Health 11 Practice: My Upcoming Health Care Visit. A theme throughout this module is to encourage communication about brain health with family members and with health care providers. This planning tool can help with that.

Engaging in Brain-Healthy Habits

We learn more every year regarding how important daily health behaviors are to memory and thinking abilities! This main part of the module

189

focuses on strategies to reduce modifiable risk factors and to support optimal cognitive functioning (Health 7–14 Learn, Health 3–10 Practice). Emphasize to your clients that it is the *combination* of healthy practices that makes the difference. Those that are key to improvement in one client are not necessarily the same as for the next. Devote session time to reviewing the information provided in Health 7 Learn: A Brain-Healthy Lifestyle: Your Daily Health Habits Matter and Health 8 Learn: Support Your Brain Health; these include the central information for this section of the module. Use Health 3 Practice: Taking Care of My Brain Health, which is an important practice form and can be repeatedly assigned between sessions to help clients develop these lifestyle habits. The sheets promoting healthy physical activity (Health 9 Learn: Be Physically Active, Health 4 Practice: My Physical Activity), nutrition (Health 10 Learn: Follow a Healthy Food and Drink Plan, Health 5 Practice: Healthy Food and Drink Log), social connections (Health 11 Learn: Stay Socially Connected to Others, Health 6 Practice: How I Felt Connected to Others), stress management (Health 12 Learn: Manage Your Stress, Health 7 Practice: Managing Stress, Health 8 Practice: My Stress Management), learning new things (Health 13 Learn: Learn New Things, Health 9 Practice: Learning New Things), and sleep (Health 14 Learn: Keep Healthy Sleep Habits, Health 10 Practice: My Healthy Sleep Habits) are additional resources to use with individual clients when special attention is needed in any of these key areas. We would not typically work our way through all of these resources with the same client.

As with the rest of this approach, you are working week by week to help your clients develop healthy habits over time, without an expectation of 100% compliance with all recommendations. You want clients to experiment with what is *possible* for them at this point, yet you can't expect them to suddenly adopt behaviors that seem utterly impossible. Over time and with effort, that list of "impossible," "possible but a stretch," and "very do-able" can shift. Throughout this module, we encourage you and your clients to return to Start 5 Practice: My Values and Strengths for a review of personal values and strengths. These are particularly important to hold on to during work on improving brain health. A focus of this treatment is having a daily life that is values-based and worth living. Help your clients make the connections between how brain health helps them hold on to these life values, and how life values help them work on their brain health.

Navigating Health Care and Managing Medications

This module also provides a number of resources for helping your clients manage medical appointments and medications; both are key to brain health! Information about the annual Medicare Wellness Visit and how to get the most from health care visits is covered in Health 15 and 16 Learn and supported by Health 11 Practice. We also address the management of prescription and over-the-counter (OTC) medications (Health 17–19 Learn, Health 12 Practice). Most older adults take a number of prescription and OTC medications, and some of these may impact brain health and cognitive functioning. Medications fall in a relative "comfort zone" and are easy to talk about for many clients. Their medication-related questions can be a helpful conduit to bringing up memory and other cognitive concerns with medical providers. You can help your clients identify such medication-related questions for their medical providers, while staying humble about your own lack of knowledge.

Clinician Note

We would like to caution you against taking an expert role regarding both prescription and OTC medications and vitamins/supplements. There are dangers in taking on the voice of authority, from acting outside of your licensed scope of practice to interfering with collaborative relationships with health care providers. Do not become prescriptive or set yourself up as an authority, and do not oversimplify what might be quite complex medical concerns across multiple comorbidities and polypharmacy.

Encourage your clients to prepare lists of questions for their medical appointments using Health 11 Practice: My Upcoming Health Care Visit and Health 12 Practice: Questions to Ask My Health Provider About Medications; ease the way for clients to discuss concerns about memory and cognitive functioning. Then, "refer and defer" to their medical provider.

Considering a Cognitive Evaluation

This section of the module is not applicable to all clients. Health 20–23 Learn cover a range of topics relevant for individuals who have concerns about their memory or thinking abilities. Societal stigma regarding neurocognitive disorders such as Alzheimer's disease has created a climate of secrecy and hesitation that was historically true of cancer before advances in treatment. Some cognitive problems *can* be treated and reversed, and that key point bears repetition as you discuss the advantages of seeking a formal evaluation of cognitive abilities and problems. There have also been significant advances in diagnosing Alzheimer's disease; early identification and diagnosis can lead to initiation of drug treatments and lifestyle changes to maximize daily functioning. Developments in neuroimaging, cerebrospinal fluid (CSF) tests, and now the breakthrough C_2N Diagnostics' PrecivityAD™ blood test all make it easier for clients and their families to obtain clarity about the source of cognitive concerns. Health 20 Learn: Why Ask for an Evaluation and Health 21 Learn: How Do You Know if You Need a Specialist? guide clients and their families to options for getting an evaluation. The following two pages (Health 22 and 23 Learn) then cover reasons (other than depression) for noticeable changes in cognitive functioning (i.e., delirium and dementia) and what specialists will consider during a differential diagnosis.

Depression (Health 5 Learn: Brain Health and Depression), delirium (Health 22 Learn: What Is Delirium?), and neurocognitive disorders, previously called dementia (Health 23 Learn: Neurocognitive Disorders (Also Called Dementia)), are all conditions that impact memory and thinking abilities, but in different ways. Most clients have not considered the number of possible explanations for cognitive complaints, and this information can often increase their level of comfort in pursuing a medical evaluation. An important point about delirium is that even after the cause of the delirium (e.g., anesthesia from surgery, infection from a urinary tract infection or COVID-19) has been removed, the brain's recovery from delirium can take months. The healthy-brain interventions across this module are also important in fostering the brain's recovery from a serious delirium. Throughout this section, we emphasize clients' use of Health 11 Practice: My Upcoming Health Care Visit to prepare for medical appointments and communicate concerns about brain health to their health care provider and involved family members.

Revising Therapy Goals, Staying Encouraged and Engaged in Treatment

Sometimes as work in this module is nearing completion, it becomes clear that more attention to brain health may be an important part of reducing depression. This is one of the modules where it is likely that some clients will develop a new goal. You can use Health 24 Learn: Setting Personal Goals Related to Brain Health in session to collaboratively decide whether there should be any changes or revisions to therapy goals. Just remember, it is important that therapy focus on addressing no more than two or three overall goals, so you won't necessarily do this with every client using this module. Health 13 Practice: My Goals for Brain Health can be used as a form to write down and rate those revised goals. Health 25 Learn: Ways to Think About Progress Toward Your Goals reminds clients of the most common pattern of change with therapy (sawtooth curve, not a straight line or stair steps). We recommend Health 14 Practice: As I Continue with Treatment: My Plan for Fully Participating for times when you have some concerns about a client's engagement in treatment, either within session or compliance with between-session practice. We suggest using Health 15 Practice: My Review of Skills for Brain Health as a way to review and consolidate key points and skills that were worked on in this module.

Suggested Progression of Content

The first step in preparing to use this module is a thorough review of all Learn pages and Practice forms so you are familiar with the content and can begin to think about the fit between different skills and specific clients. We do not expect any single client to receive this module in its entirety. We realize that behavioral health providers working within primary care may use materials from this module in very brief sessions and will select individual Learn pages and Practice forms that fit the concerns and needs of their clients. Similarly, there may be occasions within individual or group psychotherapy when clinicians choose Learn and Practice materials that appear most appropriate. You will have built a relationship with your psychotherapy clients by this point in treatment and will likely already know specific areas of interest and/or concern.

In almost all therapy cases, this module will be used after clinicians have worked on goal setting and therapy orientation in the *Skills for Getting Started* module, after facilitating emotional literacy skills in *Skills for Feeling*, and after targeting daily positive and rewarding activities in *Skills for Doing*. Sessions will use the same basic structure: (a) set an agenda, (b) review home practice, (c) select at least one topic to work on in depth, (d) summarize, (e) set up new home practice assignment, and (f) do mutual feedback. Start work on all Practice forms within session or wait for the next session to introduce them. Don't send a client home with a Practice form without a personal example already inserted. Be sure to allow time to review any Practice forms in the next session. For some of your clients, you will move directly after this module into preparation for therapy termination, in the *Skills for Wrapping Up* module.

When this module is being used with clients who desire to develop and maintain a brain-healthy lifestyle, we suggest a five-session approach that allows for several sessions devoted to reinforcing specific practices. The development of new habits takes time, and the home practice assigned often takes several weeks before any noticeable impact on quality of daily life is reported.

Table 11.1 presents the suggested sequence for this module.

Case Study Example

Because this may be a very new area of work for many behavioral health clinicians, we have included a case study to help make several key points.

Ruby is a 70-year-old African American woman with mild depression who has been referred by her primary care practitioner (PCP) for depression and "memory complaints." Your cognitive screen of Ruby (see Chapter 3) indicates that she has no significant impairment, but she did have depression scores in the moderate range (PHQ-9 = 14). She tells you that her number-one concern is worry about her memory problems, which she perceives to be a stepping stone to dementia. Ruby believes that dementia is inevitable: "You get old and that is

Table 11.1 Session Outline

Each Session: Depression Measure + Start 3 and 4 Practice

GDS-SF or PHQ-9

Start 4 Practice	Preparing for My Next Session[T]
Start 3 Practice	My Session Summary[T]

Skills for Brain Health Session 1: Progress and Psychoeducation

In Session 1: Health 1–6 Learn, Health 1 Practice (+ prior session review)

Between Sessions 1 and 2: Health 1 and 2 Practice

Health 1 Learn	Introduction to Skills for Brain Health
Health 2 Learn	Brain Health Is Important at Every Age
Health 3 Learn	Key Points About Brain Health: Cognitive Aging[T]
Health 4 Learn	How Our Brains Do and Don't Change as We Age[T]
Health 5 Learn	Brain Health and Depression
Health 6 Learn	Some Brain Changes Are Not Due to Aging
Health 1 Practice	Review of My Treatment Goals[T]
Health 2 Practice	Maintain My Physical Health by Knowing My Numbers[T]

Skills for Brain Health Session 2: Guided Discussion of Brain-Healthy Practices

In Session 2: Health 7 and 8 Learn

Between Sessions 2 and 3: Health 2 and 3 Practice

Health 7 Learn	A Brain-Healthy Lifestyle: Your Daily Health Habits Matter[T]
Health 8 Learn	Support Your Brain Health
Health 2 Practice	Maintain My Physical Health by Knowing My Numbers[T]
Health 3 Practice	Taking Care of My Brain Health[T]

Skills for Brain Health Session 3: Continued Discussion of Brain-Healthy Practices

In Session 3: Choice among Health 8–14 Learn

Between Sessions 3 and 4: Choice among Health 3–10 Practice

Health 8 Learn	Support your Brain Health[T]
Health 9 Learn	Be Physically Active[T]
Health 10 Learn	Follow a Healthy Food and Drink Plan[T]

(continued)

Table 11.1 Continued

Health 11 Learn	Stay Socially Connected to Others[T]
Health 12 Learn	Manage Your Stress[T]
Health 13 Learn	Learn New Things[T]
Health 14 Learn	Keep Healthy Sleep Habits[T]
Health 3 Practice	Taking Care of My Brain Health[T]
Health 4 Practice	My Physical Activity[T]
Health 5 Practice	Healthy Food and Drink Log[T]
Health 6 Practice	How I Felt Connected to Others[T]
Health 7 Practice	Managing Stress[T]
Health 8 Practice	My Stress Management
Health 9 Practice	Learning New Things[T]
Health 10 Practice	My Healthy Sleep Habits[T]

(Note: The following part of the module can be expanded to multiple sessions.)

Skills for Brain Health Session 4: Managing Health Care and Medications

In Session 4: Health 15–19 Learn

Between Sessions 4 and 5: Health 11 and 12 Practice

Health 15 Learn	Your Annual Medicare Wellness Visit[T]
Health 16 Learn	Preparing for Health Care Visits[T]
Health 17 Learn	Organizing Medications[T]
Health 18 Learn	Over-the-Counter (OTC) Medication Use
Health 19 Learn	Managing Medication Side Effects
Health 11 Practice	My Upcoming Health Care Visit[T]
Health 12 Practice	Questions to Ask My Health Provider About Medications

Skills for Brain Health Session 5: Review and Assessment

In Session 5: Health 24 and 25 Learn, Health 13 Practice

After Session 5: Health 13–15 Practice:

Health 24 Learn	Setting Personal Goals Related to Brain Health[T]
Health 25 Learn	Ways to Think About Progress Toward Your Goals[T]

Table 11.1 Continued

Health 13 Practice	My Goals for Brain Health[T]
Health 14 Practice	As I Continue with Treatment: My Plan for Fully Participating
Health 15 Practice	My Review of Skills for Brain Health[T]

[T] Identified as particularly appropriate for telehealth sessions.

what happens." After working on the Skills for Getting Started *and* Skills for Feeling *modules, Ruby's revised number-one goal for treating her depression is "To go to bed at night knowing that I am doing what I can to prevent dementia." She asks you, "Is this even possible?" Ruby is a very appropriate client for this module! You make the decision to go directly from* Skills for Feeling *to this* Skills for Brain Health *module, skipping over* Skills for Doing *and* Skills for Thinking. *Ruby begins to work with you in this module and benefits from psychoeducation about normal age-related changes in memory (Health 3–5 Learn). Her PHQ-9 scores begin to move but stay in the moderate range (PHQ-9 = 11), and she indicates that she is very motivated to work on her particular dementia risk factors to modify them.*

After psychoeducation, you review Health 7 Learn *and* Health 8 Learn *in session and ask Ruby which of those specific lifestyle behaviors she is not doing, or is doing but is not satisfied with how they are going. Since becoming depressed, Ruby reduced her engagement in physical activities and began eating more "junk food" as she increased her TV viewing time. She is not aware of her cholesterol levels and current blood pressure numbers, both of which are crucial for monitoring heart (and brain) health. Starting with* Health 2 Practice *is a good way to get concrete about what "improving brain health" means! Knowing this information, plus the information you have about Ruby's lifestyle, guides your selection of specific topics to work on within this module. Likely candidates would be physical activity (Health 9 Learn, Health 4 Practice) and healthy eating (Health 10 Learn, Health 5 Practice).*

As she makes progress in these areas, Ruby's depression moves into the mild range (PHQ-9 = 9), and she reports that she is more socially withdrawn due to stress over finances and has sleep issues that she didn't mention earlier but would now like to work on. These become three "micro-goals" for her therapy and involve her working to feel more socially connected to others

(*Health 11 Learn, Health 6 Practice*), *managing stress* (*Health 12 Learn, Health 7 Practice*), *and beginning to collect information about her sleep problems* (*Health 14 Learn, Health 10 Practice*). *She struggles with healthy sleep habits and with identifying and engaging in activities that help her feel connected to others. This leads you to select some materials from* Skills for Healthy Sleep *and* Skills for Doing; *these are done "in the service of" improving her brain health because that is Ruby's main reason for being in treatment. You help Ruby (and yourself) stay on track in this complex module by reviewing the brain-health goals that she developed using* Health 13 Practice. *This helps both of you assess the progress she is making and consider any needed adjustments. Her PHQ-9 scores are now in the 6-to-8 range, which is mildly depressed.*

At Session 10, Ruby tells you that she has a PCP appointment in 2 weeks but does not feel prepared; she has questions regarding her medications but is not sure what to say or ask. Together, you evaluate her progress on reducing her risk factors for dementia and decide to move into a new area covered in Health 15–19 Learn *and* Health 11 *and* 12 Practice. *This material is intended to help you work collaboratively to help Ruby prepare for her PCP appointment and bring up the questions of most importance to her. Not all of those Learn pages were relevant, but Ruby was able to look at, discuss, and pick out the ones that she found most helpful for her concerns.*

Your work with Ruby in this module concludes with a review of what she learned using Health 15 Practice, *and Ruby is able to describe and list the specific behaviors and strategies that she wants to continue to work on outside of therapy. At this point her PHQ-9 score is ranging from 2 to 5, and you jointly decide to transition to the* Skills for Wrapping Up *module to begin the process of terminating treatment.*

Not Included in This Treatment

OTC Medications Promoted for Brain Health

We encourage behavioral health clinicians to avoid giving any advice regarding the use of medications, whether prescription or nonprescription. Such advice amounts to dispensing medical advice without a license to practice medicine. It can be tempting to offer your own opinions about the advisability of adding, retaining, or discontinuing medications or vitamins purported to help or hurt brain health. If clients are interested in some change to their use of prescription or OTC medications, encourage them to make an appointment with their PCP to discuss this.

Neuropsychological Assessment for Cognitive Functioning

We cover issues related to screening and assessment of cognitive complaints in Chapter 3 of this guide and refer you to that section. In this *Skills for Brain Health* module, we have not included specific recommendations for evaluating neurocognitive disorders. This is an area of specialization that clinicians without formal training in this area should avoid. In addition to referring clients back to their PCP, you can explain that geriatricians and neurologists are two different types of medical doctors who work in this area.

Professional Development Opportunities in Brain Health

Because it is an area of genuine interest for so many older adults, many clinicians find themselves enjoying the work they do in the area of brain health. This is an aspect of life that is important for all of us, and helping individuals improve their brain health can be very rewarding. For clinicians who would like more professional development, there are a range of opportunities for learning more (see the "Additional Resources for Clinicians" list). Some clinicians decide to train as volunteer community educators in brain health for nonprofit organizations such as the Alzheimer's Association. The training and resources provided to community health educators can be one way of gaining both knowledge and credibility within your local community.

Additional Resources for Clinicians

Adames, H. Y., & Tazeau, Y. N. (Eds.). (2020). *Caring for Latinxs with dementia in a globalized world: Behavioral and psychosocial treatments*. Springer Nature.

Mast, B. T., & Yochim, B. P. (2018). *Alzheimer's disease and dementia*. Hogrefe Press.

Yeo, G., Gerdner, L., & Gallagher-Thompson, D. (2019). *Ethnicity and the dementias* (3rd ed.). Routledge Press.

Measure in Appendix D Related to This Module

AD8 (Recommendations for use are provided in Chapter 3 of this clinician guide.)

CHAPTER 12

Module 6: Skills for Managing Chronic Pain: Improving Daily Life

This personalized module of the workbook is focused on the skills of:

1. Monitoring therapy progress and fine-tuning treatment goals
2. Understanding the experience of chronic pain
3. Applying the gate control model of chronic pain
4. Revising therapy goals, staying encouraged and engaged in treatment

This chapter is provided to help you use the *Skills for Managing Chronic Pain* module of the workbook with your clients. We begin with a brief overview, followed by some practical tips based on the most common questions we hear from clinicians during professional trainings. The bulk of this chapter is devoted to reviewing skills to manage chronic and persistent pain conditions, with a description of the specific Learn pages and Practice forms available for your use in sessions. We provide recommendations for a standard progression of material (i.e., Learn pages and Practice forms that typically go with each other in the same session, estimates of how much can be accomplished in a given session), with the understanding that this may vary quite a bit depending upon your practice setting and specific client needs. We end the chapter with some comments about related topics that are not included in this treatment approach, and point readers to some resources for additional professional development in chronic pain management.

Overview

You are likely to have some clients with depression who struggle with chronic pain. Chronic pain and depression are bidirectionally related: Chronic pain contributes to the development of later-life depression, and depression increases the difficulty of implementing pain management strategies. There are a number of health conditions in middle-aged and older adults that lead to chronic pain. This means that some middle-aged and older adults will present in primary care and behavioral health settings with chronic pain concerns. For all of these reasons, clinicians across a range of treatment settings are likely to work with clients in this area.

In the context of treating later-life depression, it is important to have first engaged clients in therapy orientation and treatment planning (*Skills for Getting Started*). The psychoeducation and skills developed within this *Skills for Managing Chronic Pain* module are grounded in an understanding of the cognitive-behavioral model, which is presented and discussed in *Skills for Getting Started*. The values clarification work done at the beginning of treatment is especially key to pain management. Clients may put some parts of life "on hold" during acute pain, but it is especially important for them to reconnect with their priorities in life if they live with chronic pain. The resources for emotional literacy, savoring of positive emotions, and relaxation in *Skills for Feeling* are all very relevant to the work in this module.

Encourage your clients to increase awareness of positive emotions; this is helpful as long as you also validate the reality of their experiences of pain. Behavioral activation (*Skills for Doing*) continues to be critically important as clients develop a repertoire of pain management strategies. Physical and social activities are a vital part of having each day include positive and rewarding experiences, despite the presence of chronic pain.

All of this work is framed within the context of their personal life values and strengths to ensure that treatment goals and strategies are consistent with these. There are important culture-specific beliefs about illness and pain that can also shape your client's coping efforts. Because expectations about aging are embedded within culture, awareness of the facets of diversity most important to specific clients is very important. Throughout this entire module, you are implementing culturally sensitive ways for clients to share their interests and concerns about their pain with family members and health care providers.

When to Use This Module

If the intake interview suggests that pain predated the first onset of depressive symptoms and has had a chronic course since then, refer the client to a pain clinic or provider who can offer CBT for Chronic Pain. This may take time. Clinicians and clients can use some of this module while waiting for the client to begin treatment for chronic pain, or decide which other personalized modules within this treatment approach may also be useful. You may be treating depression in a client who is also working with a pain management team or behavioral health clinician. In these cases of concurrent services, communication and collaboration is a must. Screening and assessment of pain-related concerns are addressed in Chapter 3 of this guide, and we refer you to that section for details.

The materials in this module will be sufficient for many middle-aged and older clients who need some attention to managing chronic pain as a part of their depression treatment. There are particularly close associations among depression, chronic pain, and sleep concerns. Listen carefully to clients' narratives of how they understand the interrelationships among pain, sleep, and depression. Collaboratively discuss and decide together whether to begin with sleep or with pain management. It might be that the work in this chronic pain module leads to some work in the *Skills for Healthy Sleep* module afterwards.

Pay Attention to Sudden Changes in Pain Experiences

Many clients experience chronic pain that varies over time and can intensify with flare-ups. This cycle feels familiar to them and is a part of their living with chronic pain. If, however, pain changes very quickly and dramatically, or is a new sensation or in a new area of the body, this requires medical attention. Whenever you are uncertain about clients' reports of a sudden change in their pain, you should encourage them to contact their medical provider immediately.

Validate, Validate, Validate

Strong interpersonal and clinical skills are especially key for your work with clients experiencing chronic pain. Many individuals living with chronic pain have experienced the ignoring or dismissal of their pain by family members, friends, or health care providers. Use of core validation strategies is particularly helpful when working with this population. You want to take a "yes/and" approach in which you both validate the very real challenges of living with chronic pain (the "yes" part) and emphasize that this is why you want to help them develop some strategies that can help in their situation (the "and" part). There are many ways to validate the realities of chronic pain without reinforcing or agreeing with unhelpful beliefs, thoughts, or behaviors. A client may say, "I was in so much pain yesterday that I couldn't do anything at all other than spend the entire day in my chair watching boring TV and feeling miserable." There is much in that statement for you to validate without agreeing that spending the day in a chair feeling miserable was the only option. You will not, however, win the argument if this turns into a debate.

Your work with individuals with chronic pain requires strong clinical skills in validation while also helping to advance the development of pain management skills. You will find the discussions of validation provided in Dialectical Behavior Therapy (DBT) to be very applicable to your work with pain patients (Fruzzetti & Ruork, 2019; Koerner, 2012). Your clinical stance is one of humility regarding your ability to fully know your clients' experience of pain combined with confidence that there are some things that will help. This involves both respect and optimism. It is very helpful to repeat the emphasis on taking baby steps and maintaining an approach of collaborative empiricism (i.e., *"Let's find out together what works best for you"*). When you find yourself stuck in this work, stop and ask yourself whether you have been providing sufficient and genuine validation for how difficult it is to live with chronic pain.

Emphasize Values-Consistent Behaviors over Distraction

Although distraction may be helpful during acute pain episodes, it does not appear to be effective in the management of chronic pain (Van Ryckeghem et al., 2018). Our approach emphasizes a focus on values-based activities rather than mere cognitive distraction. There is a significant difference between your clients engaging in activities that they hope will distract them enough to "make the pain go away" and your helping them identify and participate in activities that are meaningful and related to their life values and goals. These activities are then to be scheduled and done, in some fashion, regardless of pain. Pacing is important, with a focus on consistent and moderate involvement in meaningful and valued activities. Help your clients develop ground rules for doing something rather than basing their activity on how they feel on a certain day. This will lead your clients to have a life worth living despite the pain (e.g., "I may have pain, but it doesn't have me"). When this module is effective, pain is more livable and is in the background rather than guiding daily life.

When you find either yourself or your clients using distraction language, gently shift to discussing how daily activities fit with their personal values and goals. These are to be fostered in a way that is compatible with their specific physical conditions, despite the pain (i.e., not merely as a way to decrease the experience of pain).

Support the Hard Work of Physical Therapy

Many of your clients with chronic pain are likely to have had at least one cycle of physical therapy (PT) in the early phases of their physical condition. Clients may have begun that PT with the belief or hope that it would make the pain go away. This is especially true when clients have had previous successful experience with PT in acute rehabilitation following an injury or surgery. When it becomes clear in new circumstances that PT is not going to eliminate chronic pain, some individuals become disenchanted and discontinue both PT sessions and PT exercises at home. We have found that sometimes work with clients using this module leads to renewed interest in the question of whether PT may help support their daily routines and personal goals (i.e., instead of the goal of PT making the pain go away). As is true for any related questions on physical interventions, your response can be to encourage clients to discuss their interest in PT with their health care provider or the triage nurse at their doctor's office. Our experience is that many primary care providers are happy to write a new prescription for a cycle of physical therapy to support daily functioning. Most health insurance plans include a co-pay for PT, so this may be more or less of an option depending upon the insurance coverage and financial resources of specific clients. If your client is currently in PT or has finished PT with a list of recommended exercises for use at home, then those may be reasonable things to add to daily strategies in the Practice forms provided in this module.

Attend to Pain-Related Cognitions

Anxiety and pain experiences feed off of and intensify each other. Some clients with particularly strong anxiety may engage in pain catastrophizing ("This pain is absolutely terrible, and it is never going to get any better"; "Something is broken in my body and is going to kill me"; "I can't make it through another day with this much pain"). We avoid using the term "catastrophizing" with clients in session because of the potential for them to hear this as invalidating. For these clients, we suggest that you begin work in this module and closely monitor depression scores and progress on therapy goals. If depression scores do not significantly decrease across work in this module, transition to the *Skills for Thinking* module and focus specifically on modifying pain-related cognitions.

Monitoring Therapy Progress and Fine-Tuning Treatment Goals

This module begins with the orientation provided in Pain 1 Learn: Introduction to Skills for Managing Chronic Pain and the important reminder to have a "state of therapy" discussion about therapy goals and progress. This is a good time to review the overall pattern of depression scores, using whichever weekly measure of depression is a part of this feedback-informed treatment. Complete and review Pain 1 Practice: Review of My Treatment Goals during session so that overall therapy goals stay in the forefront, even while you are spending several sessions working on pain-related concerns. Determine whether the treatment goals need to be refined to be useful in treatment moving forward. This may be a point in therapy where clients have made significant progress on one of their therapy goals and wish to revise it or replace it with another.

Understanding Chronic Pain and Reviewing Therapy Progress

In our experience, many clients are very interested in learning about and discussing ways to improve their experiences of chronic pain. Across Pain 1–4 Learn, we provide resources as you listen to clients' specific pain narrative, educate them about acute versus chronic pain, and discuss the complex relationships between chronic pain and depression. More than other areas, it is especially important to allow for sufficient session time for individuals with chronic pain to describe their pain-related experiences and challenges. *This is a good investment of session time because clients who feel heard and validated regarding the legitimacy of their pain will be more open to moving on to a focus on pain management strategies.* When clients feel invalidated or believe that the reality of their pain is being ignored, they are less engaged in treatment and are unlikely to develop and use these new skills. The more a client believes that you understand the nature of their problem and what they are going through, the more confident they will feel in your ability to help them. This confidence increases the likelihood that they will follow your recommendations for treatment.

The first session devoted to pain will likely include some time following up with ongoing behavioral activation efforts and/or work related to whichever module came before. Pain 2 Learn: Understanding Your Chronic Pain is a vehicle for you to use to collect information about clients' specific pain experiences and for them to tell you their pain narrative. Take time and be fully present for this "storytelling" about the history and current details about their pain and pain treatment. The information about acute versus chronic pain in Pain 3 Learn: Short-Term vs. Long-Term Pain sets the stage for why special attention is needed to developing new strategies for managing chronic pain. In Pain 4 Learn: Understanding Pain and Depression, we help link depression and pain concerns with each other. When you review that page with your clients, help them discuss their own history of how chronic pain and depression are related. Personalizing the details for each client sets the foundation for the strategies outlined throughout the rest of this module. Also, when clients disclose a history of chronic pain that predates their depression, this is clinically significant and indicates a need for formal treatment for chronic pain. In these cases, we strongly suggest communication with their primary care physician and referral for work with a CBT clinician who is a pain specialist, if available. You may be treating depression in a client who is also working with a pain management team or a behavioral health clinician. In these cases of concurrent services, communication and collaboration is a must.

Applying the Gate Control Model of Chronic Pain

Pain 5–8 Learn and Pain 2–8 Practice are focused on learning and applying the gate control model of chronic pain and represent the central interventions of this module. We provide simplified language and images for use with clients who have mild cognitive impairment. The essential point of gate control theory is that pain signals from various parts of the body travel through the spinal cord to be processed and recognized in the brain. These pain signals travel up to the brain; at the same time, the brain is busy sending other signals down the spinal cord to the rest of the body. We all have the ability to make it harder for pain signals to reach the brain (i.e., "close the gate") through physical, cognitive, and emotional strategies that enlist our bodies and brains. Various behaviors, thoughts, and emotions also "open the gate," thus increasing the brain's awareness of pain.

Your clients will find it helpful to talk through specific examples of their physical (Pain 6 Learn), cognitive (Pain 7 Learn), and emotional (Pain 8 Learn) factors. Pain is a real physical experience, and you should begin with attention to physical factors that increase ("open the pain gate") or reduce pain ("close the pain gate") before moving on to cognitive and emotional strategies. In one session, we can usually discuss Pain 5 Learn: Gate Control Theory of Pain, apply it to physical factors (Pain 6 Learn: Opening and Closing Your Pain Gate: Physical/ Behavioral Factors), and begin to list specific physical activities (Pain 2 and 3 Practice)—but don't try to cover any more than this. Pain 7 Learn: Opening and Closing Your Pain Gate: What You Think Counts! (cognitive factors) and Pain 8 Learn: Opening and Closing Your Pain Gate: Emotional Factors fit well together; for many clients, it is possible to review these together in a single session. Other clients will either struggle with the concepts or have so many examples that these will need to be divided up into separate sessions.

The initial practice sheets (Pain 2–5 Practice) are all designed for personalized attention to specific factors at work in the pain experiences of individual clients. These should always be discussed together and begun in session before sending them home with clients to continue to observe, list, and experiment on their own. Pain 6 Practice: My Checklist of Pain Management Strategies and Pain 7 Practice: Managing My Pain This Week are lists of common strategies for clients who find it easier to have reminders. Pain 8 Practice: Tracking Pain Management Strategies allows you to then pull these together in a "top strategies" list that is individualized for each client.

As with the rest of this approach, you are working week by week to help your clients develop healthy habits over time, without an expectation of 100% compliance with all recommendations. You want clients to experiment with what is *possible* for them at this point, yet you can't expect them to suddenly adopt behaviors that seem utterly impossible. Over time and with effort, those pain management strategies that are perceived as "impossible," "possible but a stretch," and "very do-able" can shift. Baby steps, chunking, and pacing are all key in terms of behavioral goals and strategies; in addition, there is a cognitive component to these strategies in terms of clients' expectations and ability to stay encouraged. We provided some additional ideas earlier in this chapter in the "Tips for Clinicians" section.

Throughout this module, we encourage you and your clients to return to Start 5 Practice: My Values and Personal Strengths for a review of personal values and strengths. These are particularly important to hold on to during work on chronic pain. A focus of this treatment is having a daily life that is values-based and worth living. Discussion of how these life values can be applied in day-to-day life, even with pain, helps with this.

Revising Therapy Goals, Staying Encouraged and Engaged in Treatment

Pain 9 Learn: Pain Management Strategies vs. Formal Treatment Programs for Chronic Pain is an optional page for when you've decided a client should consider engaging in CBT for Chronic Pain with a specialist. With the appropriate signed release in place, that recommendation can be supported with a faxed communication to the primary care provider. Sometimes as you are nearing completion of this module, it becomes clear that more attention to developing pain management skills is important to depression treatment. Pain 10 Learn: Setting Personal Goals Related to Your Pain can be used in session to collaboratively decide whether there should be any changes or revisions to therapy goals. Just remember, it is important for therapy to focus on addressing no more than two or three overall goals. You will not set new pain management goals with every client who uses this module. Pain 9 Practice: My Goals for Managing My Chronic Pain can be used as a form to write down and rate those revised goals. Pain 11 Learn: Ways to Think About Progress Toward Your Goals reminds clients of the most common pattern of change with therapy (sawtooth curve, not a straight line or stair steps). We recommend Pain 10 Practice: As I Continue with Treatment: My Plan for Fully Participating for times when you have some concerns about a client's engagement in treatment, either within session or in compliance with between-session practice. Use Pain 11 Practice: My Review of Skills for Chronic Pain to review and consolidate key points and skills that you worked on in this module.

The first step in preparing to use this module is a thorough review of all Learn pages and Practice forms so you are familiar with the content and can begin to think about the fit between different skills and specific clients. We realize that behavioral health providers working within primary care may use materials from this module in very brief sessions, and will select individual Learn pages and Practice forms that fit the concerns and needs of their clients. Similarly, there may be occasions within individual or group psychotherapy when clinicians choose specific Learn and/or Practice materials.

We suggest a four-session approach that allows for several sessions devoted to reinforcing specific pain management practices. The development of new habits takes time, and the home practice assigned often takes several weeks before any noticeable impact on quality of daily life is reported.

In almost all therapy cases, this module will be used after clinicians have worked on goal setting and therapy orientation in the *Skills for Getting Started* module, after facilitating emotional literacy skills in *Skills for Feeling*, and after targeting daily positive and rewarding activities in *Skills for Doing*. Sessions will use the same basic structure: (a) set an agenda, (b) review home practice, (c) select at least one topic to work on in depth, (d) summarize, (e) set up new home practice assignment, and (f) do mutual feedback. Begin work on all Practice forms within session or wait for the next session to introduce them. Don't send a client home with a Practice form without a personal example already inserted. Be sure to allow time to review any Practice form in the next session.

For some of your clients, you will move directly after this module into preparation for therapy termination in *Skills for Wrapping Up*. There will also be times when you have finished *Skills for Chronic Pain*, have started work with clients in another module, and will find yourself coming back to key Learn and Practice materials in this module to continue to reinforce pain management strategies. This may be especially true for clients using materials in the *Skills for Healthy Sleep* module.

When this module is being used in its entirety to address chronic pain as a part of individual psychotherapy for depression in middle-aged and older adults, we suggest following the outline presented in Table 12.1.

Table 12.1 Session Outline

Each Session: Depression Measure + Start 3 and 4 Practice

GDS-SF or PHQ-9

Start 4 Practice	Preparing for My Next Session[T]
Start 3 Practice	My Session Summary[T]

Skills for Pain Session 1: Psychoeducation About Chronic Pain and Review of Therapy Goals

In Session 1: Pain 1–4 Learn, Pain 1 Practice (+ prior session review)

Between Session 1 and 2: Pain 1 Practice

Pain 1 Learn	Introduction to Skills for Managing Chronic Pain
Pain 2 Learn	Understanding Your Chronic Pain
Pain 3 Learn	Short-Term vs. Long-Term Pain
Pain 4 Learn	Understanding Pain and Depression[T]
Pain 1 Practice	Review of My Treatment Goals[T]

Skills for Pain Session 2: Gate Control Theory and Physical Activities

In Session 2: Pain 5 and 6 Learn

Between Session 2 and 3: Choose from Pain 2, 3, 6, 7, 8 Practice

Pain 5 Learn	Gate Control Theory of Pain[T]
Pain 6 Learn	Opening and Closing Your Pain Gate: Physical/Behavioral Factors[T]
Pain 2 Practice	Gate Control Practice
Pain 3 Practice	Gate Control Practice: Physical Activity[T]
Pain 6 Practice	My Checklist of Pain Management Strategies[T]
Pain 7 Practice	Managing My Pain This Week[T]
Pain 8 Practice	Tracking Pain Management Strategies

Skills for Pain Session 3: Gate Control: Cognitive and Emotional Strategies

In Session 3: Pain 7 and 8 Learn, Start 5 Practice

Between Session 3 and 4: Choose from Pain 4, 5, 6, 7, 8 Practice

Pain 7 Learn	Opening and Closing Your Pain Gate: What You Think Counts[T]
Pain 8 Learn	Opening and Closing Your Pain Gate: Emotional Factors[T]
Start 5 Practice	My Values and Strengths[T]

Table 12.1 Continued

Pain 4 Practice	Gate Control Practice: Cognitive Activity[T]
Pain 5 Practice	Gate Control Practice: Emotions[T]
Pain 6 Practice	My Checklist of Pain Management Strategies[T]
Pain 7 Practice	Managing My Pain This Week[T]
Pain 8 Practice	Tracking Pain Management Strategies

Skills for Pain Session 4: Problem Solving and Treatment Goals

In Session 4: Pain 9–11 Learn, Pain 9–11 Practice

After Session 4: Pain 6–8 Practice and/or Pain 9–11 Practice

Pain 9 Learn	Pain Management Strategies vs. Formal Treatment Programs for Chronic Pain
Pain 10 Learn	Setting Personal Goals Related to Your Pain[T]
Pain 11 Learn	Ways to Think About Progress Toward Your Goals[T]
Pain 6 Practice	My Checklist of Pain Management Strategies[T]
Pain 7 Practice	Managing My Pain This Week[T]
Pain 8 Practice	Tracking Pain Management Strategies
Pain 9 Practice	My Goals for Managing My Chronic Pain[T]
Pain 10 Practice	As I Continue with Treatment: My Plan for Fully Participating
Pain 11 Practice	My Review of Skills for Chronic Pain[T]

[T] Identified as particularly appropriate for telehealth sessions.

Not Included in This Treatment

Pain Prescription and Over-the-Counter (OTC) Medications

We encourage behavioral health clinicians to avoid giving any advice regarding the use of medications, whether prescription or nonprescription, including the use of cannabis for pain. These discussions amount to dispensing medical advice without a license to practice medicine. It can be tempting to offer your own opinions about the advisability of adding, retaining, or discontinuing specific pain medications. If clients have interest in making some change to their use of prescription or OTC pain medications, encourage them to make an appointment with their primary care provider to discuss the matter. In light of the variability in laws and health care practices across different regions, keep your personal opinions about the usefulness of cannabis for pain to yourself. You can support your clients' compliance with prescribed medications and assist them in obtaining the information needed to maximize their usefulness. We provide resources for this in the *Skills for Brain Health* module (Health 18–20 Learn; Health 13 Practice).

Physical Devices for Pain Management

Some clients may ask your opinion about surgical neuromodulation (e.g., pain pumps and other devices), transcutaneous electrical nerve stimulation (TENS), or assistive devices (e.g., canes, walkers, electric beds, power reclining chairs). For the same reasons we give for not providing advice about medications, we would like to actively discourage you from giving any opinions on possible costs or benefits associated with these therapies. The best response is something to the effect of:

I don't know whether _____ would be helpful or not in your specific case. This sounds like something you should discuss with your doctor and/or physical therapist. I am happy, however, to help you sort through your list of pros and cons to see if that process helps you with your decision-making.

You can support your clients' compliance with physician-recommended devices and help them prepare questions to learn more.

Additional Resources for Clinicians

Otis, J. (2007). *Managing chronic pain: A cognitive-behavioral therapy approach*. Oxford University Press.

Thorn, B. E. (2017). *Cognitive therapy for chronic pain: A step-by-step guide*. Guilford Publications.

CHAPTER 13

Module 7: Skills for Healthy Sleep: Resting Better and Longer

This personalized module of the workbook is focused on the skills of:

1. Monitoring therapy progress and fine-tuning treatment goals
2. Understanding sleep to shape expectations
3. Using circadian rhythms to support healthy sleep
4. Building sleep debt
5. Reducing nighttime arousal
6. Revising therapy goals, staying encouraged and engaged in treatment

This chapter is provided to help you use the *Skills for Healthy Sleep* module of the workbook with your clients. We begin with a brief overview, followed by some practical tips based on the most common questions we hear from clinicians during professional trainings. The bulk of this chapter is devoted to reviewing skills to regulate sleep patterns and promote sleep-healthy practices, with a description of the specific Learn pages and Practice forms available for your use in sessions. We provide recommendations for a standard progression of material (i.e., Learn pages and Practice forms that typically go with each other in the same session, estimates of how much can be accomplished in a given session), with the understanding that this may vary quite a bit depending upon your practice setting and specific client needs. We end the chapter with some comments about related topics that are not included in this treatment approach, and point readers to resources for professional development in CBT for Insomnia (CBT-I).

Overview

Attention to sleep can be very helpful when treating depression. Sleep concerns (especially insomnia) and depression are bidirectionally related (Li et al., 2018). Clinical depression can disrupt sleep patterns, and chronic insomnia contributes to the development of later-life depression (Poole & Jackowska, 2018). Chronic insomnia is also a predictor of suicide attempts (Kay et al., 2016). Health problems in middle-aged and older adults are also related to sleep disturbances due to chronic pain, polypharmacy, and fatigue leading to increased daytime napping. Even in the absence of depression and chronic health conditions, there are changes in sleep that occur with increasing age (McCrae et al., 2015, 2016). This means that some middle-aged and older adults will present in primary care and behavioral health settings with sleep disruptions and complaints. For all of these reasons, clinicians across a range of treatment settings are likely to work with clients on sleep concerns. This is especially true when treating aging clients with depression (Webb et al., 2018).

In the context of treating later-life depression, it is important to have first engaged clients in therapy orientation and treatment planning (*Skills for Getting Started*), emotional literacy (*Skills for Feeling*), and behavioral activation (*Skills for Doing*). Physical and social activities are an important part of keeping daytimes sufficiently filled with positive experiences and preventing unplanned naps and dozing (Tighe et al., 2016). The psychoeducation and skills developed within this module are grounded in an understanding of the cognitive-behavioral model, which is presented and discussed in *Skills for Getting Started*. We want to support your work with clients to both manage expectations and improve sleep, while also staying within your scope of practice. For clinicians who do not yet have formal training and certification in CBT-I (which is a more involved treatment than this module), this is achieved by staying focused on sleep education and sleep hygiene practices specifically customized for middle-aged and older adults. The *Skills for Healthy Sleep* module provides you with the clinical tools to do just that.

All of this work is framed within the context of the client's personal life values and strengths to ensure that treatment goals and strategies are consistent with these. There are important culture-specific beliefs about sleep that can shape your clients' use of skills in this module. Because expectations about aging are embedded within culture, awareness of the facets of diversity most important to specific clients is very important. Throughout this entire module, you are implementing culturally sensitive ways for individuals to share their interests and concerns about their sleep with family members and health care providers.

When to Use This Module

The materials in this module will be sufficient for many middle-aged and older clients who need a little work on their sleep routines and related behaviors. We consider behavioral health clinicians who work within this personalized module to be "sleep coaches." In Chapter 3 of this guide, we provide recommendation for the screening and assessment of sleep concerns and refer you to that chapter for details.

We caution you not to label work within this module as CBT-I, which is more involved than the basic education and tips provided in this module. If any of your clients continue to have significant sleep concerns after working for several weeks on this material, then it is advisable to refer out to a CBT-I provider. If the intake interview suggests that insomnia predated the first onset of depressive symptoms and has had a chronic course since then, a referral to a sleep clinic or provider who can offer a full CBT-I program to address the insomnia is clearly indicated. Clinicians and clients can then discuss which other personalized modules within this treatment approach may be useful. Any focus on sleep or sleep behaviors for such clients should be avoided/deferred to that CBT-I specialist. Untrained clinicians are at risk for diluting the intensity of that work, with clients mistakenly thinking that what they are getting is CBT-I.

Tips for Clinicians

Emphasize the Difference Between Planned and Unplanned Naps

It may be ideal to eliminate all daytime naps. It is also true that some middle-aged and older adults, especially those with acute medical illnesses and chronic health conditions, experience fatigue during the day and can benefit from a period of rest or a short nap. In these cases, the goal is to completely eliminate all *unplanned* naps—episodes of dozing or snoozing in an armchair or couch while reading or watching television. Work with your clients to identify the patterns of dozing, and begin by moving those into planned naps. For generally healthy middle-aged and older adults, schedule planned naps approximately 7 to 9 hours from waking time; these should be in bed, with an alarm set for no more than 1 hour from lying down. For individuals who have severe fatigue because they are recovering from a serious illness, it may be necessary to begin with two planned naps to be taken in bed (late morning and mid-afternoon). Setting an alarm for 1 hour each time remains important.

Understand Sources of Caffeine

Many individuals with chronic health concerns have previously received medical advice to reduce or eliminate caffeine intake. Thus, suggestions regarding caffeine intake are unlikely to be entirely new to middle-aged and older adults. What may be new is information about the range of products that contain caffeine (hot chocolate, ice cream or other desserts that contain chocolate, some "decaf" coffees, etc.). One source of information about products containing caffeine (and the amounts) is available from the National Sleep Foundation at https://www.sleep.org/articles/foods-with-caffeine/. Older adults who drink some caffeinated beverages across the day may need to experiment with the timing of when to discontinue (e.g., individuals who currently "cut off" caffeine

4 hours before bedtime may need to move that to 6 hours before bedtime). Older adults also lose some sensation of being thirsty and so are commonly also dehydrated. For clients who describe drinking caffeinated beverages continuously throughout the day as their main source of liquids, one strategy is to work on decreasing that amount slowly through alternating with glasses of water.

Intervene When Client Sleeps with Radio or Television On

Especially for middle-aged and older adults who live alone, or who have had chronic insomnia, bedtimes are a trigger for increased anxiety. Over time, some of these individuals have developed a habit of sleeping every night with their radio or TV on. They will often report that this helps them fall asleep and that it does not disturb their rest during the night. It may be true that having a distraction right at the point of falling asleep can be useful for individuals who are highly anxious at bedtime. Waking up with the TV or radio on is comforting, as they may feel less alone in the middle of the night. Unfortunately, data from research studies clearly indicate that sounds (radio, TV) and/or light flickers (TV) are registered by the brain and disrupt the ability to progress into deeper sleep stages, leading to disrupted sleep. The ideal situation is when the radio or television has a timer and turns off after a set length of time (i.e., it is on and helps the individual to relax enough to fall asleep but is completely off during the rest of the night). When that is not feasible, it is possible to work with clients in a very slow and gradual way to wean them from that unhealthy habit. The important part is going *very* slowly, staying consistent, and slowly removing cues (e.g., lowering the volume in a very gradual way over multiple weeks, putting in earplugs, having the TV on but the sound completely off by the time of falling asleep, and putting a blanket over the TV screen to block the images before finally being ready to turn it entirely off prior to falling asleep). This will take time.

Work on Sleep-Related Cognitions

Some clients with particularly strong anxiety may engage in sleep-related catastrophizing ("I am so miserable and will never get to sleep tonight";

"Tomorrow has been ruined because of my not being able to sleep at all tonight"; etc.). We avoid using the term "catastrophizing" with clients in session because of the potential for them to hear this as invalidating. The main idea is that unhelpful thoughts can vary across a continuum of extreme consequences. Anxiety and poor sleep feed off of and intensify each other. Subjective sleep complaints show a stronger relationship with depression and anxiety than objective indicators (Gould et al., 2018). For these clients, we suggest that you work in this module before *Skills for Thinking*. Then, when it becomes clear that there is a need for focused work on sleep-related thoughts, we suggest that you transition to the *Skills for Thinking* module with a specific focus on sleep-related cognitions.

Key Skills in This Module

Monitoring Therapy Progress and Fine-Tuning Treatment Goals

This module begins with the orientation provided in Sleep 1 Learn: Introduction to Skills for Healthy Sleep and the important reminder to have a "state of therapy" discussion about therapy goals and progress. This is a good time to review the overall pattern of depression scores, using whichever weekly measure of depression is a part of this feedback-informed treatment. Complete and review Sleep 1 Practice: Review of My Treatment Goals during session so that overall therapy goals stay in the forefront even while you are spending several sessions working on sleep-related concerns. Determine whether the treatment goals need to be refined to be useful in treatment moving forward. This may be a point in therapy where clients have made significant progress on one of their therapy goals and wish to revise it or replace it with another.

Understanding Sleep to Shape Expectations

In our experience, many clients are very interested in learning about and discussing ways to improve their sleep. Across Sleep 1–5 Learn, we provide resources as you educate clients about age-related changes in sleep, the complex relationships between sleep and depression, and obstructive sleep apnea (OSA). The information about sleep processes in Sleep 2 Learn: How Sleep Works sets the stage while also communicating your confidence that the strategies promoted in this module can make a difference. The first session devoted to sleep will likely include some time following up with ongoing behavioral activation efforts and/or work related to whichever module comes ahead of work on sleep.

Sleep 3 Learn: Sleep Changes with Age and Sleep 4 Learn: Clinical Depression and Sleep Problems will be very important for some of your clients. The review of changes typical with age can go a long way to address sleep expectations and normalize common complaints. We intentionally specify the goal of 6 hours of sleep each night; many aging individuals with sleep complaints are getting around 6 hours but expecting that they should be sleeping closer to 7 or 8 hours. Sometimes, helping your clients adjust that expectation can be quite helpful (e.g., "I may want 8 hours but really only need around 6 hours"). In Sleep 4 Learn, we help link depression and sleep concerns with each other. When you review that page with your clients, help them discuss their own history of how sleep and depression are related. Personalizing the details for each individual sets up the background for the strategies outlined throughout the rest of this module. Also, when clients disclose a chronic history of insomnia that predates their depression, this is clinically significant and indicates a need for formal assessment and treatment for insomnia. In these cases, we strongly suggest communication with their primary care physician, leading to a referral for work with a CBT-I clinician.

Severity of OSA is linked to increased depressive symptoms in middle-aged and older adults. Your attention to promoting the evaluation and treatment of OSA can go a long way to treating depression in your clients. Sleep 5 Learn: Obstructive Sleep Apnea (OSA) lists the symptoms and recommends a sleep evaluation when OSA is suspected. In addition to the presence of daytime sleepiness and self or partner report of snoring, *depressed mood upon waking* should be viewed as a possible sign of OSA. The first step of referral is typically to the primary care provider, who will consider the appropriateness of a sleep evaluation. Many of your clients may already have a diagnosis of OSA yet have poor compliance with using their continuous positive airway pressure (CPAP) device as instructed. Importantly, adherence to proper use of CPAP devices (including during daytime naps) reduces depressive symptoms and improves cognitive functioning in adults with OSA (Nadorff et al., 2018). Our experience with individuals who struggle to adhere to CPAP use suggests it often takes a lot of patience and troubleshooting for them to successfully adjust to the device. Some clients may need several return trips to their medical supply store to work with a staff member on issues of fit and changes of the face mask/nasal "pillow," as well as possible use of a contour bed pillow. Your support and encouragement is an important part of them persisting. Spending time in session on this is worth it! Conduct weekly check-ins on CPAP adherence, emphasize its importance, and problem solve until compliance is high.

Using Circadian Rhythms to Support Healthy Sleep

Sleep 6 and 7 Learn and Sleep 2 and 3 Practice are focused on healthy sleep routines and physical environments. You should remind clients that these are important ways to support natural sleep regulation processes that are biologically built in. Of the suggestions listed in Sleep 6 Learn: Healthy Sleep Routines (which should be used between sessions in Sleep 2 Practice: My Healthy Sleep Routines), your clients are likely to find most of these to be reasonable and then really struggle with one or two. We have the *"Which of these routines are you willing to try?"* question at the bottom of Sleep 6 Learn so that you can gauge where each client is with these strategies.

As with the rest of this approach, you are working week by week to help your clients develop healthy habits over time, without an expectation of 100% compliance with all recommendations. There is also a need to be flexible with clients who are recovering from surgery or a serious illness; some individuals may also really need a late morning nap or may be bedbound. Sometimes, their bedroom has enough space to add a comfortable chair near the bed to make it easier to have some time away from the bed. For many clients, Sleep 2 Practice is enough for a between-session assignment during this part of therapy. Sleep 7 Learn: Changing Sleep Habits provides a more in-depth opportunity to explore some of those "stuck" points, because often the sleep hygiene practices that are most challenging are related to unhealthy habits that have developed over time in an effort to improve sleep. Sleep 3 Practice: Replacing Old Sleeping Habits can be used first in session as the two of you develop ideas of how to make changes to one of these unhealthy habits, and then between sessions. You want clients to experiment with what is *possible* for them at this point, yet you can't expect them to suddenly adopt behaviors that seem utterly impossible. Over time and with effort, that list of "impossible," "possible but a stretch," and "very do-able" can shift. We provided some additional ideas earlier In this chapter in the "Tips for Clinicians" section.

Building Sleep Debt

Using Sleep 8 Learn: Ways to Promote Healthy Sleep and Sleep 4 Practice: My Ways to Promote Healthy Sleep, you are now working with clients to add in healthy behaviors that build sleep debt and promote nighttime sleepiness. We have also included attention to the ways in which eating and drinking (both timing and type of food/drink) can influence sleep. Most of your middle-aged and older patients will be familiar with these and find them nice reminders. Often, it is that pattern of physical activity/exercise that is both the most challenging and the most likely to pay off with improved sleep.

Reducing Nighttime Arousal

Sleep 9 and 10 Learn and Sleep 5 Practice together focus on behavioral and cognitive strategies for reducing the level of emotional and physiological arousal at bedtime. There are a number of common sleep-related cognitions that increase anxiety and interfere with sleep. We list several of these in Sleep 9 Learn: Stress Doesn't Help with Sleep, with some suggestions for replacement thoughts. A combination of behavioral and cognitive strategies is often most helpful for managing these. Sleep 5 Practice: My Stress Management for Healthy Sleep provides a range of suggestions for what clients can do and think as they prepare for bed. We wouldn't expect one client to implement all of these; instead, the list is provided so each individual can pick and choose. Some clients have a lifetime habit of watching the news right before bedtime; that might be something to re-examine. Others find themselves ruminating about very real life stressors and/or gearing up with anticipatory anxiety ahead of bedtime. As Sleep 10 Learn: Stress Management Skills for Healthy Sleep reminds clients, the focus is on using these skills flexibly rather than following them so strictly that they become "must do" rituals that sleep becomes dependent on. Sometimes, this portion of the *Healthy Sleep* module identifies the need for additional work in relaxation strategies (provided in the *Skills for Feeling* module) or cognitive reappraisal strategies (provided in the *Skills for Thinking* module). We provided additional suggestions in the "Tips for Clinicians" section earlier in this chapter.

Revising Therapy Goals, Staying Encouraged and Engaged in Treatment

Sleep 11 Learn: Healthy Sleep Strategies vs. Formal Treatment Programs for Insomnia is an optional page for when you've decided a client should consider engaging in CBT-I with a specialist. With the appropriate release signed by the client in place, you can communicate with the client's primary care provider to suggest such a referral. Sometimes as work in a specific module is nearing completion, it becomes clear that more attention to change in that area may be an important part of ending the depression. Sleep 12 Learn: Setting Personal Goals Related to Healthy Sleep can be used in session to collaboratively decide on whether there should be any changes or revisions to therapy goals. Just remember, it is important that therapy focus on addressing no more than two or three overall goals. Sleep 1 Practice: Review of My Treatment Goals can be used as a form to write down and rate those revised goals. Sleep 13 Learn: Ways to Think About Progress Toward Your Goals reminds clients of the most common pattern of change with therapy (sawtooth curve, not a straight line or stair steps). We recommend Sleep 6 Practice: As I Continue with Treatment: My Plan for Fully Participating for times when you have some concerns about a client's engagement in treatment, either within session or in compliance with between-session practice. Use Sleep 7 Practice: My Review of Skills for Healthy Sleep to review and consolidate key points and skills that you worked on in this module.

Suggested Progression of Content

The first step in preparing to use this module is a thorough review of all Learn pages and Practice forms so you are familiar with the content and can begin to think about the fit between different skills and specific clients. We realize that behavioral health providers working within primary care may use materials from this module in very brief sessions, and will select individual Learn pages and Practice forms that fit the concerns and needs of their clients. Similarly, there may be occasions within individual or group psychotherapy when clinicians choose specific Learn pages and/or Practice forms.

When this module is being used in its entirety to help clients improve their sleep, we suggest a four-session approach that allows for several sessions devoted to reinforcing the practice of sleep hygiene. The development of new sleep habits takes time, and the home practice assigned often takes several weeks before any noticeable impact on sleep or sleep satisfaction is reported.

In almost all therapy cases, this module will be used after clinicians have worked on goal setting and therapy orientation in the *Skills for Getting Started* module, after facilitating emotional literacy skills in *Skills for Feeling*, and after targeting daily positive and rewarding activities in *Skills for Doing*. Sessions will use the same basic structure: (a) set an agenda, (b) review home practice, (c) select at least one topic to work on in depth, (d) summarize, (e) set up new home practice assignment, and (f) do mutual feedback. Begin work on all Practice forms within session, or wait for the next session to introduce them. Don't send a client home with a Practice form without a personal example already inserted. Be sure to allow time to review any Practice form in the next session.

For some of your clients, you will move directly after this module into preparation for therapy termination, in *Skills for Wrapping Up*. There will also be times when you have finished *Skills for Healthy Sleep*, have started work with clients in another module, and will find yourself coming back to key Learn and Practice materials in this module to continue to reinforce sleep hygiene behaviors. This may be especially true for clients using materials in the *Skills for Brain Health* or *Skills for Managing Chronic Pain* modules.

When this module is being used in its entirety to address sleep problems as a part of individual psychotherapy for depression in middle-aged and older adults, we suggest following the outline presented in Table 13.1.

Table 13.1 Session Outline

Each Session: Depression Measure + Start 3 and 4 Practice

GDS-SF or PHQ-9

Start 4 Practice	Preparing for My Next Session[T]
Start 3 Practice	My Session Summary[T]

Skills for Sleep Session 1: Psychoeducation About Sleep and Review of Therapy Goals

In Session 1: Sleep 1–5 Learn, Sleep 1 Practice (+ prior session review)

Between Sessions 1 and 2: Sleep 1 Practice

Sleep 1 Learn	Introduction to Skills for Healthy Sleep
Sleep 2 Learn	How Sleep Works
Sleep 3 Learn	Sleep Changes with Age[T]
Sleep 4 Learn	Clinical Depression and Sleep Problems[T]
Sleep 5 Learn	Obstructive Sleep Apnea (OSA)[T]
Sleep 1 Practice	Review of My Treatment Goals[T]

Skills for Sleep Session 2: Sleep Hygiene Practices: Stabilizing Circadian Rhythms

In Session 2: Sleep 6 and 7 Learn

Between Sessions 2 and 3: Sleep 2 Practice and/or Sleep 3 Practice

Sleep 6 Learn	Healthy Sleep Routines[T]
Sleep 7 Learn	Changing Sleep Habits
Sleep 2 Practice	My Healthy Sleep Routines[T]
Sleep 3 Practice	Replacing Old Sleeping Habits[T]

Skills for Sleep Session 3: Building Sleep Debt and Other Sleep Hygiene Practices

In Session 3: Sleep 8 Learn

Between Session 3 and 4: Choose from Sleep 2, 3, 4 Practice

Sleep 8 Learn	Ways to Promote Healthy Sleep[T]
Sleep 2 Practice	My Healthy Sleep Routines[T]
Sleep 3 Practice	Replacing Old Sleeping Habits[T]
Sleep 4 Practice	My Ways to Promote Healthy Sleep[T]

Table 13.1 Continued

Skills for Sleep Session 4: Reducing Cognitive and Physiological Arousal at Bedtime

In Session 4: Sleep 9–13 Learn

After Session 4: Sleep 5–7 Practice

Sleep 9 Learn	Stress Doesn't Help with Sleep
Sleep 10 Learn	Stress Management Skills for Healthy Sleep[T]
Sleep 11 Learn	Healthy Sleep Strategies vs. Formal Treatment Programs for Insomnia
Sleep 12 Learn	Setting Personal Goals Related to Healthy Sleep[T]
Sleep 13 Learn	Ways to Think About Progress Toward Your Goals[T]
Sleep 5 Practice	My Stress Management for Healthy Sleep [T]
Sleep 6 Practice	As I Continue with Treatment: My Plan for Fully Participating
Sleep 7 Practice	My Review of Skills for Healthy Sleep[T]

[T] Identified as particularly appropriate for telehealth sessions.

Not Included in This Treatment

Sleep Prescription and Over-the-Counter (OTC) Medications

We encourage behavioral health clinicians to avoid giving any advice regarding the use of medications, whether prescription or nonprescription. These discussions amount to dispensing medical advice without a license to practice medicine. It can be tempting to offer your own opinions about the advisability of adding, retaining, or discontinuing sleep medications. If clients have interest in making some change to their use of prescription or OTC sleep aids, encourage them to make an appointment with their primary care provider to discuss this. You can support your clients' compliance with prescribed medications and assist them in obtaining the information needed to maximize their usefulness. We provide resources for this in the *Skills for Brain Health* module (Health 18–20 Learn; Health 12 Practice).

Light Therapy

For similar reasons, we are not providing psychoeducation or recommendations regarding light therapy. You can encourage clients who express interest in light therapy to discuss this with their primary care physician, including consideration of whether a referral to a sleep specialist is indicated.

Sleep Diaries and Sleep Compression Interventions

In this *Skills for Healthy Sleep* module, we have not included sleep diaries or resources related to sleep efficiency or sleep compression strategies. These are important components to CBT-I and can be challenging for clients (and for clinicians without formal training in that treatment). The Consensus Sleep Diary (Carney et al., 2012) is an option for those interested in learning more about the use of sleep diaries and what to include.

Clinician Note

Here is why we do not consider the Skills for Healthy Sleep *module to be a brief or light form of CBT-I. When evidence-based interventions are diluted or not applied in a clinically effective manner, this can be iatrogenic. Rather than having an attitude that "trying a little bit of an intervention couldn't hurt," we believe that weakened/diluted interventions have the danger of increasing hopelessness in an individual with depression. From a client's perspective, if an intervention has been tried and did not help, perhaps their depression is so bad that nothing will help. Because of the fatigue and pessimism that are a part of depressive syndromes, we are judiciously selecting key interventions that have the highest likelihood of success when administered by those with limited training in sleep interventions. This has led us to focus in this module on administering only the strategies that can be delivered with a sufficient dosage to be effective. In the case of sleep, we have selected psychoeducation about sleep and sleep hygiene practices and do not want this module to be referred to as "CBT for Insomnia."*

Additional Resources for Clinicians

Edinger, J. D., & Carney, C. E. (2014). *Overcoming insomnia: A cognitive-behavioral therapy approach, therapist guide.* Oxford University Press.

Edinger, J. D., & Carney, C. E. (2015). *Overcoming insomnia: A cognitive-behavioral therapy approach, workbook.* Oxford University Press.

Measure in Appendix D Related to This Module

(Recommendations for use are provided in Chapter 3 of this clinician guide.)
Glasgow Sleep Effort Scale

CHAPTER 14

Module 8: Skills for Caregiving: Reducing Stress While Helping Others

This personalized module of the workbook is focused on the skills of:

1. Monitoring therapy progress and fine-tuning treatment goals
2. Identifying as a caregiver
3. Replacing self-criticism with self-compassion
4. Applying strategies from positive psychology
5. Reappraising unhelpful thoughts about caregiving
6. Asking for help from family and friends
7. Identifying, planning, and doing positive daily activities
8. Protecting well-being
9. Revising therapy goals, staying encouraged and engaged in treatment

This chapter is provided to help you use the *Skills for Caregiving* module of the workbook with your clients. We begin with a brief overview, followed by some practical tips based on the most common questions we hear from clinicians during professional trainings. The bulk of this chapter is devoted to reviewing skills to manage caregiving-related stressors and promote well-being, with a description of the specific Learn pages and Practice forms available for your use in sessions. We provide recommendations for a standard progression of material (i.e., Learn pages and Practice forms that typically go with each other in the same session, estimates of how much can be accomplished in a given session), with the understanding that this may vary quite a bit depending upon your practice setting and specific client needs. We end the chapter with some comments about related topics that are not included in this treatment approach, and point readers to resources for professional development in family caregiving interventions.

> ### Clinician Note
>
> *As you read this chapter, we encourage you to have the workbook open so that you can refer to the specific Learn pages and Practice forms as they are described and explained. You will use these Learn pages and Practice forms during sessions, encouraging your clients to review between sessions using the Learn pages and try out/record between sessions using the Practice forms. Your reviewing these items as you read through this chapter will prepare you to make the most of the treatment materials. Using these pages and forms means more than having them available to look at or read over with your clients during sessions. Instead, you'll be engaging your clients in exploring the meaning this has to them, through discussion and careful application. Your goal each session is to help your clients apply specific Learn and Practice material to their recent experiences in daily life, and to the problems that bring them into treatment.*

Overview

Some of the clients with depression with whom you work will have family caregiving responsibilities—providing unpaid care and assistance above and beyond what's typical for most families. This care is given to either their biological family members (e.g., parent, sibling, grandchild) or "chosen family" (e.g., partner/spouse, neighbor, member of their faith community, other close members of their social network). Your clients might be caring for a spouse with Alzheimer's disease, a parent with cancer, or a sibling in hospice; some may be the primary caregiver for a grandchild. Learning about this "informal" caregiving and how to work effectively to reduce caregiving-related distress is very important for behavioral health providers (Thompson et al., 2006; Zarit & Heid, 2015).

About 70% of older adults who need assistance with daily activities live in the community and receive care solely from family members, friends, neighbors, or other informal caregivers. What do caregivers do? "Caregiving" includes a wide range of activities, from management of medications and health care appointments to hands-on tasks such as bathing and toileting. Caregivers for a family member with dementia may also be involved in "round the clock" supervision to ensure their relative's safety. Typically, tasks change over time as the conditions in question either become more stable, deteriorate, or in some instances improve. Therefore, the clinical interventions that offer the best support must also change over time (Gallagher-Thompson et al., 2020a), and caregivers benefit from learning to be flexible and consider all of their coping efforts as "experiments."

Family and friends often experience considerable stress when trying to provide extensive caregiving in addition to the other demands of their everyday lives. Although caregiving can occur in the context of *any* significant physical and/or emotional disorder or family crisis (as in the case of custodial grandparents), most of the intervention research has been conducted with relatives of older adults with Alzheimer's disease or other neurocognitive disorders (Gallagher-Thompson et al., 2012). Caregivers for a family member with dementia and family caregivers of loved ones in hospice care are likely to present with the greatest amount of emotional distress, and their depression treatment must heavily emphasize materials from our *Skills for Caregiving* module. There are a host of things that you can do in your clinical work to support these clients (Gallagher-Thompson & Thompson, 2021).

The "typical" caregiver is a woman in her 50s who is either the daughter or daughter-in-law of the impaired elder. She is often married/partnered, with teenaged children (or grandchildren) living in the home. Those who fit this demographic have been referred to as part of the "sandwich generation" because they provide care and support for both elders and young people, as well as perhaps a spouse or life partner. These middle-aged and older individuals provide vital care and assistance to persons with a wide range of serious medical problems, including Alzheimer's disease and other neurocognitive disorders, stroke, cancer, HIV/AIDS, serious mental illness, chronic musculoskeletal pain, and debilitating cardiovascular problems. Each of these conditions has its own care requirements and its own trajectory of how the illness and care demands change over time, thus differentially impacting the caregiver's mental and physical health. For example, it is now common for a person with dementia to live 10 to 20 years with their diagnosis. Stressors on the caregiver are very different at the early versus later stages. Early on, memory problems are common, along with confusion and inability to take care of many activities of daily living, such as keeping track of appointments, paying bills, taking medication when and as prescribed, and making phone calls. With time, behavior problems develop, such as wandering at night, dressing and eating inappropriately, and poor impulse control. Eventually the person with dementia loses the ability to care for their personal needs (bathing, toileting) along with recognition of the family caregiver, as well as the ability to speak and make themselves understood. For many, palliative care is needed at the end stage.

Other physical conditions, such as chronic heart disease, type 2 diabetes, and stroke, present their own challenges. To help caregiving clients with depression, clinicians must inquire as to the diagnosis of the care recipient (CR) and how that diagnosis has impacted that person's life. Obtaining that information signals that you care about your client's daily life and will help them employ several practical approaches to mitigate their stress and to learn to respond differently to challenging demands. Remember that distress and strain change considerably over time during the course of one's caregiving "career."

Several decades of research have found that depression—at either the clinical or subsyndromal level—is a very commonly reported negative impact of being a caregiver. Other troublesome emotions (such as anger, frustration, guilt, and worry about the future) are also common but often ignored; most caregivers put the CR first and downplay their own physical and mental health concerns until they become overwhelmed. These negative effects are often lumped together and called "burden." Burden is a term also commonly used by many caregivers (rather than "depression" or "anxiety") to describe their distressed state, along with feeling overwhelmed. Other indices of distress, such as family conflict over caregiving, financial hardships, and work strain, are also evident (Alzheimer's Association, 2020). Family caregivers report perceptions of poorer physical health; stress and negative affective reactions can also impact their experience of daily pain (Ivey et al., 2018). Perhaps because of the benefits of helping others, however, caregivers in fact live longer than non-caregivers (Roth et al., 2018).

Numerous interventions have been developed to address these problems. In the past decade, there have been multiple reviews to evaluate their efficacy (Burgio et al., 2016; Cheng et al., 2019, 2020; Etxeberria et al., 2020; Schulz & Eden, 2016). Psychoeducational interventions that employ a skills-based approach (derived from CBT principles and methods) are very effective and often preferred by families—whether done in individual or group therapy or during home visits. A number of studies have supported cultural adaptations for ethnically diverse caregivers (Gallagher-Thompson et al., 2001, 2003, 2007, 2008, 2010) that this *Skills for Caregiving* module draws from. This module was designed to provide information on the best ways to employ a variety of these tried-and-true skills to reduce caregiving-related distress in your clients.

In the workbook, we provide 16 Learn pages and 17 Practice forms that will help your clients develop skills, including treating oneself with kindness and compassion, managing unhelpful thoughts related to caregiving, asking for help from family and friends, increasing engagement in everyday positive activities, and self-care routines. Most caregivers benefit from working on one or more of these topics, depending on their stress level and unique circumstances.

All of this work is framed within the context of your clients' personal life values and strengths, to ensure that treatment goals and strategies are consistent with these. There are important culture-specific beliefs about health, illnesses, and family roles that shape clients' understanding of the CR's illness, expectations for their caregiving roles, and communication within families and with health care providers (Yeo et al., 2019). Because expectations about aging are embedded within culture, awareness of the facets of diversity most important to specific clients is very important. Throughout this entire module, you are implementing culturally sensitive ways for clients work on these skills while staying connected with their support network, including family members and health care providers.

When to Use This Module

For many of your caregiving clients with depression, this is a key personalized module to use after *Skills for Getting Started*, *Skills for Feeling*, and *Skills for Doing*. Learning the CBT conceptual model in *Skills for Getting Started* is important, as is the time spent orienting clients to therapy. In *Skills for Feeling*, both relaxation and anger management skills are often relevant to reduce overall stress and allow for more effective caregiving. For most of these clients, behavioral activation (implemented in *Skills for Doing*) is a central facet of successful therapy; this has a strong evidence base (Zabihi et al., 2020). We provide very basic resources in this *Skills for Caregiving* module for working with unhelpful thoughts about caregiving situations; some clients will need more and move from this module to *Skills for Thinking* for additional work on cognitive reappraisal skills.

We recommend that you consider using this module right after completing the first three core modules if caregiving burden or stress is a significant issue contributing to the client's depression. For very distressed clients who present to therapy with family caregiving concerns as their major life stressor, you may wish to consider using this module right after *Skills for Getting Started*. Emotionally distressed clients can have difficulty generalizing and may dismiss anything that is not immediately applicable to their caregiving situation. Such clients may need their treatment focus to incorporate a consideration of caregiving issues from the very beginning of therapy. You can then decide whether to circle back to material in *Skills for Feeling*, *Skills for Doing*, and *Skills for Thinking* after some initial sessions focused on caregiving concerns using the current module.

It is noteworthy that "burden" is not experienced to the same degree by all caregivers. There are significant differences by gender, role in the family, relationship to the CR, race, ethnicity, cultural values, and other aspects of diversity. Thus, "one size does not fit all" when it comes to employing CBT with distressed caregivers, which means that assessment should take a high priority. Screening and assessment of caregivers is addressed in Chapter 3 of this guide, and we refer you to that section for details.

Tips for Clinicians

Link Assessment to Conceptualization and Treatment Planning

It is very important to complete a detailed assessment. Chapter 3 includes a description of recommended assessment strategies with caregivers, and Appendix D includes a structured Caregiving Intake Assessment

Interview and key measures. There are also a number of other helpful assessment approaches that we have not had the space to cover in this treatment but that may be helpful for your clinical practice (O'Malley & Qualls, 2016). After your assessment, share your observations with the client and work collaboratively to develop one or two specific goals for this module (e.g., reduce stress, improve self-care, develop self-compassion, increase engagement in everyday positive activities). Focus therapy time on these goals. Remember, it's easy to become distracted by everyday ups and downs in the caregiver's life and turn therapy into more of a supportive (rather than skill-building) effort. Effective therapy requires *both* empathy and skill training!

Connect Clients with Community Resources

An important caregiving skill is knowing how to obtain help from community-based agencies and service providers. Because community-based long-term care services are such a patchwork, and eligibility criteria vary greatly from region to region in the United States, we provide some national resources in Care 14 Learn. Ultimately, however, there are few general clinical guidelines to recommend other than becoming knowledgeable about the services available for caregivers caring for *X, Y,* or *Z* specific illness in your community. Although it may be beyond your scope of practice to actually link clients to these services, it will be very helpful for you to be educated about them and to share this information with your clients. For most caregivers, this is an essential component to their being able to care for their CR over the long haul.

Caregivers often have a number of questions related to community resources, such as:

- "Should I talk to a social worker to see if Dad qualifies for home health care?"
- "Is my wife eligible for an adult day care program?"
- "Is there a way to get respite so I can take some time off without worrying or feeling guilty?"
- "When is the right time for mom to move to assisted living? Can we afford it?"

"What about a nursing home? Should I place him in a memory care unit?"

▪ "What if I get sick and can't care for them anymore? Who will step in?"

These are important areas of concern to many caregivers who will bring them up as topics for discussion, often asking your advice as to what to do. If possible, help your client make contact with a social worker (or other professional with this kind of experience) for detailed planning. As a behavioral health specialist, you can frame this discussion in terms of what's needed for "staying able" to provide care. In many ways that is the focus of this entire *Skills for Caregiving* module—what skills does your client need to reduce distress and depression associated with caregiving? Helping your clients get useful practical advice for decision-making is an essential part of this process.

Termination can be particularly stressful for clients who may have no one else to talk to openly and honestly about all that caregiving entails. We recommend spending time in session to educate your clients about how to search for other resources (e.g., written materials pertaining to caregiving stress and/or their CR's illness; joining an online community of persons struggling with similar problems or disorders, or attending in-person support groups specific to the chronic health problems of their CR; and searching reliable websites for workshops and lectures on key caregiving topics). Finally, as we describe in the *Skills for Wrapping Up* module, caregivers need to learn to recognize their own "danger signals" so they can seek professional assistance if needed in the future.

Understand Implications of Types of Caregiving

Studies have found that family caregivers of those with dementia are generally more distressed than caregivers of physically impaired elders. Because of the inexorable progressive decline over time in many functions, caregivers report a strong sense of having "lost" their CR while the person is still alive. Persons with dementia usually become a shadow of their former selves, so besides caregivers having to cope with behavior problems and changes in their daily living patterns, they also are coping with many losses—loss of future possibilities is how caregivers often sum it up. This intense combination of stress, depression, grief, and role overload/multiple competing time demands requires a multifaceted approach so that most (if not all) of these dimensions are addressed in treatment. Thus, in addition to this module, some clients will find helpful strategies in additional modules of the workbook, including *Skills for Thinking*, *Skills for Sleep*, and *Skills for Living with Loss*.

Attend to Caregiving-Related Cognitions

Note that the emphasis on cognitive reappraisal strategies is on the *helpfulness* of such thoughts rather than on the *evidence* "for" or "against" the thought itself. For example, the thought, "No matter what I do, it is never enough," can first be validated. It is true that whatever the client is doing on a day-to-day basis is "never enough" in the sense of curing the illness or causing remarkable improvement in the CR's physical or mental health. Help refocus the client's attention on what they are doing well to provide a good quality of life for their loved one. It is helpful to ask what they are doing daily to make life easier or more tolerable for the CR. Then listen and note the responses to aid discussion. This often results in a reappraisal of the client's efforts as, "What I'm doing is good enough for now" or "It's keeping Roberto out of the nursing home, so I must be doing some things right." You should check that the client's negative affect does in fact change as these thoughts are modified. In our experience, most caregivers are grateful to be able to see their situation from a different perspective—as long as it's clear that the clinician understands and accepts the "partial truths" in these thoughts and does not dismiss them out of hand (e.g., "Oh, I'm sure you're doing all you can").

The second most common negative thought that many caregivers have is, "Things are only going to get worse." Again, first validate that there is likely to be some truth to that statement, but it does not tell the whole story. For example, this thought can stimulate the client to do some careful planning for the future in areas they have control over (e.g., finances, living will, durable power of attorney for health care). These legal documents are much more easily crafted and executed when the CR can still understand what is happening. To the extent that this thought can generate adaptive problem-solving behavior, it can be useful and motivating rather than an unduly negative view that fuels the caregiver's depression. Another strategy when faced with this kind of thinking is to focus the client's attention on what is happening day to day. Are all days "bad"? Are there times when the CR brings a smile to the caregiver's face? Times when they both are able to relax and be in sync with one another? Usually there are "good days," and by focusing on them, clients are grounding themselves in daily life. These shifts in perspective (to more helpful ways of viewing the same situation) are crucial for therapeutic success. We also recommend that you pay attention to unhelpful thoughts that interfere with social roles and relationships; these are likely to influence daily activities and social functioning.

There may be sufficient material in this module to help clients work on their unhelpful thoughts about caregiving. When you have done that, and depression scores are not decreasing, we suggest that you transition to the *Skills for Thinking* module and use those resources while retaining a specific focus on unhelpful thoughts that are elicited in caregiving situations.

Respond to Suspected Elder Abuse

Definitions of what constitutes elder abuse or mistreatment vary from state to state, but there are several categories that are found in most states' descriptions of what constitutes an actionable situation with regard to a dependent adult. These include physical mistreatment/abuse (hitting, punching, kicking, pulling hair), emotional mistreatment (yelling at the person, belittling, shaming, escalating anxiety and tension, frequent arguing), financial exploitation (misappropriating funds, stealing from the CR, forging the CR's signature on checks, withdrawing funds from bank accounts without permission), and finally sexual abuse (unwanted sexual activity of any kind at any time). Neglect of the CR is also reportable in many states, involving such actions as denying or limiting food, leaving the CR unsupervised for many hours (to the point where it's dangerous), and not assisting with needed personal care tasks such as bathing. Since most behavioral health care providers are mandated reporters, it is imperative to know and understand the statutes that apply in the state/jurisdiction in which you are practicing, what the reporting requirements are, and what is likely to happen after a report is made.

You might be asking now: How often does this come up as a therapeutic issue in the caregiving context? That's a great question! Reliable data are hard to come by, but it's estimated that abuse is far more common in caregiving situations than one might suspect. Highly stressed clients can slip into emotional abuse or neglect fairly readily when their coping resources are overwhelmed and they have little outside support. Financial abuse seems common in families in which a family member is abusing substances and/or when the caregiver is experiencing significant financial distress due to caregiving (e.g., the client had to quit their job or reduce their hours or their insurance is not adequate to cover care-related expenses such as medications, durable equipment). This level of distress can bring caregivers into therapy; when that is the case, focusing on the skills included in this module will be helpful.

The more common situation, however, occurs when a married heterosexual caregiver is herself in her 70s or 80s, is in frail health or is petite in stature, and is caring for her strong (and often larger) husband with dementia who is behaving in ways that are verbally or physically abusive to her. In these cases, it is the caregiving client who is the victim of abuse. Clinicians need to explore the nature and extent of the abuse and determine if legal action to protect the client is required, what the risks are for it continuing, and whether a safety plan is needed and is in place.

Therapeutically it is helpful to discuss what strategies could be employed to "dial down" the situation so that the client would feel safe again. Helpful skills include the client seeking medical advice as to what medications could reduce the spouse's angry behavior, hiring in-home support to keep him occupied for several hours daily, and asking other family members to spend time with him engaging in simple positive activities that could be maintained by your client when alone with her spouse. As with the other personalized modules in this guide, we recommend that the clinician and the client collaboratively select the skills to work on and reassess progress regularly. We describe several screening tools relevant to elder abuse risk assessment in Chapter 3 of this clinician guide.

Key Skills in This Module

Monitoring Therapy Progress and Fine-Tuning Treatment Goals

This module begins with <u>Care 1 Learn: Introduction to Skills for Caregiving</u> and the important reminder to have a "state of therapy" discussion about therapy goals and progress. This is a good time to review the overall pattern of depression scores, using whichever weekly measure of depression is a part of this feedback-informed treatment. Complete and review <u>Care 1 Practice: Review of My Treatment Goals</u> during session so that overall therapy goals stay in the forefront even while you are spending time addressing caregiving-related concerns. Determine whether the treatment goals need to be refined to be useful moving forward. This may be a point in therapy where clients have made significant progress on one of their therapy goals and wish to revise it or replace it with another.

Identifying as a Caregiver

This module begins with the orientation to caregiving provided in <u>Care 1 Learn</u>. The first session devoted to caregiving will likely include some time following up with ongoing behavioral activation efforts and/or work related to whichever module came before. You will likely have already completed an assessment of caregiving issues (see Chapter 3 of this clinician guide for detailed recommendations). This means that clients have likely already had an opportunity to tell you the narrative of their caregiving situation and what they find most stressful. Be aware that LGBTQ+ clients may have additional experiences and concerns due to lack of community recognition and support for their unique caregiving situation and needs. If a client is extensively involved in family caregiving responsibilities (i.e., including for "chosen" family members) and you have not yet assessed the details of their caregiving situation, this is the time to devote a session to that assessment.

Replacing Self-Criticism with Self-Compassion

Many middle-aged and older adults grew up in households and communities where harsh criticism was used as a way to "motivate." Caregivers are especially likely to be hard on themselves. Care 2 Learn: Treat Yourself with Kindness, Not Criticism introduces the importance of self-compassion to help counter that view. Have your clients describe to you how they would encourage a very young child who is taking on something that is difficult for them. Then discuss how it might be helpful for the client to use the same approach for themselves. We all do our best in managing stressful situations when others are patient and encouraging; it is now time for your clients to apply that to themselves. Care 2 Learn and Care 3 Learn: Self-Kindness for Caregivers help clients move from a pattern of self-critical thoughts to more compassionate thoughts and actions. Care 2 Practice: Treating Myself Kindly in Caregiving Situations is provided as a possible between-session assignment to build use of self-compassionate thoughts and actions in daily life. Additional Learn pages and Practice forms related to self-compassion are in the *Skills for Thinking* module and may be helpful for some clients who need additional opportunities to practice and discuss self-compassion within session. With its focus on specific self-encouraging thoughts, Care 4 Practice: Ways to Encourage Myself as a Caregiver can also be used as a part of this work on self-compassion. We want to emphasize that clients agreeing that self-compassion is a good thing (i.e., having insight) is not at all the same as being able to apply specific self-compassionate strategies during particularly difficult times. Practicing during daily events is key to using self-compassion amid life's struggles.

Applying Strategies from Positive Psychology

There are accumulating data on the benefits of positive psychology applications for family caregivers (Cheng et al., 2017). Depending upon the preferences of your clients, the following session can focus on Care 4 Learn: Managing Caregiving Stress to highlight the positive (e.g., gratitude, kind acts, positive experiences). Clients need support and encouragement to focus on small daily positive experiences with their CR. Benefit-finding strategies can be very useful as a way to cultivate a sense of hope, as long as you are careful to also validate the very real difficulties that the client is facing. Gently encourage the client to see the positive as well as the negative aspects of caregiving. For virtually all caregivers, the experience is not entirely negative or positive. Rather, caregiving involves a balancing act of positive and negative experiences that goes on for years. As the treating clinician, your job is to help clients see this and acknowledge the value of trying to maintain a balanced perspective. Care 5 Learn: Giving Yourself Credit as a Caregiver, Care 6 Learn: Encouraging Yourself, Care 3 Practice: Managing "OK" Is Good Enough: My Examples, and Care 4 Practice: Ways to Encourage Myself as a Caregiver help clients become aware of what is going well, provide effective coping experiences, and learn to give themselves credit and encouragement. As you work with these clients to enhance their current coping efforts, remind them of existing areas of personal strength and resources. Inquire about challenging situations they have faced in the past and what coping skills they used to help survive these situations. This builds self-efficacy for coping. Many caregivers can benefit by developing the skill of encouraging themselves and giving themselves credit for small successes in caregiving.

Reappraising Unhelpful Thoughts About Caregiving

When family caregivers with depression come for therapy and also experience significant emotional distress related to their caregiving role, therapy time needs to be spent working on common negative thoughts that are very specific to the caregiving role. Examples include a strong emphasis on personal responsibility (e.g., "No matter what I do, it is never enough") and worry about the future (e.g., "Things are only going to get worse"). These can be challenging for clinicians to work with because there are elements of truth in many unhelpful thought patterns seen in family caregivers. Some habitual thoughts may be accurate but not helpful. Use Care 7 Learn: Managing Your Unhelpful Thoughts in session to discuss clients' own most common unhelpful and upsetting thoughts about caregiving. Two reappraisal questions are provided on that page to use (helpfulness and taking on the perspective of someone else). Care 5–7 Practice are all available for you to use within and between session; choose one or two of these that seem the best fit for individual clients. We know that you may decide that specific individuals need more attention to their unhelpful thoughts, especially if there is other evidence of "all or none" thinking or overgeneralizing. You have the option to use the resources provided in *Skills for Thinking* to work on these in more depth, with a focus on thoughts that come up in their daily caregiving experiences. We have also provided some additional suggestions in this chapter's "Tips for Clinicians" section.

Asking for Help from Family and Friends

Some of your clients are quite hesitant to ask family or friends for help with caregiving. Many have tried to elicit assistance and have been turned down. Most relatives and friends do not want to get "stuck" doing unpleasant caregiving tasks (e.g., feeding, toileting, or trying to go for a walk and finding that the CR is in such pain that they cannot continue and it seems that the situation has gotten worse instead of better). After a while, unfortunately, caregivers stop asking. This reinforces a vicious cycle in which caregivers try to do it all, find they cannot, become depressed and withdrawn, and are decreasingly likely to ask for assistance. You can approach this topic initially by asking, *"Who is in your support network? What do they do to support you?"* A helpful tool for getting this information in detail is the Atlas CareMap (https://atlascaremap. org), which provides a systematic way for clients to identify their caregiving needs, their support network, and where the gaps are in support (e.g., emotional, instrumental, financial, respite). We have used this tool within session with caregivers and found the process to be helpful both in terms of spelling out immediate needs and determining if additional community services are required. Care 14 Learn: National Resources for Caregivers in the United States outlines some resources; we discussed community resources earlier in this chapter in the "Tips for Clinicians" section.

Once it is clear who is a part of your client's social network and how they help (or don't help) at present, the therapy skill is to learn how to effectively ask for help. This is covered in Care 8 Learn: Asking for Help from Friends and Family and Care 8 Practice: Asking for Help with

Caregiving. In our experience, clients learn this very well when you role play in session so that you can do real-time coaching to improve the outcome. Use of role plays is also discussed in the *Skills for Relating* module in this guide. With caregivers, a key skill involves thinking through specific details of the request (e.g., 2 hours of respite care while the client goes to the dentist, 8 hours while the client attends a conference or crucial business meeting, a week while the client goes on vacation) and whether this is a one-time ask, as needed, or on an ongoing basis (e.g., every week). You can discuss these details in session to prepare for the role play. It is also important that clients are calm and reasonable while making their request rather than angry or accusatory (e.g., "You've hardly ever helped me with Mom; it's about time you did something!"). You are helping clients stay flexible in working out arrangements; they may not get all that they want, but it may be enough to make a difference. Finally, clients need to express their thanks for the help they are getting.

Identifying, Planning, and Doing Positive Daily Activities

Care 9–11 Learn and Care 9–12 Practice are focused on supporting daily positive activities. As described in *Skills for Doing* in this guide, activities should be simple and easy to incorporate into one's daily schedule (e.g., looking at flowers, having a favorite cup of tea, talking on the phone to a friend, reading a book, working on a craft project for or with a grandchild). Each client's list will be highly individualized and developed through questioning and problem solving. See *Skills for Doing* to review the methodology, which is similar here.

Along with developing new habits of regular positive activities for oneself (i.e., ones that are consciously chosen and deliberately done, not ones that just happen to occur), we also strongly recommend an additional focus. Doing shared positive activities with the CR has been shown time and again to improve mood, reduce agitation, and increase quality of life for both caregiver and CR (Bilbrey et al., 2020a). These shared activities should be simple and enjoyable for both persons. Trial and error is usually needed to figure this out. Although it may be a bit tedious to go through this process repeatedly in session, rewards are substantial, and we encourage you to keep problem solving until some new daily patterns of enjoyable activities are established.

Protecting Well-Being

Care 12 Learn: Staying Able to Provide Care, Care 13 Learn: Your "R&R" (Rest and Recuperation), Care 13: Practice: My Staying Able to Provide Care, and Care 14 Practice: My "R&R" (Rest and Recuperation) are all focused on different ways to support clients' self-care activities, including physical, social, and spiritual wellness. Care 14 Practice provides a way to personalize these through a simple weekly journal format. This component of treatment relates to the concept of taking time for oneself to recharge. We find that it is helpful to begin with very concrete issues related to physical health, because clients can usually think of some immediate problems for their family member if their own health becomes compromised.

Despite the appropriateness of the metaphor related to air travel—in which travelers are reminded to put on their own oxygen mask before helping others—we find that use of this analogy is experienced as patronizing and irritates many clients. Also note that some terminology related to "self-care" or "taking care of yourself" may be offensive to caregivers, including those from some cultural groups. Our experience with Latinx caregivers, for example, has taught us a better way to present the concept: *"This is what you need to learn to do so that you can be a better caregiver and take the best possible care of your loved one."* This view is consistent with Latinx cultural values (e.g., *familismo* or the primacy of the family's needs over the individual's needs) and therefore allows these clients to participate fully in this component of therapy (Adames & Tazeau, 2020).

Throughout this module, we encourage you and your clients to return to Start 5 Practice: My Values and Strengths for a review of personal values and strengths. Many family caregivers find their role deeply meaningful and rewarding, yet overwhelming and stressful. Importantly, these clients have experienced and coped with difficult challenges in their past. Finding a way to validate the difficulties of their present situation while noting their past use of inner strengths and personal resources can be helpful. Attention to personal values and strengths can help remind them of past successful coping efforts and can enhance self-efficacy for managing their current difficult situation. This self-efficacy has consistently been shown to be related to lower levels of depression and greater well-being in caregivers (Steffen et al., 2018).

Revising Therapy Goals, Staying Encouraged and Engaged in Treatment

Use Care 15 Learn: Setting Personal Goals Related to Your Caregiving in session to collaboratively decide on whether there should be any changes or revisions to therapy goals. Remember, it is important that therapy focus on addressing no more than two or three overall goals. You will not necessarily do this with every client using this module. Care 15 Practice: My Goals for Managing Caregiving Stress can be used as a form to write down and rate those revised goals. Care 16 Learn: Ways to Think About Progress Toward Your Goals reminds clients of the most common pattern of change with therapy (sawtooth curve, not a straight line or stair steps). We recommend using Care 16 Practice: As I Continue with Treatment: My Plan for Fully Participating for times when you have some concerns about a client's engagement in treatment, either within session on in compliance with between-session practice. We suggest Care 17 Practice: My Review of Skills for Caregiving as a way to review and consolidate key points and skills from this module.

Suggested Progression of Content

The first step in preparing to use this module is a thorough review of all Learn pages and Practice forms so you are familiar with content and can begin to think about the fit between different skills and specific clients. We realize that behavioral health providers working within primary care may be using materials from this module in very brief sessions, and will select individual Learn pages and Practice forms that fit the concerns and needs of their clients. Similarly, there may be occasions within individual or group psychotherapy when clinicians choose specific Learn and/or Practice materials.

In almost all therapy cases, this module will be used after clinicians have worked on goal setting and therapy orientation in the *Skills for Getting Started* module, after facilitating emotional literacy skills in *Skills for Feeling*, and after targeting daily positive and rewarding activities in *Skills for Doing*. Sessions will use the same basic structure: (a) set an agenda, (b) review home practice, (c) select at least one topic to work on in depth, (d) summarize, (e) set up new home practice assignment, and (f) do mutual feedback. Begin work on all Practice forms within session or wait for the next session to introduce them. Don't send a client home with a Practice form without a personal example already inserted. Be sure to allow time to review any Practice form in the next session.

For some of your clients, you will move directly after this module into preparation for therapy termination, in *Skills for Wrapping Up*. There will also be times when you have finished *Skills for Caregiving*, have started work with clients in another module such as *Skills for Thinking*, and will find yourself coming back to key Learn pages and Practice forms in this module to reinforce key strategies.

When this module is being used in its entirety to address significant levels of caregiving stress as a part of individual psychotherapy for depression in middle-aged and older adults, we suggest an eight-session approach as shown in Table 14.1.

Not Included in This Treatment

Interventions for Behavior Problems Associated with Dementia

When the CR has Alzheimer's disease or another neurocognitive disorder, there are a number of behavioral problems that significantly disrupt daily life and are very stressful. These vary over the stages of the illness. Even after a client has developed ways to address one problem (e.g., repeated questioning that transitions from mildly irritating to extremely frustrating), new problems emerge and past strategies are no longer effective. Some family caregivers of persons with dementia will benefit from the development of behavior management skills, which are very important but beyond the scope of this more general module.

Table 14.1 Session Outline

Each Session: Depression Measure + Start 3 and 4 Practice

GDS-SF or PHQ-9

Start 4 Practice	Preparing for My Next Session[T]
Start 3 Practice	My Session Summary[T]

Skills for Caregiving Session 1: Review of Therapy Goals, Self-Compassion for Caregivers

In Session 1: Care 1–3 Learn, Care 1 Practice (+ prior session review)

Between Sessions 1 and 2: Care 1 and 2 Practice

Care 1 Learn	Introduction to Skills for Caregiving
Care 2 Learn	Treat Yourself with Kindness, Not Criticism
Care 3 Learn	Self-Kindness for Caregivers[T]
Care 1 Practice	Review of My Treatment Goals[T]
Care 2 Practice	Treating Myself Kindly in Caregiving Situations[T]

Skills for Caregiving Session 2: Self-Encouragement

In Session 2: Care 4–6 Learn

Between Sessions 2 and 3: Care 3 and 4 Practice

Care 4 Learn	Managing Caregiving Stress[T]
Care 5 Learn	Giving Yourself Credit as a Caregiver[T]
Care 6 Learn	Encouraging Yourself[T]

Care 3 Practice Managing "OK" Is Good Enough: My Examples[T]

Care 4 Practice	Ways to Encourage Myself as a Caregiver[T]

Skills for Caregiving Session 3: Unhelpful Thoughts About Caregiving

In Session 3: Care 7 Learn

Between Sessions 3 and 4: Choice of Care 5, 6, 7 Practice

Care 7 Learn	Managing Your Unhelpful Thoughts[T]
Care 5 Practice	When It May Be Time to Step Back[T]
Care 6 Practice	Revising Upsetting Thoughts About Caregiving
Care 7 Practice	Revising Unhelpful Thoughts About Caregiving[T]

Table 14.1 Continued

Skills for Caregiving Session 4: Asking for Help and Continued Focus on Unhelpful Thoughts

In Session 4: Care 7 and 8 Learn

Between Sessions 4 and 5: Care 8 Practice (plus choice of Care 5, 6, or 7 Practice)

Care 7 Learn	Managing Your Unhelpful Thoughts[T]
Care 8 Learn	Asking for Help from Friends and Family[T]
Care 5 Practice	When It May Be Time to Step Back[T]
Care 6 Practice	Revising Upsetting Thoughts About Caregiving
Care 7 Practice	Revising Unhelpful Thoughts About Caregiving[T]
Care 8 Practice	Asking for Help with Caregiving[T]

(Note: Some clients will require more than two sessions to cover Care 7 Learn. At this point, you may decide to move to resources in Skills for Thinking.)

Skills for Caregiving Session 5: Behavioral Activation

In Session 5: Care 9 and 10 Learn

Between Sessions 5 and 6: Care 9–11 Practice

Care 9 Learn	Planning Positive Activities for Your Family Member[T]
Care 10 Learn	Increasing Your Daily Positive Activities
Care 9 Practice	Positive Things for My Family Member to Do
Care 10 Practice	Rewarding Activities This Week for My Family Member[T]
Care 11 Practice	My Rewarding Activities This Week

Skills for Caregiving Session 6: Shared Behavioral Activation

In Session 6: Care 11 Learn

Between Sessions 6 and 7: Care 12 Practice

Care 11 Learn	Planning Shared Positive Activities for the Two of You[T]
Care 12 Practice	Our Shared Activities This Week[T]

Skills for Caregiving Session 7: Staying Able to Provide Care (Physical Health)

In Session 7: Care 12 Learn

Between Sessions 7 and 8: Care 13 Practice

Care 12 Learn	Staying Able to Provide Care[T]
Care 13 Practice	My Staying Able to Provide Care[T]

(continued)

Table 14.1 Continued

Skills for Caregiving Session 8: Self-Care as "R&R" (Psychosocial Self-care) and Review

In Session 8: Care 13 - 16 Learn

After Session 8: Care 14 - 17 Practice

Care 13 Learn	Your "R&R" (Rest and Recuperation)[T]
Care 14 Learn	National Resources for Caregivers in the United States[T]
Care 15 Learn	Setting Personal Goals Related to Your Caregiving[T]
Care 16 Learn	Ways to Think About Progress Toward Your Goals[T]
Care 14 Practice	My "R&R" (Rest and Recuperation)[T]
Care 15 Practice	My Goals for Managing Caregiving Stress[T]
Care 16 Practice	As I Continue with Treatment: My Plan for Fully Participating
Care 17 Practice	My Review of Skills for Caregiving[T]

[T] Identified as particularly appropriate for telehealth sessions.

Readers are referred to Burgio and Wynn (2021) for evidence-based and very practical resources for helping dementia family caregivers.

Caregiver Family Therapy

Caregiving does not impact just one family member, and many clinicians are interested in working with family dyads or larger number of family members. This is an important and complex area, involving changes in family roles and dynamics and an additional set of clinical assessment and intervention skills (Qualls, 2016). We would like to refer clinicians to Qualls and Williams (2013) for guidance in this.

Care at the End of Life

You may find yourself working with clients who are caring for a family member at the end of life. This is important work and merits more attention than we can provide in just a portion of this specific module.

For that reason, we have decided not to attempt a superficial coverage of end-of-life issues. There are several excellent approaches that are available for your work with these clients. These include recommendations by Allen and colleagues (2016, 2018) and the CBT approach developed by Satterfield (2008), among others.

Additional Resources for Clinicians

Burgio, L. D., & Wynn, M. J. (2021). *The REACH OUT Caregiver Support Program: A Skills Training Program for Caregivers of Persons with Dementia, Clinician Guide.* Oxford University Press.

Lorig, K., Laurent, D., Schreiber, R., Gecht-Silver, M., Gallagher-Thompson, D., Minor, M., Gonzalez, V., Sobel, D., & Lee, D. (2018). *Building better caregivers.* Bull Publishing.

Mace, N. L., & Rabins, P. V. (2017). *The 36-hour day.* Johns Hopkins Press.

Pot, A. M., Gallagher, T. D., Xiao, L. D., Willemse, B. M., Rosier, I., Mehta, K. M., Zandi, D., & Dua, T. (2019). iSupport: A WHO global online intervention for informal caregivers of people with dementia. *World Psychiatry, 18*(3), 365–366. https://doi-org.ezproxy.umsl.edu/10.1002/wps.20684

Spencer, B., & White, L. (2015). *Coping with behavior change in dementia: A family caregiver's guide.* Whisppub.

Measure in Appendix D Related to This Module

Elder Abuse Suspicion Index (EASI)
Caregiving Intake Assessment Interview
REACH II Risk Appraisal Measure (RAM)
Caregiver Abuse Screen (CASE)

CHAPTER 15

Module 9: Skills for Living with Loss: Bereavement and Grief

This personalized module of the workbook is focused on the skills of:

1. Monitoring therapy progress and fine-tuning treatment goals
2. Understanding grief reactions
3. Supporting self-care, routines, and taking care of life
4. Responding to upsetting thoughts associated with bereavement
5. Managing grief following specific losses (e.g., pet, home, or treasured objects)
6. Revising therapy goals, staying encouraged and engaged in treatment

This chapter is provided to help you use the *Skills for Living with Loss* module of the workbook with your clients. We start with a brief overview, followed by some practical tips based on the most common questions we hear from clinicians during professional trainings. The bulk of this chapter is devoted to reviewing skills to validate normal grieving and support self-care by your bereaved clients. Descriptions are provided for the specific Learn pages and Practice forms that are available for your use in sessions. We make recommendations for a standard progression of material (i.e., Learn pages and Practice forms that typically go with each other in the same session, estimates of how much can be accomplished in a given session), with the understanding that this may vary quite a bit depending upon your practice setting and specific client needs. We end the chapter with some comments about related topics that are not included in this treatment approach, and point readers to resources for professional development in the area of grief and loss.

Overview

You are very likely to work with depressed clients who have had a recent loss or combination of losses. Deaths become more common with increasing age, including the deaths of pets, close friends, parents, siblings, and life partners. Other important losses can be related to retirement, declining health (of the client or someone they care for), a move, and/or loss of roles/activities that have been important parts of personal identity. These losses often result in sadness, the "pangs of grief," and temporary disruptions to physical, cognitive, and social functioning. Loss events do not, however, typically lead to clinical depression in most middle-aged and older adults. Some individuals with a history of depression are more vulnerable to the effects of these losses. Other clients are hit particularly hard by a single loss or a cascade of losses that precipitate or coincide with late-onset depression. For all of these individuals, your knowledge of how older adults respond to bereavement is important (Thompson et al., 2004).

It can be especially helpful for you as the clinician to be aware that there are a number of different trajectories for how bereavement and depression are (and sometimes are not) related to each other (Neimeyer & Holland, 2015). Figure 15.1 shows that some individuals are depressed prior to

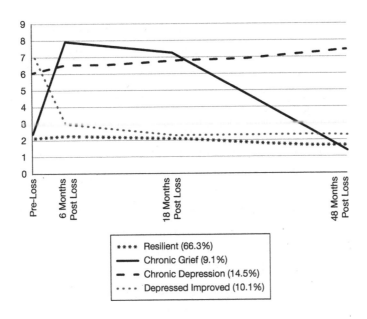

Figure 15.1

Heterogeneity in Depression Following Loss in Older Adults

Reprinted from Galatzer-Levy & Bonanno (2012). Beyond normality in the study of bereavement: Heterogeneity in depression outcomes following loss in older adults. *Social Science & Medicine*, 74(12), p. 1992, with permission from Elsevier.

the death, and depression scores remain relatively stable from before to after bereavement. For others who are in the resilient pattern, depressive symptoms remain relatively low over the course of adjusting to the death of someone important. Still others develop a chronic pattern of depression following the death that takes several years to abate.

For all of these reasons, clinicians across a range of treatment settings are likely to work with clients who are grieving different types of loss, with or without significant depressive symptomatology. As will be seen throughout the *Living with Loss* module, this work involves being present to and normalizing common grief reactions while also supporting clients' management of daily life functioning and tasks. You will also need to be alert to indications of complicated grief and possibly manage referrals for specialized treatment. This *Living with Loss* module has been developed to help you with all of these.

Refer back to Figure 2.1: Model of Depression in Older Adults, shown on page 21 of this guide, where we see that daily activities are key to the link between bereavement and clinical depression. On the left side of

Figure 2.1, we see life circumstances that may have created the context for depression, including bereavement and other losses. These losses are possible contributors, but they affect depression indirectly—largely through decreases in daily meaningful and rewarding activities (including those that connect us with others). The right side of the figure shows how these decreases in daily activities play an especially strong role in perpetuating the cycle of depression in middle-aged and older adults. For that reason, even as you are lending support to someone overwhelmed by their grief, a priority is working to help them return to daily meaningful and valued activities and relationships. Some of your clients will also have overly generalized and negative thoughts that contribute to maintaining their depression; these thoughts can interfere with their ability to live a rewarding life. As is true throughout your work with aging individuals with depression, therapy focused on revising these thoughts will focus especially on those that are self-critical and interfere with connections with others.

In the context of treating later-life depression, it is important to first engage clients in therapy orientation and treatment planning (*Skills for Getting Started*). The psychoeducation and skills developed within this *Skills for Living with Loss* module are grounded in an understanding of the cognitive-behavioral model, which is presented and discussed in *Skills for Getting Started*. The values clarification work done at the beginning of treatment is especially key to living with loss. Clients may put some parts of life on hold following a bereavement, but it is important for them to feel grounded by their life values and personal strengths during the pain of grief. Resources for emotional literacy and the savoring of positive emotions in *Skills for Feeling* are all very relevant to the work in this module. And behavioral activation (*Skills for Doing*) continues to be critically important as clients cope with the aftermath of their losses.

All of this work is framed within the context of their personal life values and strengths to ensure that treatment goals and strategies are consistent with these. There are important culture-specific beliefs about death and grief that shape your clients' experiences and coping responses. Because responses to loss are embedded within culture, your awareness of the facets of diversity most important to specific clients is very important. Throughout this entire module, you are implementing culturally sensitive ways for clients to share their experiences and concerns about loss and grief with their existing support network.

When to Use This Module

The materials in this module will be sufficient for many middle-aged and older clients who have experienced a recent loss or series of losses and who express interest in this module. You may be in the middle of treatment with a client who experiences an anticipated or unanticipated loss. Some of the psychoeducation about grief and support for self-care is certainly appropriate for use in those circumstances, without necessarily using the entire module. Because we provide resources for a range of losses (e.g., death of a loved one, death of a pet, losses related to declining health or retirement, a move), no one client would receive all of the material in this module. Screening and assessment of grief reactions are addressed in Chapter 3 of this guide, and we refer readers to that section for details.

Tips for Clinicians

Inquire About Spiritual and Religious Concerns

Spiritual and religious beliefs and practices may be comforting for some clients but unhelpful or distressing for others. Some individuals experience a rupture in their relationship with God and/or their spiritual community; this has been referred to as complicated spiritual grief (Burke & Neimeyer, 2014). We encourage you not to oversimplify spiritual concerns, nor to assume that religious clients will find their religion a source of support and comfort. Some will but others will not. When appropriate, refer clients to faith leaders in their community or other sources of spiritual direction compatible with their faith traditions and interests. You should also be prepared to integrate themes and concerns of spirituality and religion into treatment, as appropriate for the client. The format of this integration can vary depending on the preferences of the client. Religiously Integrated Cognitive Behavioral Therapy (RCBT) is a manualized approach to support the work of integrating religious beliefs into a cognitive-behavioral framework (Pearce et al., 2015). Spiritually Integrated Psychotherapy is another evidence-based and clinically useful approach for working with such issues in depth (Pargament, 2011).

Validate Cognitive Complaints in Bereaved Clients

Grief interferes with concentration and executive functions such as organization and decision-making. As a part of receiving psychoeducation on grief, some clients ask for specific recommendations on managing those cognitive symptoms associated with grief reactions. In these circumstances, we suggest consideration of the pages within the *Skills for Brain Health* module that best reflect the specific concerns of that individual.

Work with Your Clients on Their Grief-Related Cognitions

It is quite common for bereaved individuals to have some regrets and upsetting thoughts related to a death or relationship. These thoughts are most often centered around decisions made during the last illness, events surrounding the actual death, or relationship issues that were unresolved at the time of death (Boelen & Lensvelt-Mulders, 2005). Such thoughts are fairly common yet upsetting and can lead to strong feelings of guilt; some clients will wish to address these in therapy. Clients may also have a range of thoughts and beliefs about their interactions with others since the death, leading to increasing withdrawal and social isolation. We recommend that you prioritize thoughts that directly interfere with social roles and relationships (e.g., "I was married to Carol for 40 years and all of our friends are couples; they won't really want to spend time with me now that I am alone," or other thoughts that involve not fitting into social networks anymore). These have a strong likelihood of influencing daily activities and social functioning. If it becomes clear that there is a need for detailed work on loss and grief-related thoughts, transition to the *Skills for Thinking* module and use those skills to examine and reappraise the most salient loss-related thoughts that interfere with relationships (i.e., within the *Skills for Thinking* module, stay focused on grief- and loss-related unhelpful thoughts).

Key Skills in This Module

Monitoring Therapy Progress and Fine-Tuning Treatment Goals

This module begins with the orientation provided in <u>Loss 1 Learn: Introduction to Skills for Living with Loss</u> and the important reminder to have a "state of therapy" discussion about therapy goals and progress. This is a good time to review the overall pattern of depression scores, using whichever weekly measure of depression is a part of this feedback-informed treatment. Complete and review <u>Loss 1 Practice: Review of My Treatment Goals</u> during session so that overall therapy goals stay in the forefront even while you are spending time addressing loss-related concerns. Determine whether the treatment goals need to be refined to be useful in treatment moving forward. This may be a point in therapy where clients have made significant progress on one of their therapy goals and wish to revise or replace it with another.

Understanding Grief Reactions

Across <u>Loss 1–4 Learn</u>, we provide resources to help you (1) listen to clients' specific experience of loss; (2) educate clients about the wide range of normal grief reactions; and (3) give clients an opportunity to share culturally specific traditions, beliefs, and personal preferences for expressing grief. It is especially important to allow sufficient session time for bereaved individuals to describe their loss or losses and share their grief reactions, *if this is what they wish to do*. This is a good investment of session time; clients who feel heard and validated will be more open to also spending time on self-care and other coping efforts. Telling the story of their loss can also create a sense of coherence during a time that is very disruptive to many facets of personal identity.

The first session devoted to loss will likely include some time following up with ongoing behavioral activation efforts and/or work related to whichever module came before. <u>Loss 2 Learn: There Are Many Types of Losses</u> is a way for you to better understand your clients' specific loss experiences and for them to tell you the story of their most important loss or recent losses. Take time and be fully present for this storytelling. Especially when the loss was unexpected, or followed a long and complicated illness, some clients want to tell you all the details that surrounded the actual death or other loss. Let them talk with minimal interruptions or questions; family and friends may not have allowed them the opportunity to tell that story. In addition, LGBTQ+ older adults may have lost a partner or member of their chosen family, with experiences of disenfranchised grief (i.e., loss not acknowledged through typical societal practices and supports). This is a time for you to listen and be a witness to their loss, without asking too many questions or turning this into an interview or assessment.

The information about myths versus facts of grief in <u>Loss 3 Learn: Grief Looks Different for Everyone</u> is an important way to validate the legitimacy of grief and normalize a wide range of grief reactions. Many clinicians find this discussion of myths versus facts to be particularly helpful in countering beliefs that grief *should* look a certain way or follow a specific pattern. Using <u>Loss 4 Learn: Traditions, Beliefs, and Preferences</u>, help clients discuss their own, many of which will be linked to their cultural identities (e.g., ethnic, religious, familial). Together, this sequence of loss narrative; psychoeducation; and sharing of cultural traditions, beliefs, and preferences may take one, two, or several sessions, depending upon the complexity of your clients.

The main thing to emphasize is respect and support of each client's personal preferences for what they share and do not share, and how they grieve. This is not the time for you to initiate additional grief work to address trauma or assign specific grief-related practices. Research studies have demonstrated that such grief-specific interventions can be iatrogenic (i.e., lead to short- and long-term negative outcomes for some individuals). For this reason, avoid suggesting any grief-work activities that are your idea (e.g., writing a letter to the deceased, creating specific rituals, organizing photo albums). Support whatever is spontaneously mentioned by clients as something that they would like to do to honor their dead loved one, as long as it is safe and contributes to the client's self-care.

Supporting Self-Care, Routines, and Taking Care of Life

Loss 5–7 Learn and Loss 2–5 Practice are all focused on different ways to support clients' self-care at various phases after the loss. You would not necessarily use all of these with all bereaved clients. Loss 5 Learn: Your Self-Care Is Important and Loss 2 Practice: My Self-Care This Week list a wide range of self-care ideas, including physical, social, and spiritual wellness. Loss 3 Practice: My Weekly Self-Care Journal provides a way to personalize these through a simple weekly journal format. The essential point of Loss 6 Learn: Routine Changes and Loss 4 Practice: My Routines is that some losses (deaths, moves, retirements, etc.) disrupt the rhythms of daily life. Devote time to developing new routines; this helps to stabilize clients.

Clients often indicate that they are overwhelmed by specific tasks or projects that are difficult or complicated or require new skills. Your ability to help them focus and problem solve the details of that task or project can relieve significant anxiety. Loss 7 Learn: Taking Care of Life and Loss 5 Practice: Taking Care of Life Tasks with DEEDS are provided to assist with this process, using the DEEDS model of five-step problem solving. DEEDS was first presented in Do 16 Learn in *Skills for Doing*. Chapter 8 of this clinician guide includes a discussion of working with clients on problem-solving skills and is worth reviewing prior to doing this work with bereaved clients.

Throughout this *Skills for Living with Loss* module, we encourage you and your clients to return to Start 5 Practice: My Values and Strengths to review personal values and strengths. These are particularly important to focus on at this time to foster the development of a daily life that is values-based and worth living. Importantly, your clients have experienced and coped with difficult losses in their past. Find a way to validate their current pain while noting their past use of inner strengths and personal resources. Attention to personal values and strengths will remind them of past successful coping efforts and will enhance self-efficacy for managing their current difficult situation.

Responding to Upsetting Thoughts Associated with Bereavement

Loss 8–12 Learn and Loss 6 Practice will be relevant for some, but not all, clients using this module. These materials involve attention to more complex emotional, cognitive, and behavioral aspects of grief reactions. By listening carefully during earlier sessions focused on grief and loss, you may hear repeated themes of feeling pressure to move on (Loss 8 Learn: Managing Pressure to "Move On"), loss of personal identity (Loss 9 Learn: Losing a Part of Your Identity and Continuing to Grow as a Person), social isolation (Loss 10 Learn: Staying Connected to Others; Loss 6 Practice: Thoughts About My Loss), as well as regrets and unfinished business (Loss 11 Learn: Living with Regrets and Unfinished Business; Loss 6 Practice: Thoughts About My Loss). Our experience is that we can work on *one* of these areas in a given session, but rarely more. It is very important to have your clients write down their responses to the questions on these Learn pages *during session*. That is a key part of working on these thoughts, because it allows clients to go back and review across multiple weeks; this repetition is important. A good between-session assignment is for clients to reread the specific Learn page several times between session.

Grief-related cognitions that create or reinforce social isolation are the most important to prioritize and address. In addition to using Loss 8–11 Learn, we introduce a simplified three-column thought record using Diane's and Joe's examples in Loss 12 Learn: Thoughts About My Loss: Examples. This may be the first time that clients see a thought record if they have not yet used the *Skills for Thinking* module. Point out that upsetting feelings are triggered by thoughts that happen in the context of specific situations. Diane and Joe were each alone when they had their strongest upsetting feelings and negative thoughts; that may or may not be true for a specific client. Clients can then use Loss 6 Practice: Thoughts About My Loss between sessions to develop skills in responding to these unhelpful thoughts (especially those that maintain social isolation). It is very important for you and your clients to talk through a specific example from their own recent life (ideally in the past week or two). Clients need to have a full example completed for Loss 6 Practice (all three columns filled out) before you send them home with that as a between-session assignment.

Clinician Note

In this section of the Skills for Living with Loss *module, we refer several times to* Skills for Thinking. *Transitioning from the loss module to work on self-compassion and reappraisal skills may be especially helpful for clients who find themselves stuck in a cycle of regret or other thoughts that perpetuate social isolation and suboptimal daily functioning.*

When strength of negative feelings is high (i.e., 75% or greater), it means that the thoughts associated with those feelings are also strong and likely to require the kind of focused attention found in Skills for Thinking. *If, however, a client's feelings are milder or more moderate, complete* Loss 6 Practice: Thoughts About My Loss, *with special attention to generating more helpful thoughts and actions in session (i.e., in the third column). That strategy may resolve the issue without needing to delve into the* Skills for Thinking *module. This is a clinical decision based on the client's response to this approach. If distress and social withdrawal are significantly reduced through developing more adaptive thoughts as part of this module, then there is no need to go further into this domain. We made additional suggestions for working with loss-related cognitions earlier in this chapter in the "Tips for Clinicians" section.*

Managing Grief Following Specific Losses (e.g., Pet, Home, or Treasured Objects)

For many adults, especially if they have been living alone, pets hold a very special place in their social world and daily life. A beloved pet provides important emotional support and requires daily care and attention that create an important role and set of daily routines and responsibilities. Your clients may be grieving a pet's death or loss due to their own declining health or a recent move. Especially when a move to assisted living or another form of residential care is unplanned (e.g., a fall led to an emergency hospitalization followed by rehab and discharge directly to residential care), the sudden loss of a pet can be experienced as tragic. Loss 13 Learn: Losing a Beloved Pet and Loss 7 Practice: Coping with the Loss of My Pet are provided as companion sheets for such clients. Loss 13 Learn is used in session to help clients share their reactions to the loss, with sufficient time allowed for processing of thoughts and emotions.

In the same session, use the second half of Loss 13 Learn to support ways to honor the pet and cope with the loss. You should encourage the client to actually write in their responses to the two questions provided ("What are some of the things that you miss the most, as you cope with the loss of your pet?" and "Are there some specific ways that you currently remember and honor your pet?"). Clients can review their written responses between sessions, which can be a helpful source of validation. In the same session, use Loss 7 Practice to either activate coping responses or provide a reminder to clients that they are already engaged in healthy coping. One way to do this is to complete Loss 7 Practice together in session based on the client's past week. Then provide the completed version plus a clean copy of Loss 7 Practice for the time between the current session and the next scheduled session. This process may be used in one or several sessions.

Some of your older clients may be grieving a recent relocation or a future planned move. Especially when a move is unplanned (e.g., a fall led to an emergency hospitalization followed by rehab and discharge directly to a family member's home or assisted living), the sudden loss of their home and/or treasured objects can be extremely disorienting and upsetting. Loss 14 Learn: Losing Your Home or Treasured Objects, Loss 8: Practice: Preparing to Move, and Loss 9 Practice: Coping with the Loss of My Home are provided as companion sheets for such clients. Use Loss 14 Learn in session to help the client share their reactions to the loss, allowing sufficient time for processing of thoughts and emotions. You should encourage the client to actually write in their responses to the two questions provided ("What are some of the most important parts of your move or loss of treasured objects?" and "What are some of the things that you miss now, or will miss in the future?"). The client can review their written responses between sessions, which can be a helpful source of validation. In the same session, use either Loss 8 Practice: Preparing to Move or Loss 9 Practice: Coping with the Loss of My Home to either activate coping responses or provide a reminder to clients that they are already engaged in healthy coping. One way to do this is to complete Loss 8 or 9 Practice together in session based on the client's past week. Then provide the completed version plus a clean copy for the time between the current session and the next scheduled session. This process may be used in one or several sessions.

Revising Therapy Goals, Staying Encouraged and Engaged in Treatment

You can use Loss 15 Learn: Setting Personal Goals Related to Living with Loss in session to collaboratively decide whether to change or revise therapy goals. Remember, it is important that therapy focus on addressing no more than two or three overall goals. You will not necessarily do this with every client using this module. You can use Loss 1 Practice: Review of My Treatment Goals to write down and rate those revised goals. Loss 16 Learn: Ways to Think About Progress Toward Your Goals reminds clients of the most common pattern of change with therapy (sawtooth curve, not a straight line or stair steps). We recommend using Loss 10 Practice: As I Continue with Treatment: My Plan for Fully Participating for times when you have some concerns about a client's engagement in treatment, either within session or in compliance with between-session practice. Use Loss 11 Practice: My Review of Skills for Living with Loss to review and consolidate key points and skills from this module.

Suggested Progression of Content

The first step in preparing to use this module is a thorough review of all Learn pages and Practice forms so you are familiar with the content and can begin to think about the fit between different skills and specific clients. We realize that behavioral health providers working within primary care may use materials from this module in very brief sessions, and will select individual Learn pages and Practice forms that fit the concerns and needs of their clients. Similarly, there may be occasions within individual or group psychotherapy when clinicians choose specific Learn and/or Practice materials.

In almost all therapy cases, this module will be used after clinicians have worked on goal setting and therapy orientation in the *Skills for Getting Started* module, after facilitating emotional literacy skills in *Skills for Feeling*, and after targeting daily positive and rewarding activities in *Skills for Doing*. Sessions will use the same basic structure: (a) set an agenda, (b) review home practice, (c) select at least one topic to work on in depth, (d) summarize, (e) set up new home practice assignment, and (f) do mutual feedback. Start work on all Practice forms within session, or wait for the next session to introduce them. Don't send a client home with a Practice form without a personal example already inserted. Be sure to allow time to review any Practice form in the next session.

For some of your clients, you will move directly after this module into preparation for therapy termination, in *Skills for Wrapping Up*. There will also be times when you have finished *Skills for Living with Loss*, have started work with clients in another module, and will find yourself coming back to key Learn pages and Practice forms in this module to reinforce key strategies.

When this module is being used to support clients in normative grief reactions, we suggest a four-session approach that allows for several sessions devoted to normalizing grief and reinforcing personal strengths and healthy coping. When this module is being used to support grieving clients, we suggest following the outline presented in Table 15.1.

Not Included in This Treatment

Treatment Strategies for Traumatic Grief and Prolonged Grief Disorder

Our treatment approach is focused on helping clinicians work with middle-aged and older adults who have experienced a range of losses, in the context of treating depression. By the time they have reached 55, approximately 80% of adults will have experienced at least one traumatic life event, yet rates of posttraumatic stress disorder in older adults are low (Monson et al., 2016). Not all of your clients who have experienced a traumatic loss require trauma-focused interventions. When over- or misapplied, some trauma-focused interventions can be iatrogenic and

Table 15.1 Session Outline

Each Session: Depression Measure + Start 3 and 4 Practice

GDS-SF or PHQ-9

Start 4 Practice	Preparing for My Next Session[T]
Start 3 Practice	My Session Summary[T]

Skills for Living with Loss Session 1: Review of Therapy Goals and Psychoeducation About Grief

In Session 1: Loss 1–4 Learn, Loss 1 Practice (+ prior session review)

Between Sessions 1 and 2: Loss 1 Practice

Loss 1 Learn	Introduction to Skills for Living with Loss
Loss 2 Learn	There Are Many Types of Losses
Loss 3 Learn	Grief Looks Different for Everyone[T]
Loss 4 Learn	Traditions, Beliefs, and Preferences[T]
Loss 1 Practice	Review of My Treatment Goals[T]

(Note: Some clients will require more than one session to cover Loss 1–4 Learn.)

Skills for Living with Loss Session 2: Self-Care During Grief

In Session 2: Loss 5 Learn

Between Sessions 2 and 3: Loss 2 Practice and/or Loss 3 Practice

Loss 5 Learn	Your Self-Care Is Important[T]
Loss 2 Practice	My Self-Care This Week[T]
Loss 3 Practice	My Weekly Self-Care Journal[T]

Skills for Living with Loss Session 3: Routines and Taking Care of Life

In Session 3: Loss 6 and 7 Learn

Between Sessions 3 and 4: Loss 4 Practice and/or Loss 5 Practice

Loss 6 Learn	Routine Changes[T]
Loss 7 Learn	Taking Care of Life[T]
Loss 4 Practice	My Routines[T]
Loss 5 Practice	Taking Care of Life Tasks with DEEDS[T]

(continued)

Table 15.1 Continued

(Note: Clients may need several sessions for Loss 7 Learn/Loss 5 Practice.)

Skills for Living with Loss Session 4: Problem Solving and Treatment Goals

In Session 4: Loss 15 and 16 Learn, Loss 10 and 11 Practice

After Session 4: Loss 10 and 11 Practice

Loss 15 Learn	Setting Personal Goals Related to Living with Loss
Loss 16 Learn	Ways to Think About Progress Toward Your Goals[T]
Loss 10 Practice	As I Continue with Treatment: My Plan for Fully Participating
Loss 11 Practice	My Review of Skills for Living with Loss[T]

[T] Identified as particularly appropriate for telehealth sessions.

lead to increased depression and poorer daily functioning. A number of different forms of traumatic loss, however, may call for specific intervention practices for some clients, including suicide loss survivors (Jordan & McGann, 2017). This *Living with Loss* module will be helpful for a range of grief reactions, but it is not a treatment for complicated or traumatic grief. We discuss strategies for screening for complicated grief in Chapter 3. To refer clients to a clinician trained in complicated grief, or to become trained yourself in that approach, see: https://complicatedgrief.columbia.edu/professionals/complicated-grief-professionals/overview/.

End-of-Life Concerns and Anticipatory Grief

You may find yourself working with clients who have a life-threatening illness or who are caring for a family member at the end of life. This is important work and merits more attention than we can provide in just a portion of this specific module. For that reason, we have decided not to attempt a superficial coverage of end-of-life issues. There are several excellent approaches that are available for your work with these clients. These include Meaning-Centered Psychotherapy for Cancer Patients (Breitbart, 2017), Dignity Therapy (Chochinov, 2012), and the CBT approach developed by Satterfield (2008).

Additional Resources for Clinicians

Neimeyer, R. A. (Ed.). (2012). *Techniques of grief therapy: Creative practices for counseling the bereaved*. Routledge Press.

Neimeyer, R. A. (Ed.). (2015). *Techniques of grief therapy: Assessment and intervention*. Routledge Press.

Measures in Appendix D Related to This Module

(Recommendations for use are provided in Chapter 3 of this clinician guide.)

Traumatic Grief Inventory-SR (TGI-SR)

Unfinished Business in Bereavement Scale (UBBS)

CHAPTER 16

Module 10: Skills for Relating: Getting Along and Communicating Your Needs

This personalized module of the workbook is focused on the skills of:

1. Monitoring therapy progress and fine-tuning treatment goals
2. Understanding communication styles
3. Developing communication skills
4. Enhancing social connections
5. Practicing skills using role plays
6. Revising therapy goals, staying encouraged and engaged in treatment

This chapter is provided to help you use the *Skills for Relating* module of the workbook with your clients. We start with a brief overview, followed by some practical tips based on the most common questions we hear from clinicians during professional trainings. The bulk of this chapter is devoted to reviewing communication skills, with descriptions of the specific Learn pages and Practice forms that are available for your use in sessions. We provide recommendations for a standard progression of material (i.e., Learn pages and Practice forms that typically go with each other in the same session, estimates of how much can be accomplished in a given session), with the understanding that this may vary quite a bit depending upon your practice setting and specific client needs. We end the chapter with some comments about related topics that are not included in this treatment approach, and point readers to resources for professional development in helping clients develop communication skills.

As you read this chapter, we encourage you to have the workbook open so that you can refer to the specific Learn pages and Practice forms as they are described and explained. You will use these Learn pages and Practice forms during sessions, encouraging your clients to review between sessions using the Learn pages and try out/record between sessions using the Practice forms. Your reviewing these items as you read through this chapter will prepare you to make the most of the treatment materials. Using these pages and forms means more than having them available to look at or read over with your clients during sessions. Instead, you'll be engaging your clients in exploring the meaning this has to them, through discussion and careful application. Your goal each session is to help your clients apply specific Learn and Practice material to their recent experiences in daily life, and to the problems that bring them into treatment.

Overview

Depression creates difficulties with interpersonal communication and relationships. We've created this module to help clients use specific skills to improve communication with the people in their lives. These skills rely on the client knowing the basics of CBT; we expect that psychotherapy clients will have already completed the core modules (*Skills for Getting Started, Skills for Feeling,* and *Skills for Doing*) and have spent some time developing those core skills. All of this work is framed within the context of their personal life values and strengths to ensure that treatment goals and strategies are consistent with those. Because communication and other interpersonal skills are embedded within culture, awareness of cultural influences on communication and how this applies to specific clients is important. We encourage you to collaboratively focus on culturally appropriate behaviors and responses and avoid encouraging behaviors that conflict with clients' reported cultural norms.

When to Use This Module

With some middle-aged and older clients who have experienced depression on and off throughout their adulthood, we find that either they are frequently in conflict with family and/or friends or they are estranged from them and wish they could have more contact. Often that distance is rooted in long-term disagreements and stress. (An example would be a 70-year-old mother who disapproved of her son's marriage 20 years ago and has had problems relating to her daughter-in-law and their subsequent children. Now, she realizes how cut off she has been from their lives and the lives of her grandchildren, and she would like to remedy this.) This module may be appropriate for such clients. This is not, however, a module that explicitly targets social isolation. We do have experience using these strategies to help clients achieve modest gains in social connections that can improve the quality of their daily lives. Sometimes small changes in social connectedness can decrease loneliness and reduce the risks associated with social isolation.

Tips for Clinicians

Start with Small to Medium-Level Current Difficulties That Have Practical Implications

As you work with clients to identify situations in their present-day lives that may benefit from this module, we suggest you start with a focus on moderate/intermediate-level issues. The situations should be current and feel important enough to your clients to spend time in therapy discussing but should not involve the most difficult/conflicted relationships in their lives. Use a metaphor that fits with the client's life to emphasize the value in starting small (e.g., if you were just beginning to walk daily, you wouldn't start with a 5-mile hike). As they begin to practice communication skills, prepare clients for both a positive and a negative outcome; remember, we do not have control over the other person's responses. In our experience, repairing conflicted relationships takes time and effort. Often, the first attempt is rebuffed, so you need to prepare the client for this and encourage them to try again (which they will want to do anyway, if it is really important). When current interpersonal difficulties are identified as important in maintaining or worsening your client's depression, however, these skills need to be rehearsed with practice in managing alternative scenarios.

Help Clients Focus on Strategy

An important feature of the broken record and other techniques used to handle conflicted interactions is that it keeps your client in a strategic mode of communication and focused on their present life. This helps them avoid becoming emotionally flooded, which most often results in counterproductive communications, or simply rehashing past grievances without any focus on the present. Once clients experience success in using such strategies in their daily lives, it encourages them to be more observant of what is really transpiring in the communication. We refer to it as "going to the meta level" or "above oneself" to observe the context and the impact of the interaction. Older clients often report that this helps keep them from getting angry or becoming anxious and depressed. As mentioned in Chapter 4 as well as in this chapter's section on *Suggested Progression of Content*, CBT routinely includes end-of-session feedback, during which you specifically ask clients for details about what worked in that session and whether there was anything that you said or did that was upsetting or didn't work. This routine solicitation of feedback in CBT sessions (along with your nondefensive and curious responses to negative feedback) helps to prevent and heal ruptures in the therapeutic alliance, leading to stronger, warmer, and more effective therapeutic relationships (Castonguay et al., 2010). We've also provided in Appendix D the five-item version of the Agnew Relationship Measure (ARM-5; Cahill et al., 2012) for your client to complete periodically across different phases of treatment. Both of these approaches to therapy feedback provide examples as you help clients refine their communication skills. Remind your clients of occasions when they were effective in sharing with you their concerns or requests related to therapy. Highlight the strategy that was used so that they can generalize this skill to other interpersonal relationships.

Return to Problem-Solving Skills Using DEEDs

Middle-aged and older adults can experience a number of interpersonally related life stressors that pose true difficulties in daily life. Some of these stressors may tax existing coping abilities, especially in clients with depression who experience poor concentration and/or cognitive limitations. In *Skills for Doing* (<u>Do 16–18 Learn</u> and <u>Do 6 Practice</u>), we have provided the DEEDS clinical tool to use as clients learn problem-solving skills. This is different than merely having session time filled with solving the problem of the week (which can take up entire sessions and the bulk of psychotherapy if you and your client fall into that pattern). The DEEDS tool in *Skills for Doing* is designed to be used repeatedly, across different problems that involve their interpersonal relationships, to reinforce clients learning and then using problem-solving skills on their own. This will take multiple repetitions.

Start with Existing Contacts for Socially Isolated Clients

Resist the urge to focus on development of friendships with entirely new individuals, or on using therapy time to discuss past reasons for a longstanding pattern of social isolation. Research suggests that it takes most adult relationships 1 to 2 years before they transition from acquaintance to friend—if then. The perception of being socially connected to others, in contrast to feeling lonely, can be impacted by a range of activities and interventions. It is possible to increase level of contact and social activities with acquaintances in a way that matters for socially isolated older adults, without expecting these to all become close intimate friendships. So, start with existing contacts and work to broaden and deepen these, keeping expectations modest.

Support Use of Hearing Aids

Hearing limitations can create interpersonal conflict within older couples and families and are also linked to social isolation and cognitive impairment. When finances allow, support hearing-related evaluations and interventions. Some insurance plans include at least modest support for hearing aids, so that should be explored. Also support efforts to maintain ear health (e.g., removal of accumulated wax) and keep hearing aids in working order (clean to remove wax, use of heating devices to remove moisture overnight, replace batteries, periodic maintenance where hearing aid was purchased). This can be a valuable contribution to your clients' quality of daily life.

Monitoring Therapy Progress and Fine-Tuning Treatment Goals

This module begins with the orientation provided in <u>Relate 1 Learn: Introduction to Skills for Relating to Others</u> and the important reminder to have a "state of therapy" discussion about therapy goals and progress. This is a good time to review the overall pattern of depression scores, using whichever weekly measure of depression is a part of this feedback-informed treatment. Complete and review <u>Relate 1 Practice: Review of My Treatment Goals</u> during session so that overall therapy goals stay in the forefront even while you are spending several sessions working on interpersonal skills. Determine whether the treatment goals need to be refined to be useful in treatment moving forward. This may be a point in therapy where clients have made significant progress on one of their therapy goals and wish to revise or replace it with another.

Understanding Communication Styles

You will use <u>Relate 2 Learn: Communication Styles</u> to explain to clients that there are different *styles* of communication (i.e., passive, assertive, and aggressive) that exist across a continuum. What style of communication one adopts often varies from person to person (e.g., the client may communicate one way with their spouse but another way with business associates or friends outside the home). Sometimes a small increase or decrease in use of a specific style can make a difference, so we are looking to help build flexibility. The decision to use this module typically means that the client is having interpersonal difficulties and may be overusing either passive or aggressive styles, or both. You want to help clients focus on the style or manner of interacting that is giving them the most trouble in the present. Clients have the option to complete <u>Relate 2 Practice: Recognizing Communication Styles</u> and/or <u>Relate 3 Practice: Tweaking Communication Styles</u> to have experience labeling these using concrete examples.

<u>Relate 3 Learn: Passive Communication</u> helps you discuss the core features of passive communication, and <u>Relate 4 Learn: Aggressive Communication</u> helps you discuss the core features of aggressive

communication. Ask clients which style they use more often and have them describe details of a recent encounter illustrating that. The cost–benefit analysis is very important to help the client see that the costs outweigh the benefits—if not in the short term, then clearly in the long term.

Relate 5 Learn: Assertive Communication covers assertive communication and is helpful to use with most clients who are learning communication skills. In contrast to the passive and aggressive styles, communicating effectively involves expressing oneself clearly and honestly while considering both one's personal rights and feelings and the rights and feelings of others. Effective, expressive statements are those communications that are done without humiliating, dominating, or insulting the other person. This is not as easy as it sounds, because the other person in the interaction may hear or interpret what one is saying differently from what one's meaning is.

It can be very useful to discuss the last time the client believes they communicated effectively with someone. This can be an example from another domain of the client's life, such as a volunteer position, when giving feedback to you during a therapy session, or it can be an example from a time when the client communicated effectively with a person with whom they are now in conflict. (The latter can have more educational value, since it gives you a better idea of how the other person actually responds in real-life situations.) Sum up this part of the module by encouraging clients to consider the following issues before they are going to have an interpersonal interaction with someone with whom they are, or have been, in conflict:

1. What is the goal or objective of your message?
2. How might alternative methods of communication help you reach your goal?
3. Pick the communication style that will most likely provide the best outcome.

Developing Communication Skills

There are specific strategies you can focus on to help your clients communicate effectively. Relate 6 Learn: Ways to Communicate Effectively covers the key strategies of using "I" statements and staying flexible.

Using "I" statements (instead of "you" did this and that, and it's "your fault" or "you should do X or Y") helps to ground the person in the interaction and helps to clarify what it is they are really seeking from the interaction. For example: If a 90-year-old widowed woman living alone says, "Why don't you come over more to visit?" to her adult children, she is not likely to get many visitors. That kind of statement tends to make the other person defensive or may sound accusatory. Instead, she could state clearly: "Arnetta and Marlene, I am lonely, and I miss spending time with you. Can we figure out a day and time when you can drop by and spend an hour with me?" This is a definite invitation instead of a vague demand, and so is more likely to result in a positive response. Again, stating clearly what one wants or needs is an integral part of communicating effectively. You will also work with clients on developing specific requests that are do-able. In the above example, asking for someone to "spend an hour with me" is better than "come over for a visit," which could be perceived as a more involved experience.

Relate 6 Learn also addresses the need to stay flexible, which involves learning how to negotiate and compromise and "developing options if I can't get exactly what I want." An emphasis on flexibility is a very good intervention for those whose thinking tends to run in "all or none" terms. Such clients seem to think that if they can't have it all, then why bother? Explain that placing that kind of interpersonal demand on other people usually does not result in their going along with the client; more often, they tend to back away, since the demand is too extreme. This emphasis on flexibility is also relevant to the material provided in Relate 7 Learn: Making Requests/Asking for Help and Relate 4 Practice: Listing My Needs and Wants, Then Asking for Help!

Relate 7–11 Learn and Relate 4 and 5 Practice focus on requesting help and use of the "broken record technique." Together, these clinical materials help clients develop the ability to say "no" and skills to ask for things that are needed (i.e., asking repeatedly in a calm manner and remaining steadfast, assuming the request is reasonable). The broken record technique is particularly effective when dealing with obstinate people who may be pressuring the client to do something they would rather avoid. This technique is also a useful way for the client to get something that they want, depending on the other person's willingness to respond. The basics are provided in Relate 9 Learn: Broken Record Technique. Then, a case study is provided in Relate 10 Learn: Understanding the Broken Record Technique, with some opportunities in Relate 11 Learn: Brainstorming Your Broken Record Technique to practice developing statements within session. Relate 5 Practice: Using the Broken Record Technique is available for between-session skill development.

Some clients with depression have a range of nonverbal behaviors that interfere with social relationships. Relate 12 Learn: Nonverbal Communication and Depression and Relate 6 Practice: My Nonverbal Communication Skills are available for you to use with specific clients who need to attend to and modify their nonverbal communication.

Enhancing Social Connections

Relate 13–15 Learn and Relate 7 and 8 Practice are provided as tools to use with clients who are socially isolated and wish to reach out to people, or who are in conflict and want to re-establish a stronger connection. Due to loss of spouse or partner, friends dying or moving away, and changes in health that may preclude their continuing to do shared hobbies, some older adults find that their social networks have shrunk considerably. Often, this is a gradual process that takes place over a number of years and may not even be noticed until it has reached rather extreme proportions. Role playing can be used as part of a skill set to increase the likelihood that a person who is interpersonally isolated will begin to reach out to other people and develop satisfying relationships. One effective method is the "triple role play" technique:

1. The clinician takes on the role of a person in the client's life with whom there is current distance and simulates an exchange that helps the client develop alternative thoughts and actions.
2. Roles are then reversed: The client plays the other person, while the clinician plays the client, thereby being a model and helping them experience how a different style of interaction might work.
3. Roles are switched back so that the client can practice using a new style of interacting with the socially distant person. This can be extremely beneficial.

Clients' development of new communication patterns will be supported by discussing these roles and what the client learned from each part of the experience. The more often this exercise is repeated, the more likely it is that clients will be effective in changing their interactive pattern with specific individuals.

Practicing Skills Using Role Plays

We provide <u>Relate 14 Learn: Role Playing: 3-Part Exercise</u> and <u>Relate 8 Practice: My Role Play</u> to support your clinical work using role plays with your clients. To set the stage, the client delineates a particular interpersonal situation that is causing them distress and describes it in some detail to the clinician (so that you can get into the role). Role-play segments should not be long and detailed or else they may become too stressful to foster new learning and change. Processing the client's feelings and thoughts after each role-play segment is extremely important in helping them get a better perspective on how to change their habitual interactive pattern used in distant or problematic relationships. Further practice usually strengthens its effectiveness.

Clinicians must be sensitive to the possibility that for some clients, this "triple role play" technique may be too challenging. However, in our experience, we have found this technique to be effective with many older clients who are experiencing emotionally distant or conflictual relationships with significant others.

As noted earlier, in the first part of this technique, clients play themselves and the clinician plays the other person in the interaction. Enacting the situation as closely as possible to what the client described actually happened helps both individuals become aware of the thoughts, feelings, and actions that probably occurred and sets the stage for the next two parts of the role play. The role play should go on for no more than 5 minutes or so, with about 10 additional minutes spent processing the feelings and thoughts that the client is aware of.

Next, the client plays the other person and the clinician plays the client, but here, you play the client *communicating effectively*. Before doing the second role play, it is helpful to ask the client to predict how the interaction is going to go. This usually produces a spate of negative thoughts that can be challenged before or after the second role play, with the object being to help the client realize that negative expectations for the interaction can lead to self-fulfilling prophecies. On the other hand, by encouraging a positive problem-solving attitude, you can empower the client. If clients grasp that even briefly, they will want more time to practice! After this 5-minute second role play, again spend about 10 minutes processing the client's thoughts and feelings. Often at this time, the client is developing more of an awareness of how they were coming across, and how that can be improved upon. Presumably, you have been able to role model more effective communication in this segment, thereby showing the client some alternative ways that have a good chance of turning out better than in the first interaction.

In the third part of the role play, clients again play themselves and the clinician again plays the other person. In this exchange, encourage the client to practice other ways of communicating their needs or requests so that they have the chance to develop options and to try them out in a safe environment, with a coach right there to give feedback. Usually, this is a more successful experience than the first role play, and this contrast is in itself informative. After about 5 minutes again of role play, spend another 10 minutes or so processing what was said, how it felt, what thoughts were associated with it, and what the resulting feelings were. Generally, by now, the client has had the chance to practice, literally, different ways of making the request and can learn from the role play how these different ways of presenting the request may be received by the other person.

For the client to get the most out of this exercise, you need to be prepared with some alternative responses (so that you can model them), and you need to monitor timing so that the entire process can be completed in one full session. Generally, this leads to the home practice assignment of actually talking with the identified person and then reporting back next time how it went. Whether or not to make this the assignment depends on your judgment: If you think the client is ready for the interaction and will in fact be able to implement what was learned, and if there appears to be a reasonable chance for success, then it is an excellent assignment. Whether the client gets what they want or not, they will learn something from the experience. However, if you think that there is a high probability of failure, or if the client did not really seem to understand how to proceed, then it is not advisable. Home practice then could be to select a less challenging situation and to practice effective communication in that situation.

For some clients, role playing is very effective: They are able to get into it, and they learn through modeling, practice, and feedback. For others, it is extremely difficult to get them to participate. In those cases, it is not worth struggling with clients to get them to do this. If they are reluctant, then it is necessary to find other ways to help them restructure their interpersonal interactions so that they are more effective. In such cases, preparing 3-by-5 or 4-by-6 "coping cards" may be effective: The client writes the stressful interpersonal situation on one side and lists several verbatim responses and reminders to themselves on the other side.

Revising Therapy Goals, Staying Encouraged and Engaged in Treatment

Relate 16 Learn: Setting Personal Goals for Relating to Others provides the option for you and your client to collaboratively decide on whether there to make any changes or revisions to therapy goals. Again, it is important that therapy can focus on addressing no more than two or three overall goals. Sometimes as work in a specific module is nearing completion, it becomes clear that focused work on change in one area is likely to be an important part of ending the depression. You can use Relate 1 Practice: Review of My Treatment Goals as a form to write down and rate those revised goals. Relate 17 Learn: Ways to Think About Progress Toward Your Goals reminds clients of the most common pattern of change with therapy (sawtooth curve, not a straight line or stair steps). We recommend using Relate 9 Practice: As I Continue with Treatment: My Plan for Fully Participating for times when you already have some concerns about a client's engagement in treatment, either within session on in compliance with between-session practice. We suggest using Relate 10 Practice: My Review of Skills for Relating as a way to review and consolidate key points and skills that were worked on in this module.

Suggested Progression of Content

The first step in preparing to use this module is a thorough review of all Learn pages and Practice forms so you are familiar with the content and can begin to think about the fit between different skills and specific clients. We realize that behavioral health providers working within primary care may use materials from this module in very brief sessions, and will select individual Learn pages and Practice forms that fit the concerns and needs of their clients. Similarly, there may be occasions within individual or group psychotherapy when clinicians choose specific Learn and/or Practice materials.

When this module is being used in its entirety to help clients improve their interpersonal effectiveness in daily life, we suggest using six to eight sessions, including several devoted to role playing challenging conversations. Role playing and processing of the role plays take time, and the home practice assigned often takes several weeks before results are observed. Thus, this can be a very appropriate component for the middle phase of treatment, when you are focusing on skill development with clients who struggle with their communication style and interpersonal effectiveness.

In almost all therapy cases, this module will be used after clinicians have worked on goal setting and therapy orientation in the *Skills for Getting Started* module, after facilitating emotional literacy skills in *Skills for Feeling*, and after targeting daily positive and rewarding activities in *Skills for Doing*. Sessions will use the same basic structure: (a) set an agenda, (b) review home practice, (c) select at least one topic to work on in depth, (d) summarize, (e) set up new home practice assignment, and (f) do mutual feedback. Start work on all Practice forms within session or wait for the next session to introduce them. Don't send a client home with a Practice form without a personal example already inserted. Be sure to allow time to review any Practice form in the next session.

For some of your clients, you will move directly after this module into preparation for therapy termination, in *Skills for Wrapping Up*. There will also be times when you have finished *Skills for Relating,* have started work with clients in another module, and will find yourself coming back to key Learn pages and Practice forms in this module to continue to reinforce effective interpersonal behaviors and communication strategies. This may be especially true for family caregivers who are using materials in the *Skills for Caregiving* module.

When this module is being used in its entirety to address communication problems as a part of individual psychotherapy for depression in middle-aged and older adults, we suggest following the outline presented in Table 16.1.

Table 16.1 Session Outline

Each Session: Depression Measure + Start 3 and 4 Practice

GDS-SF or PHQ-9

Start 4 Practice	Preparing for My Next Session[T]
Start 3 Practice	My Session Summary[T]

Skills for Relating Session 1: Assess Progress and Psychoeducation

In Session 1: Relate 1 and 2 Learn, Relate 1 Practice (+ prior session review)

Between Sessions 1 and 2: Relate 2 Practice

Relate 1 Learn	Introduction to Skills for Relating to Others
Relate 2 Learn	Communication Styles[T]
Relate 1 Practice	Review of My Treatment Goals[T]
Relate 2 Practice	Recognizing Communication Styles[T]

Skills for Relating Session 2: Communication Styles

In Session 2: Relate 3 or 4 Learn, Relate 5 Learn

Between Sessions 2 and 3: Relate 3 Practice

Relate 3 Learn	Passive Communication
Relate 4 Learn	Aggressive Communication
Relate 5 Learn	Assertive Communication
Relate 3 Practice	Tweaking Communication Styles[T]

Skills for Relating Session 3: Making Requests

In Session 3: Relate 6–8 Learn

Between Sessions 3 and 4: Relate 4 Practice

Relate 6 Learn	Ways to Communicate Effectively[T]
Relate 7 Learn	Making Requests/Asking for Help[T]
Relate 8 Learn	Tips on Asking for Help[T]
Relate 4 Practice	Listing My Needs and Wants, Then Asking for Help![T]

Table 16.1 Continued

Skills for Relating Session 4: Broken Record Technique

In Session 4: Relate 9–11 Learn

Between Sessions 4 and 5: Relate 5 Practice

Relate 9 Learn	Broken Record Technique[T]
Relate 10 Learn	Understanding the Broken Record Technique
Relate 11 Learn	Brainstorming Your Broken Record Technique
Relate 5 Practice	Using the Broken Record Technique[T]

Skills for Relating Session 5: Connecting with Others

In Session 5: Relate 12–14 Learn

Between Sessions 5 and 6: Relate 6, 7, or 8 Practice

Relate 12 Learn	Nonverbal Communication and Depression
Relate 13 Learn	Connecting with Others
Relate 14 Learn	Role Playing: 3-Part Exercise
Relate 6 Practice	My Nonverbal Communication Skills
Relate 7 Practice	Visualizing My Interactions with Others
Relate 8 Practice	My Role Play

Skills for Relating Session 6: Connecting with Others

In Session 6: Relate 12–14 Learn

Between Sessions 6 and 7: Relate 6, 7, or 8 Practice

Relate 12 Learn	Nonverbal Communication and Depression
Relate 13 Learn	Connecting with Others
Relate 14 Learn	Role Playing: 3-Part Exercise
Relate 6 Practice	My Nonverbal Communication Skills
Relate 7 Practice	Visualizing My Interactions with Others
Relate 8 Practice	My Role Play

(continued)

Table 16.1 Continued

Skills for Relating Session 7: Connecting with Others

In Session 7: Relate 12–14 Learn

Between Sessions 7 and 8: Relate 6, 7, or 8 Practice

Relate 12 Learn	Nonverbal Communication and Depression
Relate 13 Learn	Connecting with Others
Relate 14 Learn	Role Playing: 3-Part Exercise
Relate 6 Practice	My Nonverbal Communication Skills
Relate 7 Practice	Visualizing My Interactions with Others
Relate 8 Practice	My Role Play

Skills for Relating Session 8: Review and Assessment

In Session 8: Relate 15–17 Learn, Relate 10 Practice

After Session 8: Relate 9 or 10 Practice

Relate 15 Learn	INVEST in Your Relationships
Relate 16 Learn	Setting Personal Goals for Relating to Others[T]
Relate 17 Learn	Ways to Think About Progress Toward Your Goals[T]
Relate 9 Practice	As I Continue with Treatment: My Plan for Fully Participating
Relate 10 Practice	My Review of Skills for Relating[T]

[T] Identified as particularly appropriate for telehealth sessions.

Not Included in This Treatment

Treatment for Social Anxiety

We provide some initial support to work with mild social anxiety, but do not expect this module to be sufficient for individuals who meet criteria for a social anxiety disorder. For many of these individuals, this is a lifelong problem that may well have increased with losses to their existing social network. Readers are referred to Hope et al. (2019a, 2019b) for an evidence-based approach to working with socially anxious clients.

Social Skills Training in Appropriate Self-Disclosure

Social norms for self-disclosure do not typically change dramatically over the adult years. For this reason, clinical resources to help clients who have significant social skills deficits are beyond the scope of this module. We provide resources in the "Additional Resources for Clinicians" section for clinicians who are looking for tools in social effectiveness training. For clients who may meet criteria for a personality disorder, we refer readers to the works of Videler and colleagues (2018) and Lynch and colleagues (2007) for further suggestions.

Additional Resources for Clinicians

McKay, M., Davis, M., & Fanning, P. (2018). *Messages: The communication skills book* (4th ed.). New Harbinger Press.

Van Orden, K. A., Bower, E., Lutz, J., Silva, C., Gallegos, A. M., Podgorski, C. A., Santos, E. J., & Conwell, Y. (2020). Strategies to promote social connections among older adults during "social distancing" restrictions. *American Journal of Geriatric Psychiatry.* doi:10.1016/j.jagp.2020.05.004

Measure in Appendix D Related to This Module

(Recommendations for use are provided in Chapter 3 of this clinician guide.)
Agnew Relationship Measure-5 (ARM-5)

Afterword: Professional Development

After reviewing this clinician guide and the accompanying client workbook, you are ready to use them in your therapeutic work with middle-aged and older adults. We invite you to take an additional step: namely, to reflect on your current clinical skill set and consider obtaining additional education, training, and/or consultation to enhance your therapeutic work. This is particularly relevant if much of your practice consists of middle-aged and older adults with depression, as this is a rapidly evolving field. We make a number of recommendations for professional development in this afterword and have listed additional resources in Appendix A.

Several psychological organizations have collaborated to bring together updates on resources for education and training that are intended to help clinicians hone their practice skills. These include the American Psychological Association (APA)'s Division 12, Section II (Society of Clinical Geropsychology), APA Division 20 (Adult Development & Aging), and the APA Committee on Aging (CONA). APA's Careers in Aging Roadmap is a step-by-step guide to help undergraduate and graduate students, and those at the postdoctoral or post-licensure level, think about a variety of ways to gain both academic and practical experience in the field of mental health and aging. More information is available at the "Exploring Careers in Aging" roadmap (https://www.apa.org/pi/aging/resources/careers). A common issue that this roadmap addresses is: *"My training/practice setting doesn't have a geropsychology or geriatric mental health specialty. What should I do?"* Examples of recommended avenues for education and training include taking courses in psychological assessment and evidence-based treatment methods (at the graduate level). At the postgraduate level, specific fellowships (with stipends) may be appropriate. Many of these are in VA settings as the VA is a major employer of persons with geriatric mental health training and experience. Post-licensure, there are numerous continuing education opportunities as well as opportunities to obtain supervised experience and/or clinical case consultation from experts in the field.

Two other important professional organizations are the Council of Professional Geropsychology Training Programs (CoPGTP) and Psychologists in Long-Term Care (PLTC). The CoPGTP is a very active group that lists a variety of educational and health care institutions that offer training relevant to geriatric mental health at all levels, including the post-licensure level. Their website (https://copgtp.org/training/graduate-training/) is updated regularly and is another recommended "go-to" spot for many practicing clinicians in the field who want advanced training and/or supervised experience. PLTC (http://www.pltcweb.org/index.php) is a professional organization dedicated to the advancement of psychological practice in long-term and skilled nursing care. Functionally, cognitively, ethnically, and culturally, older adults as a clinical population are by their nature some of the most diverse clientele a clinician can work with. The members of this network of practitioners (and scholars and researchers) have a strong interest in serving the increasingly diverse population of adults in long-term care settings. This organization provides opportunities to be mentored by experts in the field as well as networking sessions and a very active listserv that addresses common clinical issues arising when attempting to provide CBT and related treatments for depression in long-term care settings.

All of these professional organizations have collaborated on developing a standardized set of professional guidelines, referred to as the "Pikes Peak model" of competencies. This is described in detail in the Pikes Peak Geropsychology Knowledge and Skill Assessment Tool, which can be downloaded from https://gerocentral.org/competencies/competencies-tool-online. Due to limited space, we are unable to describe this in more detail, but we invite clinicians to consult this self-evaluation tool as part of the process of continual learning and practice enhancement.

At all levels, clinicians can join organizations that focus on geriatric mental health issues, such as the American Society on Aging (ASA) and the Gerontological Society of America (GSA), both of which have special interest groups on these topics. The ASA (https://www.asaing.

org) promotes careers in aging, hosts an online jobs posting service, and supports professional development in a range of areas, including elder abuse prevention, dementia services, and disability access in local communities. The GSA (https://www.geron.org) supports professional development in gerontological science and practice in a wide range of disciplines, including behavioral health. We have featured one of their products in this clinician guide (i.e., the KAER Toolkit for early identification of dementia). Professional organizations from other fields, such as nursing, social work, and a variety of counseling specialties, can also be consulted to determine if they have special interest groups and training experiences related to geriatric mental health.

Beyond professional organizations, there are a number of key resources that can help you keep up to date as a busy clinician. There are several professional journals that focus on geriatric mental health issues. These are peer-reviewed and publish papers from multiple disciplines (not just psychiatry or psychology). These include *Aging and Mental Health*, *American Journal of Geriatric Psychiatry*, *Clinical Gerontologist* (which publishes case reports as well as empirical research), *Generations* (published by the ASA; practitioner oriented), *International Psychogeriatrics*, and the *Journal of Mental Health and Aging*. Regularly scanning the contents of these journals (and others that are more specialized, such as *Cognitive and Behavioral Practice*, which focuses on innovations in the CBT field) enables you to incorporate new methods into your therapeutic work.

We also invite you to check out the GeroCentral website (https://gerocentral.org/), which provides "one-stop shopping" for many clinicians. This site contains excellent resources, along with training recommendations and opportunities at all levels of practice. The "Training & Career" section provides training resources for each level of professional psychology as well as for those who are post-licensure— see https://gerocentral.org/training-career for details. Their list of continuing education options will continue to grow as new opportunities emerge. GeroCentral also plans to develop its own series of webinars on timely topics of interest to practicing clinicians. The site provides opportunities for mentoring at any level of training or career development, which can be particularly helpful for clinicians who are relatively new to working with persons in the second half of life.

Finally, there are independent groups that provide focused CBT training and consultation—including both didactic and clinical/experiential components—to interested providers. Clinicians seeking training and consultation can be either individuals or small groups of clinicians in mental health clinics and community-based organizations. One example is the Optimal Aging Center in Los Altos, California, which has active training and consultation programs in CBT and in caregiver-focused interventions (www.optimalagingcenter.com).

Professional Development Resources

Professional Training Opportunities

Training in CBT with Middle-Aged and Older Clients

Optimal Aging Center: www.optimalagingcenter.com

Training in CBT with Adults

Academy of Cognitive and Behavioral Therapies: www.academyofct.org
Association for Behavioral and Cognitive Therapies (USA): http://www.abct.org
Beck Institute of Cognitive and Behavioral Therapies: https://beckinstitute.org

Professional Associations Across the Globe (Continuing Education Opportunities)

Asian Association for Cognitive Behaviour Therapy: https://asiancbt.weebly.com
Association for Behavioral and Cognitive Therapies (USA): http://www.abct.org
Australian Association for Cognitive and Behaviour Therapy: https://www.aacbt.org.au
British Association for Behavioural and Cognitive Psychotherapies: https://www.babcp.com
European Association for Behavioural and Cognitive Therapies: https://eabct.eu
Indian Association for Cognitive Behaviour Therapy: http://iacbt.org/message.html

Module 5: Skills for Brain Health

Alzheimer's Association: alz.org/help-support/brain_health

Alzheimer's Disease Education and Referral (ADEAR) Center: www.nia.nih.gov/health/about-adear-center

American College of Sports Medicine: www.ACSM.org

American College of Sports Medicine's Physical Activity Readiness Questionnaire: https://www.acsm.org/docs/default-source/files-for-resource-library/par-q-acsm.pdf

American Heart Association's Brain Health Resources: www.heart.org/en/health-topics/brain-health

Brain Basics: www.ninds.nih.gov/disorders/patient-daregiver-education/Know-Your-Brain.org

Cleveland Clinic Healthy Brains: www.healthybrains.org

Gerontological Society of America's KAER Toolkit: www.geron.org/images/gsa/kaer/gsa-kaer-toolkit.pdf

National Institute on Aging's Exercises and Physical Activity: www.nia.nih.gov/health/exercise-physical-activity

Nutrition and Brain Health: www.nutritionletter.tufts.edu; www.eatright.org

World Health Organization (WHO): Recommendations on physical activity for health: www.who.int/publications-detail/global-recommendations-on-physical-activity-for-health

Module 6: Skills for Managing Chronic Pain

International Association for the Study of Pain: www.iasp-pain.org

National Institute of Health's National Center for Complementary and Integrative Health: www.nccih.nih.gov/health/chronic-pain-in-depth

National Register of Health Providers: https://www.findapsychologist.org (Clients can enter their ZIP code and enter the keyword "pain" to find a behavioral health clinician who specializes in pain management.)

U.S. Department of Veterans Affairs, Pain Management Resource Center: www.va.gov/PAINMANAGEMENT/Veteran_Public/CHRONIC_PAIN_101.asp

Module 7: Skills for Healthy Sleep

Board of Behavioral Sleep Medicine (credentialing via diplomate in behavioral sleep medicine): www.bsmcredential.org
International Directory of CBT-I Providers: https://cbti.directory
Society of Behavioral Sleep Medicine, online training: www.behavioralsleep.org

Module 8: Skills for Caregiving

Professional Development Opportunities in Family Caregiving

Family Caregiver Alliance: www.caregiver.org
Optimal Aging Center: www.optimalagingcenter.com
Rosalyn Carter Institute: www.rosalynncarter.org

Information and Referral Resources

AARP Caregiving Support: https://www.aarp.org/home-family/caregiving
Alzheimer's Association: www.alz.org
Alzheimer's Association, Los Angeles Chapter: www.alzheimersla.org
Alzheimer's Disease and Referral (ADEAR) Center: www.nia.nih.gov/health/about-adear-center
Alzheimer's Disease International: www.alz.co.uk
National Association of Area Agencies on Aging: www.n4a.org
National Center on Caregiving:www.caregiver.org/national-center-caregiving
National Eldercare Locator: https://eldercare.acl.gov/Public/Index.aspx
National Institute on Aging: www.nia.nih.gov/health/caregiving
U.S. Department of Veterans Affairs, Caregiver Support: www.caregiver.va.gov
World Health Organization (WHO) Global Network for Aging-Friendly Cities and Communities: www.who.int/ageing/projects/age_friendly_cities_network/en
World Health Organization (WHO): I-Support for Dementia Program: www.who.int/publications-detail/isupport-for-dementia

Module 9: Skills for Living with Loss

Association for Death Education and Counseling: https://www.adec.org
Center for Complicated Grief: https://complicatedgrief.columbia.edu
National Institute of Aging: https://www.nia.nih.gov/health/mourning-death-spouse

Module 10: Skills for Relating

AARP's Connect2Affect website: https://connect2affect.org
COVIA's Well Connected Program (free telephone-based social activities for older adults): (877) 797-7299; https://covia.org/services/well-connected
Institute on Aging's 24-hour toll-free Friendship Line: (800) 971-0016; https://www.ioaging.org/services/all-inclusive-health-care/friendship-line

Appendix B

Recommendations for Group Treatments

Open-Ended Format for Inpatient and Partial Hospitalization Settings

For clinicians who work with aging patients with depression in psychiatric settings, there are Learn pages and Practice forms that fit a variety of open therapy groups. Instead of recommending set materials for specific group sessions, it is more appropriate to identify a range of materials that can be considered (e.g., depending upon variability of patient functioning, length of stay, and issues in the current treatment milieu).

Repetition, especially repeated use of the same Practice forms, is very valuable because patients' mental status can change from session to session. Lower-functioning patients also benefit from repetition. These are merely suggestions; as you become more familiar with the resources provided within the workbook, you may identify additional materials that are a fit for your group and treatment setting.

Module 1: Skills for Getting Started: Planning Your Treatment

Start 4 Learn: What to Expect from Cognitive-Behavioral Therapy (CBT)
Start 5 Learn: Rules for Our Group
Start 6 Learn: Overview of Clinical Depression
Start 8 Learn: What Is Clinical Depression?
Start 9 Learn: Antidepressant Medications
Start 10 Learn: Your Life Values and Personal Strengths
Start 13 Learn: What Is the Cognitive-Behavioral Model?
Start 17 Learn: Ways to Think About Progress Toward Your Goals
Start 2 Practice: One Daily Exception
Start 5 Practice: My Values and Strengths
Start 6 Practice: The Cognitive-Behavioral Model of My Depression
Start 12 Practice: Ways to Encourage Myself

Module 2: Skills for Feeling: Recognizing and Managing Strong Emotions

Feel 2 Learn: Understanding Emotions
Feel 3 Learn: Emotional Literacy
Feel 5 Learn: Feelings Are Just the Tip of the Iceberg
Feel 6 Learn: The ABC Model
Feel 7 Learn: Nurturing Positive Emotions
Feel 8 Learn: Highlighting the Positive
Feel 11 Learn: Awareness of Tension
Feel 12 Learn: Relaxation Is Important
Feel 13 Learn: How to Relax
Feel 2 Practice: My Mood Scale
Feel 4 Practice: ABC Form
Feel 5 Practice: Recognizing Positive Emotions
Feel 11 Practice: Relaxation Diary
Feel 12 Practice: My Relaxation Practice Log

Module 3: Skills for Doing: Values-Based Living and Solving Problems

Module 4: Skills for Thinking: Self-Compassion and Helpful Thoughts

Coping with the Blues: 6-Week Class

Begin each week's class with Start 5 Learn: Rules for Our Group. For an 8-week class format, add two classes to review the content of Weeks 5 and 6 and problem solve barriers.

Week 1
Class
Start 7 Learn:	Recognizing Common Signs of Depression
Start 10 Learn:	Your Life Values and Personal Strengths
Start 11 Learn:	Celebrating Diversity

Assignments
Start 1 Practice:	My Depressive Symptoms
Start 5 Practice:	My Values and Strengths
Start 12 Practice:	Ways to Encourage Myself (Encourage use for rest of class)

Week 2
Class
Feel 2 Learn:	Understanding Emotions
Feel 3 Learn:	Emotional Literacy
Feel 6 Learn:	The ABC Model

Assignments
Feel 2 Practice:	My Mood Scale
Feel 4 Practice:	ABC Form

Week 3
Class
Feel 7 Learn:	Nurturing Positive Emotions
Feel 8 Learn:	Highlighting the Positive

Assignments
Feel 5 Practice:	Recognizing Positive Emotions
Feel 6 Practice:	Growing Positive Emotions

Week 4
Class
Do 2 Learn:	Activities Affect Your Mood
Do 3 Learn:	What Are Positive Activities?
Do 4 Learn:	Snapshot of Where You Are Right Now
Do 5 Learn:	Using the First Steps

Assignments

Do 2 Practice: First Steps

Do 3 Practice: First Steps Instructions

Week 5

Class

Do 8 Learn: The Importance of Doing

Do 9 Learn: Making Your List

Do 15 Learn: Example of Positive Activities Log

Assignments

Do 4 Practice: List of Positive Activities

Do 5 Practice: PAL: Positive Activities Log

Week 6

Do 11 Learn: Using Values and Purpose

Do 12 Learn: Physical Activity Is Important

Do 13 Learn: Your Plan for Physical Activity

Do 14 Learn: Schedule Your Activities

Brain-Healthy Living: 6-Week Class

Begin each week's class with Start 5 Learn: Rules for Our Group. For an 8-week class format, add two classes to review the content of Weeks 3 through 6 and problem solve barriers.

Week 1
Class
Health 3 Learn:	Key Points About Brain Health: Cognitive Aging
Health 4 Learn:	How Our Brains Do and Don't Change as We Age
Health 15 Learn:	Your Annual Medicare Wellness Visit

Assignments
Health 2 Practice:	Maintain My Physical Health by Knowing My Numbers
Health 11 Practice:	My Upcoming Health Care Visit

Week 2
Class
Health 7 Learn:	A Brain-Healthy Lifestyle: Your Daily Health Habits Matter
Health 8 Learn:	Support Your Brain Health
Health 9 Learn:	Be Physically Active

Assignments
Health 3 Practice:	Taking Care of My Brain Health
Health 4 Practice:	My Physical Activity

Week 3
Class
Health 9 Learn:	Be Physically Active
Health 10 Learn:	Follow a Healthy Food and Drink Plan

Assignments
Health 3 Practice:	Taking Care of My Brain Health
Health 5 Practice:	Healthy Food and Drink Log

Week 4
Class
Health 11 Learn:	Stay Socially Connected to Others
Health 12 Learn:	Manage Your Stress

Assignments

Health 3 Practice:	Taking Care of My Brain Health
Health 6 Practice:	How I Felt Connected to Others
Health 7 Practice:	Managing Stress

Week 5

Class

Health 13 Learn:	Learn New Things
Health 14 Learn:	Keep Healthy Sleep Habits

Assignments

Health 9 Practice:	Learning New Things
Health 10 Practice:	My Healthy Sleep Habits

Week 6

Health 7 Learn:	A Brain-Healthy Lifestyle: Your Daily Health Habits Matter

Coping with Caregiving: 6-Week Class

Begin each week's class with Start 5 Learn: Rules for Our Group. For an 8-week class format, add two classes to review the content of Weeks 3 through 6 and problem solve barriers.

Week 1
Class
Care 3 Learn:	Self-Kindness for Caregivers
Care 4 Learn:	Managing Caregiving Stress

Assignments
Care 2 Practice:	Treating Myself Kindly in Caregiving Situations
Care 3 Practice:	Managing OK Is Good Enough: My Examples

Week 2
Class
Care 5 Learn:	Giving Yourself Credit as a Caregiver
Care 6 Learn:	Encouraging Yourself

Assignments
Care 3 Practice:	Managing OK Is Good Enough: My Examples
Care 4 Practice:	Ways to Encourage Myself as a Caregiver

Week 3
Class
Care 7 Learn:	Managing Your Unhelpful Thoughts
Care 8 Learn:	Asking for Help from Friends and Family

Assignments
Care 5 Practice:	When It May Be Time to Step Back
Care 6 Practice:	Revising Upsetting Thoughts About Caregiving
Care 8 Practice:	Asking for Help with Caregiving

Week 4
Class
Care 9 Learn:	Planning Positive Activities for Your Family Member
Care 11 Learn:	Planning Shared Positive Activities for the Two of You

Assignments

Care 10 Practice: Rewarding Activities This Week for My Family Member
Care 12 Practice: Our Shared Activities This Week

Week 5

Class

Care 12 Learn: Staying Able to Provide Care
Care 13 Learn: Your "R&R" (Rest and Recuperation)

Assignments

Care 13 Practice: My Staying Able to Provide Care
Care 14 Practice: My "R&R" (Rest and Recuperation)

Week 6

Care 14 Learn: National Resources for Caregivers in the United States
Care 16 Learn: Ways to Think About Progress Toward Your Goals
Care 17 Practice: My Review of Skills for Caregiving

California Older Person's Positive Experiences Schedule-Revised (COPPES-R)

Scoring Information and Instructions

Increasing daily rewarding, meaningful, and valued activities is a priority in treatment for depression. When clients cannot think of things on their own that are do-able and that improve mood, they benefit from completing the COPPES-R (Rider et al., 2016) to help "prime the pump." Along with the information provided in this appendix, additional resources for the COPPES-R, including an online administration and scoring tool, are provided at the Optimal Aging Center's website (www.optimalagingcenter.com). The actual COPPES-R scale is provided in the client workbook.

Most older adults with depression significantly reduce their frequency of engagement in everyday positive activities due to symptoms of anhedonia and fatigue. Some would like to do more of what they think will make them feel better but are unsure about where to start and how to "get going." Others start out feeling hopeless and convinced that nothing they do will make a difference in their depression. It is helpful for clients to reflect on the kinds of activities they have enjoyed in the past or might enjoy doing at this point in their lives, emphasizing small things (watching a favorite TV show, enjoying a special cup of tea, talking on the phone with a friend) that are do-able with minimal resources. The COPPES-R contains 46 items covering a broad range of simple everyday activities, such as "listening to sounds of nature." It is not an exhaustive list, however, and was created over a decade ago. The revised version provided here has been updated. There are no blank spaces built in to the questionnaire where unique individualized activities can be added—however, these individualized activities are crucial to the success of this behavioral activation approach, so ask clients to make note of them as well. Finally, some clients are unwilling or unable to complete COPPES-R; in those cases, it is wise to use alternative methods to obtain similar information (discussed later in this appendix).

For each COPPES-R item, the client is asked to give two ratings:

- The first is for how often the activity occurred in the past month: 0 = not at all, 1 = 1 to 6 times, and 2 = 7 or more times. If this seems confusing, you can reframe it this way: 0 = didn't happen; 1 = a few times, maybe once a week; and 2 = generally twice a week or more often, in the past month.
- The second is for how positive, rewarding, or valued it was, or would have been if it had happened. So even if frequency = 0 (it wasn't actually experienced), the client rates their likely level of experiencing the event as positive: 0 = not at all, 1 = somewhat, and 2 = very much. It can be easier to do the second rating if you explain it this way: 0 = was not (or would not have been) positive if it occurred; 1 = was (or would have been) somewhat positive; and 2 = was (or would have been) very positive.

We recommend that clinicians start doing the COPPES-R *in session* so that clients understand the instructions and are able to then complete it for home practice. Clients are also asked to note which items really strike them as appropriate and relevant, and to record activities they think might be rewarding or valued that come to their mind while completing COPPES-R. Ask clients to bring all of this with them to the next session so you can review the content in detail. If the client expresses reluctance, ask them to consider this to be an "experiment" to find out what will make them feel better. Their responses to the COPPES-R will then be used to encourage them to do these activities most or all days of the week. This is a tried-and-true method of improving depression in older adults. For most, that explanation is sufficient.

For clients who are unwilling to comply at this point, use alternative methods to generate information about potentially positive everyday activities. These include:

1. Asking what activities the client experienced as positive in the past ("even if you haven't done that activity in a long long time"). You can also ask why the client thinks they don't do x or y much anymore, noting barriers and then making plans to address them. Knowing their past employment and family histories is helpful to encourage discussion if the client is not able to generate much on their own.
2. Asking what the client can recall doing in the past week that "brings a smile to their face." Again, note responses and inquire how often these things are done currently, and gently explore what prevents these from being done more often. If the client cannot recall much, you can ask them to describe a "more or less good day" from the past week, which usually brings at least some positive activities to light.
3. Clinicians can start reading items from COPPES-R and recording responses in session. This is a very effective way to get the information without having a tug-of-war with the client over home practice.

In our experience, any or all of these methods can be effective as long as the clinician does them in the service of generating a personalized list of activities for the client to do more or less daily, to improve mood.

For those using the COPPES-R as part of treatment, we recommend that clinicians review the following information about how to interpret results before the next session and allow most (if not all) of a typical 45-minute session for review and discussion. The goals are (1) to create together an individualized list of potentially positive activities for clients to plan in their schedules and actually do before next session and (2) to begin to problem solve barriers and obstacles to their being able to do so.

1. Review which items (if any) are scored both 2 for frequency and 2 for being positive. These are things the person is doing fairly regularly to uplift their mood. It is good to note them and encourage the client to continue doing them but indicate they are not the focus for discussion.
2. Review the most productive pattern: Some of the COPPES-R items may be scored 0 for frequency and 2 for positivity. These are things the client would really like to be doing but isn't doing now. *These are key items to focus on.* Some of these activities will become targets to increase once it is clear what gets in the way of clients doing them. Often, discussing these activities (and associated barriers) stimulates discussion about related things the client might enjoy doing that aren't on the list and that are unique to them. The goal is to encourage the development of a list of positive activities that are highly individualized for each client.
3. Review the "in between" pattern: items that are scored 0 or 1 for frequency and 1 for positivity. These are "so-so," and the client's mood may possibly improve if these activities were included. Because these items are not as clear-cut, it is important to discuss these to understand their relevance.
4. Review items where frequency is 2 and positivity is 0. These are activities you can encourage the client to consider decreasing because they are not positive, rewarding, valued, or meaningful. Our focus here is on activities to *increase*. Do not attempt to problem-solve these items with the aim of increasing their perceived value. Depending upon the client's situation, you may focus on some of these items with the goal of reducing their frequency.

Clinician Note

Some clients do not complete the COPPES-R in its entirety—they may say that instructions were confusing or that they started it but were not able to finish. When that happens, we recommend that the COPPES-R be completed in session. Spend the remaining session time to begin to discern patterns of response, to be continued at next session.

During or after this review of response patterns, it is helpful to consider the items as fitting into five face-valid categories (Rider et al., 2016): socializing, relaxing, contemplating/reflecting, being effective, and being active (doing things). This can guide discussion about which domains are most meaningful for each client. In our experience, many clients observe that something they particularly like to do (whether or not they are actually doing it now) is missing from COPPES-R. For example, clients with a history of building or making things and organizing projects might not view any of the items as similar. But, given that background, it is likely they would enjoy "doing things" that they can still do. In those cases, these clients can be encouraged to think about what specifically could be built, created, or repaired at home or elsewhere, and what obstacles or barriers there might be to tackling such projects.

Some clients comment about the lack of items specific to family members—such as talking with their adult children or visiting with grandchildren. These are not explicit in the "socializing" domain but are likely to be important to clients for whom family has been a source of emotional support. Typically, these clients have stopped reaching out (or responding) to their families, and this emotional withdrawal is associated with their depression. Here again, the COPPES-R can be a springboard for discussion about this domain of activities. If activities in this category (ones that clients think of as positive, rewarding, or valued) are not on the list, you can add them to the individualized list of positive activities that will be generated as part of the plan for behavioral activation (Module 3: *Skills for Doing*).

Exactly which activities each client will choose to increase in order to improve mood is only learned by discussing not only COPPES-R items and activities that are not on COPPES-R but also those that the client brings up. Remember that the goal is to develop a daily tracking list of up to 10 potentially positive everyday activities that the client is likely to be able to do and/or increase (if already doing x or y but not often). To facilitate this, problem solving is essential. For example, if the client would enjoy "having a daily plan" but doesn't do that now, possible obstacles would be the belief that they are so poorly organized that it just won't work. Clearly, this activity will not be done/increased until the interfering thoughts of inadequacy and future failure are addressed. Reviewing the problem-solving approach recommended in Module 3: *Skills for Doing* will help with this, as well as keeping in mind that COPPES-R is not an "end in itself" but a "means to an end"—that end being increasing engagement in everyday positive activities. How these positive activities are identified is not as important as the fact that they *are* identified and are discussed sufficiently that the client feels "ready, willing, and able" to take some first small steps towards behavioral activation.

Clinical Tools and Measures

ADDRESSING Model Worksheet for Case Conceptualization

<u>Start 11 Learn: Celebrating Diversity</u> can be used with your clients to assess their most salient identities. Use this worksheet to aid in your case conceptualization for each client.

Definitions of ADDRESSING framework	Client name: *Record client information in each section below.*
Age and generational influences	
Disability status (developmental disability)	
Disability status (acquired physical / cognitive / psychological disabilities)	
Religion and spiritual orientation	
Ethnic and Racial identity	
Socioeconomic status	
Sexual orientation	
Indigenous heritage	
National origin	
Gender	

Client Initials: _____   Date:_____

GDS-SF

Circle the answer that best describes how you felt over the <u>past week</u>.

Yes   No   1. Are you basically satisfied with your life?*

Yes   No   2. Have you dropped many of your activities and interests?

Yes   No   3. Do you feel that your life is empty?

Yes   No   4. Do you often get bored?

Yes   No   5. Are you in good spirits most of the time?*

Yes   No   6. Are you afraid that something bad is going to happen to you?

Yes   No   7. Do you feel happy most of the time?*

Yes   No   8. Do you often feel helpless?

Yes   No   9. Do you prefer to stay at home, rather than going out and doing things?

Yes   No   10. Do you feel that you have more problems with memory than most?

Yes   No   11. Do you think it is wonderful to be alive now?*

Yes   No   12. Do you feel worthless the way you are now?

Yes   No   13. Do you feel full of energy?*

Yes   No   14. Do you feel that your situation is hopeless?

Yes   No   15. Do you think that most people are better off than you are?

Total Score: _____

(* items reverse scored)

Client Initials: _____   Date:_____

GAD-7

Please respond to each question or statement by selecting the option that fits you best. Over the past <u>*2 weeks,*</u> *how often have you been bothered by the following problems?*

	Not at all	Several days	More than half the days	Nearly half every
1. Feeling nervous, anxious or on edge	0	1	2	3
2. Not being able to stop or control worrying	0	1	2	3
3. Worrying too much about different things	0	1	2	3
4. Trouble relaxing	0	1	2	3
5. Being so restless that it is hard to sit still	0	1	2	3
6. Becoming easily annoyed or irritable	0	1	2	3
7. Feeling afraid as if something awful might happen	0	1	2	3

Client Initials: _____   Date:_____

_____

AD8
_____

Remember, "Yes, a change" indicates that you think there has been a change in the last several years caused by cognitive (thinking and memory) problems.

Circle your choice of "Yes, a change," "No, no change," "DK, Don't know."

Yes No DK   Problems with judgment (e.g. falls for scams, bad financial decisions, buys gifts inappropriate for recipients)

Yes No DK   Reduced interest in hobbies/activities

Yes No DK   Repeats questions, stories or statements

Yes No DK   Trouble learning how to use a tool, appliance or gadget (e.g. computer, microwave, remote control)

Yes No DK   Forgets correct month or year

Yes No DK   Difficulty handling complicated financial affairs (e.g. balancing checkbook, income taxes, paying bills)

Yes No DK   Difficulty remembering appointments

Yes No DK   Consistent problems with thinking and/or memory

Total Score: _____

Client Initials: _____   Date:_____

EASI-sa

These questions ask you about events that may occur in the daily lives of adults. All you have to do is circle Yes or No to answer each question.

<u>Over the last 12 months</u>

1. Have you relied on people for any of the following: bathing, dressing, shopping, banking or meals?   *Yes   No*

2. Has anyone prevented you from getting food, clothes, medication, glasses, hearing aids or medical care, or from being with people you wanted to be with?   *Yes   No*

3. Have you been upset because someone talked to you in a way that made you feel shamed or threatened?   *Yes   No*

4. Has anyone tried to force you to sign papers or to use your money against your will?   *Yes   No*

5. Has anyone made you afraid, touched you in ways that you did not want, or hurt you physically?   *Yes   No*

Yaffe, M. J., Weiss, D., & Lithwick, M. (2012). Seniors' self-administration of the Elder Abuse Suspicion Index (EASI): A feasibility study. *Journal of Elder Abuse & Neglect, 24*(4), 277–292. Reprinted by permission of the publisher (Taylor & Francis, LTD, https://www.tandfonline.com).

Client Initials: _____   Date:_____

SMAST-G

Directions: Circle Yes or No for these questions based on the <u>past year</u>.

1. When talking with others, do you ever underestimate how much you actually drink?	Yes	No
2. After a few drinks, have you sometimes not eaten or been able to skip a meal because you didn't feel hungry?	Yes	No
3. Does having a few drinks help decrease your shakiness or tremors?	Yes	No
4. Does alcohol sometimes make it hard for you to remember parts of the day or night?	Yes	No
5. Do you usually take a drink to relax or calm your nerves?	Yes	No
6. Do you drink to take your mind off your problems?	Yes	No
7. Have you ever increased your drinking after experiencing a loss in your life?	Yes	No
8. Has a doctor or nurse ever said they were worried or concerned about your drinking?	Yes	No
9. Have you ever made rules to manage your drinking?	Yes	No
10. When you feel lonely, does having a drink help?	Yes	No

Total SMAST-G Score (0–10): _____

Reprinted by permission from Springer Nature Customer Service Centre GmbH: Springer Nature, by Blow, F. C., & Barry, K. L. (2012). Alcohol and substance misuse in older adults. *Current Psychiatry Reports, 14*(4), 310–319.

Client Initials: _____   Date:_____

GSES

The following seven statements relate to your night-time sleep pattern in the past week. Please indicate by circling one response how true each statement is for you.

1. I put too much effort into sleeping when it should come naturally	Very much	To some extent	Not at all
2. I feel I should be able to control my sleep	Very much	To some extent	Not at all
3. I put off going to bed at night for fear of not being able to sleep.	Very much	To some extent	Not at all
4. I worry about not sleeping if I cannot sleep	Very much	To some extent	Not at all
5. I am no good at sleeping	Very much	To some extent	Not at all
6. I get anxious about sleeping before I go to bed	Very much	To some extent	Not at all
7. I worry about the consequences of not sleeping	Very much	To some extent	Not at all

Republished with permission of John Wiley & Sons from Broomfield, N. M., & Espie, C. A. (2005). Towards a valid, reliable measure of sleep effort. *Journal of Sleep Research, 14*(4), 401–407; permission conveyed through Copyright Clearance Center, Inc.

Client Initials: _____   Date:_____

Caregiving Intake Assessment Interview

(Clinician administered)

1. What is the caregiver's current living situation (e.g., with care recipient, other family members)? How many people are in the household? How many people does the caregiver provide care for (e.g., minor children, spouse, aunt, etc.)?
2. Is caregiver employed? Is there financial strain? Does care recipient have adequate income/insurance to support additional care if needed?
3. How distressed is the caregiver at this time? What words do they use to describe their distress? What emotions are expressed? Is there any mention of positive aspects of caregiving (as well as the negative ones)?
4. What are the primary diagnoses/problems of the care recipient? How do these impact daily life and daily demands for the caregiver?
5. How does the caregiver describe their coping strategies (e.g., problem solving, avoidance, cognitive reappraisal, self-care, activities outside of the home, exercise, overeating, alcohol misuse)?
6. How do the caregiver's cultural values and beliefs provide support or present obstacles (e.g., increased sense of burden, guilt) to effective caregiving?
7. How much support does the caregiver get from others on a regular basis? Who is in their social network? Who helps, and in what ways? What help is needed that the caregiver is not getting?
8. What kind of help and support does the caregiver believe would be most beneficial for their mental health and well-being (i.e., not just capacity to provide excellent care)?

Client Initials: _____   Date:_____

REACH II Risk Appraisal

(CR = Care recipient)

1. Do you have written information about memory loss, Alzheimer's Disease, or dementia?			
No	Yes		
1	0		

2. Can (CR) get to dangerous objects (e.g., loaded or unlocked gun, or sharp objects)?			
No	Yes		
0	1		

3. Do you ever leave (CR) alone or unsupervised in the home?			
Never	Sometimes	Often	Very Often
0	1	2	3

4. Does (CR) try to leave the home and wander outside?			
Never	Sometimes	Often	Very Often
0	1	2	3

5. Does (CR) drive?			
Never	Sometimes	Often	Very Often
0	1	2	3

6. Overall, how satisfied have you been in the past month with the help you have received from family members, friends, or neighbors?			
Not at all	A little	Moderately	Very
3	2	1	0

7. In the past month, have you had trouble falling asleep, staying asleep, or waking up too early in the morning?			
Never	Sometimes	Often	Very Often
0	1	2	3

8. In the past month, how satisfied have you been with the support, comfort, interest and concern you have received from others?			
Not at all	A little	Moderately	Very
3	2	1	0

9. In general, would you say your health is:

Excellent	Very good	Good	Fair	Poor
0	1	2	3	4

10. In the past week, have you felt depressed, sad, had crying spells or felt like you often needed to cry?

Rarely/None of the time (<1 day)	Sometimes (1-2 days)	Often (3-4 days)	Most or almost all of the time (5-7 days)
0	1	2	3

11. How often in the past six months have you felt like screaming or yelling at (CR) because of the way he/she behaved?

Never	Sometimes	Often	Very Often
0	1	2	3

12. How often in the past six months have you had to keep yourself from hitting or slapping (CR) because of the way he/she behaved?

Never	Sometimes	Often	Very Often
0	1	2	3

13. Do you feel stressed between caring for (CR) and trying to meet other responsibilities (work/family)?

Never	Sometimes	Often	Very Often
0	1	2	3

14. Do you feel strained (i.e. stressed, tense, or anxious) when you are around (CR)?

Never	Sometimes	Often	Very Often
0	1	2	3

15. Is it hard or stressful for you to help (CR) in basic daily activities, like bathing, changing clothes, brushing teeth, or shaving?

Never	Sometimes	Often	Very Often
0	1	2	3

16. Has providing help to (CR) made you feel good about yourself?

Disagree a lot	Disagree a little	Neither agree nor disagree	Agree a little	Agree a lot
4	3	2	1	0

Reproduced with permission from Czaja et al. (2009).

Scoring and interpretation: The RAM is a 16-item validated measure based on the REACH II 59-item baseline battery (Czaja et al., 2009). It targets six risk domains: depressive symptomatology, caregiver burden, self-care and healthy behaviors, social support, patient problem behaviors, and safety.

Total possible scores range from 0 to 40, with higher scores indicating a higher-risk caregiver. Depressive symptomatology is assessed by having the caregiver (CG) rate the degree to which they felt depressed in the last week (#10). Burden is assessed by having the CG rate the stress associated with caregiving responsibilities and the degree to which they feel good as a result of caregiving (#13, #14, #16). Self-care and healthy behaviors is assessed by asking the CGs about their own health or problems with sleep (#7, #9). Social support is assessed by having the CG rate their satisfaction with support from others (#6, #8). Patient problem behaviors is assessed by asking the caregiver if he/she has information about Alzheimer's disease and the degree to which difficulties are experienced trying to help the patient with basic activities (#1, #15). Two dimensions of safety are assessed: risk associated with the caregiver's behaviors (#11, #12) and risk associated with the patient's impairment (#2–#5).

Client Initials: _____   ᵃ Date:_____

CASE

Directions: Answer the following questions as helper or caregiver. Circle Yes or No.

1. Do you sometimes have trouble making (____) control his or her temper or aggression?   Yes   No

2. Do you often feel you are being forced to act out of character or do things that you feel bad about?   Yes   No

3. Do you find it difficult to manage (____'s) behavior?   Yes   No

4. Do you sometimes feel that you are forced to be rough with (____)?   Yes   No

5. Do you sometimes feel you can't do what is really necessary or what should be done for (____)?   Yes   No

6. Do you often feel you need to reject or ignore (____)?   Yes   No

7. Do you often feel so tired and exhausted that you cannot meet (____'s) needs?   Yes   No

8. Do you often feel you have to yell at (____)?   Yes   No

Reis, M., & Nahmiash, D. (1995). Validation of the Caregiver Abuse Screen (CASE). *Canadian Journal on Aging / La Revue Canadienne Du Vieillissement, 14*(S2), 45–60. Reproduced with permission by Cambridge University Press.

Client Initials: _____   Date: _____

TGI-SR

Instructions: This questionnaire contains two parts. Part 1 asks about the losses of loved ones you have been confronted with and Part 2 asks to what extent you experience grief reactions related to your most distressing loss.

Part 1: List the **most important** people in your life who have died.

- Write down the date (approximate) that the deceased persons died
- Indicate if these persons died by violent causes by circling Yes or No
  (death due to homicide, suicide or some unnatural cause)

Name: _____ Relationship: _____ Death date: _____ Violent? Yes No

Name: _____ Relationship: _____ Death date: _____ Violent? Yes No

Name: _____ Relationship: _____ Death date: _____ Violent? Yes No

Name: _____ Relationship: _____ Death date: _____ Violent? Yes No

Name: _____ Relationship: _____ Death date: _____ Violent? Yes No

Name: _____ Relationship: _____ Death date: _____ Violent? Yes No

Part 2: From the persons who died, listed in Part 1, please select one person whose death is currently mostly on your mind or is currently most distressing you. Write down the name of this person.

The loss that is currently mostly on my mind/distressing is the death of:_____

*Please circle a choice for how often you have experienced each reaction in the **past month**, in response to the death of this person:* _____

(N = Never, R = Rarely, S = Sometimes, F = Frequently and A = Always)

1. I had intrusive thoughts/images related to the person who died.   N   R   S   F   A

2. I experienced intense emotional pain, sadness or pangs of grief.   N   R   S   F   A

3. I found myself longing or yearning for the person who died.   N   R   S   F   A

4. I experienced confusion about my role in life or
   a diminished sense of self.   N   R   S   F   A

5. I had trouble accepting the loss.   N   R   S   F   A

6. I avoided places/objects or thoughts that reminded me
   that the person I lost has died.   N   R   S   F   A

7. It was hard for me to trust others.   N   R   S   F   A

8. I felt bitterness or anger related to his/her death.   N   R   S   F   A

9. I felt that moving on (e.g., making new friends, pursuing
   new interests) was difficult for me.   N   R   S   F   A

10. I felt emotionally numb.   N   R   S   F   A

11. I felt that life is unfulfilling or meaningless without him/her.   N   R   S   F   A

12. I felt stunned, shocked, or dazed by his/her death.   N   R   S   F   A

13. I noticed significant reduction in social, occupational, or other   N   R   S   F   A
    important areas of functioning as a result of his/her death.

14. I had intrusive thoughts and images associated with the   N   R   S   F   A
    circumstances of his/her death.

15. I had difficulty with positive reminiscing about the lost person.   N   R   S   F   A

16. I had negative thoughts about myself in relation to the   N   R   S   F   A
    loss (e.g., thoughts about self-blame).

17. I had a desire to die in order to be with the deceased.   N   R   S   F   A

18. I felt alone or detached from other individuals.   N   R   S   F   A

Boelen, P. A., Djelantik, A. M. J., de Keijser, J., Lenferink, L. I. M., & Smid, G. E. (2019). Further validation of the Traumatic Grief Inventory-Self Report (TGI-SR): A measure of persistent complex bereavement disorder and prolonged grief disorder. *Death Studies, 43*(6), 351–364. Reprinted by permission of the publisher (Taylor & Francis, LTD, https://www.tandfonline.com).

Client Initials: _____   Date:_____

Brief UBBS

*Directions: Circle your answer for how distressed you have been by this issue in the <u>**past month**</u>.*

	Not at all Distressed				Extremely Distressed
1. I wish we did more things together.	1	2	3	4	5
2. There were secrets in our relationship that should have been discussed.	1	2	3	4	5
3. I should have told him/her "I love you" more often.	1	2	3	4	5
4. I never got closure on some important issue or conflict in our relationship.	1	2	3	4	5
5. I wish I had told _____ how much s/he meant to me.	1	2	3	4	5
6. I feel that I need _____'s permission to live fully since s/he died.	1	2	3	4	5
7. I wish I would have taken my chance to say goodbye.	1	2	3	4	5
8. I feel a deep sense of anger toward _____ that I don't know how to resolve now that s/he is gone.	1	2	3	4	5

Holland, J. M., Klingspon, K. L., Lichtenthal, W. G., & Neimeyer, R. A. (2020). The Unfinished Business in Bereavement Scale (UBBS): Development and psychometric evaluation. *Death Studies, 44*(2), 65–77. Reprinted by permission of the publisher (Taylor & Francis, LTD, https://www.tandfonline.com).

Client Initials: _____   Date:_____

ARM-5

Thinking about today's meeting, circle the number for how strongly you agree or disagree with each item.

	Strongly Disagree	Disagree	Slightly Disagree	Neutral	Slightly Agree	Agree	Strongly Agree
1. My therapist is supportive.	1	2	3	4	5	6	7
2. My therapist and I agree about how to work together.	1	2	3	4	5	6	7
3. My therapist and I have difficulty working jointly as a partnership.	1	2	3	4	5	6	7
4. I have confidence in my therapist and her/his techniques.	1	2	3	4	5	6	7
5. My therapist is confident in her/himself and her/his techniques.	1	2	3	4	5	6	7

Cahill, J., Stiles, W. B., Barkham, M., Hardy, G. E., Stone, G., Agnew-Davies, R., & Unsworth, G. (2012). Two short forms of the Agnew Relationship Measure: The ARM-5 and ARM-12. *Psychotherapy Research, 22*(3), 241–255. Reprinted by permission of the publisher (Taylor & Francis, LTD, https://www.tandfonline.com).

Ann M. Steffen, PhD, ABPP, is a professor in the Department of Psychological Sciences at the University of Missouri-St. Louis, where she has spent her career in teaching, research, supervision, and direct clinical services focused on the needs of older adults and family caregivers. She earned her PhD in clinical psychology from Indiana University-Bloomington and completed a postdoctoral fellowship in clinical geropsychology at Stanford University School of Medicine. Dr. Steffen is a faculty clinician at the UM-St. Louis Community Psychological Service and is frequently invited to present professional training workshops on the most recent advances in cognitive-behavioral treatments with middle-aged and older adults. Dr. Steffen is a dual certified Diplomat in Behavioral and Cognitive Psychology (ABBCP) and a Diplomat in Geropsychology (ABGERO) of the American Board of Professional Psychology.

Larry W. Thompson, PhD, ABPP, is an emeritus professor from Stanford University School of Medicine, where he served as faculty for 20 years following faculty appointments at both Duke University School of Medicine and University of Southern California's Department of Psychology and Andrus Gerontology Center, where he developed the first clinical aging program in psychology. He is a pioneer in the field, having worked with academic partner and spouse (Dolores) to develop effective ways to use CBT with older adults, and to conduct several large-scale research studies, funded by NIMH, to evaluate its efficacy. During his time at the VA Palo Alto Health Care System he trained several hundred interns and postdoctoral fellows in clinical issues related to older adult mental health.

Dr. Thompson has had a stellar research career: He has published over 200 peer-reviewed articles (and given numerous presentations) documenting how well this treatment method works with this population. As well, he has collaborated with researchers in Australia, Spain, and the United Kingdom to expand the "reach" of CBT and is a senior consultant to several ongoing projects of a similar nature. He has received several prestigious awards, including the M. Powell Lawton award for lifetime contributions to the field of geropsychology.

In the past decade, Dr. Thompson has focused on training mental health clinicians in community-based clinics and organizations, and he thoroughly enjoys working with staff who are "in the trenches" when it comes to geriatric mental health. He is currently co-founder of the Optimal Aging Center (www.optimalagingcenter.com) and spends many hours giving back to the community through presentations and research consultations via that Center. He intends to continue these activities for many more years!

Dolores Gallagher-Thompson, PhD, ABPP, is currently an active emerita professor in the Department of Psychiatry and Behavioral Sciences at Stanford University School of Medicine and a Family Caregiving Institute Partner at the Betty Irene Moore School of Nursing, University of California at Davis. She has devoted her career to developing and researching innovative ways to apply CBT to the problems of middle-aged and older adults, including family caregivers of persons with Alzheimer's disease or another form of dementia. With her academic partner (and spouse) Larry, she has trained several hundred geropsychologists in the VA Palo Alto Health Care System; they were instrumental in the development of the credentialing process for a specialty in geropsychology and are foundational board members of the ABPP Geropsychology Specialty Board (ABGERO).

Dr. Gallagher-Thompson has over 200 peer-reviewed publications in professional journals and has given countless presentations on the "nuts and bolts" of doing CBT with older adults and their families. She has received numerous awards for her work, including the M. Powell Lawton award for lifetime contributions to the field of geropsychology.

She is co-founder of the Optimal Aging Center, a virtual platform for training professionals and providing education to the public (www. optimalagingcenter.com), as well as a senior consultant on several research programs related to family caregiving in diverse populations. And, she is always eager to mentor young investigators with similar research and clinical interests!

References

Adames, H. Y., & Tazeau, Y. N. (Eds.). (2020). *Caring for Latinxs with dementia in a globalized world: Behavioral and psychosocial treatments.* Springer Nature.

Aguilera, A., Garza, M. J., & Muñoz, R. F. (2010). Group cognitive behavioral therapy for depression in Spanish: Culture-sensitive manualized treatment in practice. *Journal of Clinical Psychology, 66*(8), 857–867.

Allen, R. S., Noh, H., Beck, L. N., & Smith, L. J. (2016). Caring for individuals near the end of life. In L. D. Burgio, J. E. Gaugler, & M. M. Hilgeman (Eds.), *The spectrum of family caregiving for adults and elders with chronic illness* (pp. 142–172). Oxford University Press.

Allen, R. S., Sun, F., Dorman, H. R., & Albright, A. E. (2018). Palliative and end-of-life care in the context of dementia. In G. E. Smith & S. T. Farias (Eds.), *APA handbook of dementia* (pp. 631–644). American Psychological Association.

Alzheimer's Association. (2020). Alzheimer's disease: Facts and figures. doi.org/10.1002/alz.12068

American Psychiatric Association. (2013). *Diagnostic and statistical manual of mental disorders* (5th ed.). American Psychiatric Publishing.

American Psychological Association. (2019). Clinical practice guideline for the treatment of depression across three age cohorts. https://www.apa.org/depression-guideline/guideline.pdf

Arnold, M. (2008). Polypharmacy and older adults: A role for psychology and psychologists. *Professional Psychology: Research and Practice, 39*(3), 283–289.

Ayers, C., Strickland, K., & Wetherell, J. L. (2015). Evidence-based treatment for late-life generalized anxiety disorder. In P. A. Areán (Ed.), *Treatment of late-life depression, anxiety, trauma, and substance abuse* (pp. 103–131). American Psychological Association.

Baltes, P. B., & Freund, A. M. (2003). Human strengths as the orchestration of wisdom and selective optimization with compensation. In L. G. Aspinwall & U. M. Staudinger (Eds.), *A psychology of human strengths: Fundamental questions and future directions for a positive psychology* (pp. 23–35). American Psychological Association.

Bandura, A. (1997). *Self-efficacy: The exercise of control*. Macmillan.

Barrera, T. L., Cummings, J. P., Armento, M., Cully, J. A., Bush Amspoker, A., Wilson, N. L., Mallen, M. J., Shrestha, S., Kunik, M. E., & Stanley, M. A. (2017). Telephone-delivered cognitive-behavioral therapy for older, rural veterans with depression and anxiety in home-based primary care. *Clinical Gerontologist, 40*(2), 114–123.

Beck, A. T. (1976). *Cognitive therapy and the emotional disorders*. International Universities Press.

Beck, A. T., Rush, J., & Shaw, B. (1979). *Cognitive therapy of depression*. Guilford Press.

Berking, M., Ebert, D., Cuijpers, P., & Hofmann, S. G. (2013). Emotion regulation skills training enhances the efficacy of inpatient cognitive behavioral therapy for major depressive disorder: A randomized controlled trial. *Psychotherapy and Psychosomatics, 82*(4), 234–245.

Bieling, P. J., McCabe, R. E., & Antony, M. M. (2009). *Cognitive-behavioral therapy in groups*. Guilford Press.

Bilbrey, A., Cassidy-Eagle, E., & Gallagher-Thompson, D. (2020a). Working with depressed caregivers: Behavioral activation. In L. B. Dunn & E. Cassidy-Eagle (Eds.), *Practical strategies in geriatric mental health: Cases and approaches* (pp. 31–41). American Psychiatric Association Press.

Bilbrey, A. C., Laidlaw, K., Cassidy-Eagle, E., Thompson, L. W., & Gallagher-Thompson, D. (2020b). Cognitive behavioral therapy for late-life depression: Evidence, issues, and recommendations. *Cognitive and Behavioral Practice*. https://doi.org/10.1016/j.cbpra.2020.02.003

Blackburn, I. M., James, I. A., Milne, D. L., Baker, C., Standart, S., Garland, A., & Reichelt, F. K. (2001). The Revised Cognitive Therapy Scale (CTS-R): Psychometric properties. *Behavioural and Cognitive Psychotherapy, 29*, 431–446.

Blazer, D. G., & Steffens, D. C. (2015). Depressive disorders. In D. C. Steffens, D. G. Blazer, & M. E. Thakur (Eds.), *The American Psychiatric Publishing textbook of geriatric psychiatry* (5th ed., pp. 243–282). American Psychiatric Publishing, Inc.

Blazer, D. G., & Wallace, R. B. (2016). Cognitive aging: What every geriatric psychiatrist should know. *American Journal of Geriatric Psychiatry, 24*(9), 776–781.

Blazer, D. G., Yaffe, K., & Liverman, C. T. (Eds.) (2015). *Cognitive aging: Progress in understanding and opportunities for action*. National Academies Press.

Blow, F. C., & Barry, K. L. (2012). Alcohol and substance misuse in older adults. *Current Psychiatry Reports, 14*(4), 310–319.

Blow, F. C., Gillespie, B. W., & Barry, K. L. (1998). Brief screening for alcohol problems in elderly populations using the Short Michigan Alcoholism Screening Test—Geriatric Version (SMAST-G). *Alcoholism: Clinical and Experimental Research*, *22*(3), 20–25.

Boelen, P. A., Djelantik, A. M. J., de Keijser, J., Lenferink, L. I. M., & Smid, G. E. (2019). Further validation of the Traumatic Grief Inventory-Self Report (TGI-SR): A measure of persistent complex bereavement disorder and prolonged grief disorder. *Death Studies*, *43*(6), 351–364.

Boelen, P. A., & Lensvelt-Mulders, G. J. (2005). Psychometric properties of the Grief Cognitions Questionnaire (GCQ). *Journal of Psychopathology and Behavioral Assessment*, *27*(4), 291–303.

Bower, E. S., Wetherell, J. L., Mon, T., & Lenze, E. J. (2015). Treating anxiety disorders in older adults: Current treatments and future directions. *Harvard Review of Psychiatry*, *23*(5), 329–342.

Braun, M. M., Karlin, B. E., & Zeiss, A. (2016). Cognitive-behavioral therapies in older adult populations. In C. M. Nezu & A. M. Nezu (Eds.), *Oxford handbook of cognitive and behavioral therapies* (pp. 349–362). Oxford University Press.

Breitbart, W. (2017). *Meaning-centered psychotherapy in the cancer setting: Finding meaning and hope in the face of suffering*. Oxford University Press.

Broomfield, N. M., & Espie, C. A. (2005). Towards a valid, reliable measure of sleep effort. *Journal of Sleep Research*, *14*(4), 401–407.

Brown, L. J. E., & Astell, A. J. (2012). Assessing mood in older adults: A conceptual review of methods and approaches. *International Psychogeriatrics*, *24*(8), 1197–1206.

Bryan, C. J., & Rudd, M. D. (2018). *Brief cognitive-behavioral therapy for suicide prevention*. Guilford Publications.

Burgio, L. D., Gaugler, J. E., & Hilgeman, M. M. (Eds.). (2016). *The spectrum of family caregiving for adults and elders with chronic illness*. Oxford University Press.

Burgio, L. D., & Wynn, M. J. (2021). *The REACH OUT Caregiver Support Program: A Skills Training Program for Caregivers of Persons with Dementia, Clinician Guide*. Oxford University Press.

Burke, L. A., & Neimeyer, R. A. (2014). Complicated spiritual grief I: Relation to complicated grief symptomatology following violent death bereavement. *Death Studies*, *38*(4), 259–267.

Byers, A. L., Covinsky, K. E., Barnes, D. E., & Yaffe, K. (2012). Dysthymia and depression increase risk of dementia and mortality among older veterans. *American Journal of Geriatric Psychiatry*, *20*(8), 664–672.

Cahill, J., Stiles, W. B., Barkham, M., Hardy, G. E., Stone, G., Agnew-Davies, R., & Unsworth, G. (2012). Two short forms of the Agnew Relationship Measure: The ARM-5 and ARM-12. *Psychotherapy Research, 22*(3), 241–255.

Carney, C. E., Buysse, D. J., Ancoli-Israel, S., Edinger, J. D., Krystal, A. D., Lichstein, K. L., & Morin, C. M. (2012). The consensus sleep diary: Standardizing prospective sleep self-monitoring. *Sleep, 35*(2), 287–302.

Castanho, T. C., Amorim, L., Zihl, J., Palha, J. A., Sousa, N., & Santos, N. C. (2014). Telephone-based screening tools for mild cognitive impairment and dementia in aging studies: A review of validated instruments. *Frontiers in Aging Neuroscience, 6*, 16. doi:10.3389/fnagi.2014.00016

Castonguay, L. G., Constantino, M. J., McAleavey, A. A., & Goldfried, M. R. (2010). The therapeutic alliance in cognitive-behavioral therapy. In J. C. Muran & J. P. Barber (Eds.), *The therapeutic alliance: An evidence-based guide to practice* (pp. 150–171). Guilford Press.

Catalan-Matamoros, D., Gomez-Conesa, A., Stubbs, B., & Vancampfort, D. (2016). Exercise improves depressive symptoms in older adults: An umbrella review of systematic reviews and meta-analyses. *Psychiatry Research, 244*, 202–209.

Cheng, S.-T., Au, A., Losada, A., Thompson, L. W., & Gallagher-Thompson, D. (2019). Psychological interventions for dementia caregivers: What we have achieved, what we have learned. *Current Psychiatry Reports, 21*, 59. https://doi.org/10.1007/s11920-019-1045-9

Cheng, S.-T., Li, K.-K., Losada, A., Zhang, F., Au, A., Thompson, L. W., & Gallagher-Thompson, D. (2020). The effectiveness of nonpharmacological interventions for informal dementia caregivers: An updated systematic review and meta-analysis. *Psychology and Aging, 35*, 55–77.

Cheng, S.-T., Mak, E. P., Fung, H., Kwok, T., Lee, D. T., & Lam, L. C. (2017). Benefit-finding and effect on caregiver depression: A double-blind randomized controlled trial. *Journal of Consulting and Clinical Psychology, 85*(5), 521–529.

Chochinov, H. (2012). *Dignity therapy: Final words for final days.* Oxford University Press.

Clauss-Ehlers, C. S., Chiriboga, D. A., Hunter, S. J., Roysircar, G., & Tummala-Narra, P. (2019). APA Multicultural Guidelines executive summary: Ecological approach to context, identity, and intersectionality. *American Psychologist, 74*(2), 232–244.

Conti, E. C., Kraus-Schuman, C., & Stanley, M. A. (2017). Cognitive-behavioral therapy in older adults. In S. G. Hofmann & G. J. G.

Asmundson (Eds.), *Science of cognitive behavioral therapy* (pp. 223–255). Academic Press.

Coon, D. W., & Thompson, L. W. (2003). Association between homework compliance and treatment outcome among older adult outpatients with depression. *American Journal of Geriatric Psychiatry, 11,* 53–61.

Coon, D. W., Thompson, L. W., & Gallagher-Thompson, D. (2007) Adapting homework for an older adult client with cognitive impairment. *Cognitive and Behavioral Practice, 14*(3), 252–260.

Cuijpers, P., Ebert, D. D., Acarturk, C., Andersson, G., & Cristea, I. A. (2016). Personalized psychotherapy for adult depression: A meta-analytic review. *Behavior Therapy, 47*(6), 966–980.

Cuijpers, P., Karyotaki, E., Pot, A. M., Park, M., & Reynolds III, C. F. (2014). Managing depression in older age: Psychological interventions. *Maturitas, 79*(2), 160–169.

Cuijpers, P., Karyotaki, E., Reijnders, M., & Huibers, M. J. H. (2018). Who benefits from psychotherapies for adult depression? A meta-analytic update of the evidence. *Cognitive Behaviour Therapy, 47*(2), 91–106.

Cuijpers, P., van Straten, A., Smit, F., & Andersson, G. (2009). Is psychotherapy for depression equally effective in younger and older adults? A meta-regression analysis. *International Psychogeriatrics, 21*(1), 16–24.

Czaja, S. J., Gitlin, L. N., Schulz, R., Zhang, S., Burgio, L. D., Stevens, A. B., Nichols, L. O., & Gallagher-Thompson, D. (2009). Development of the risk appraisal measure: a brief screen to identify risk areas and guide interventions for dementia caregivers. *Journal of the American Geriatrics Society, 57*(6), 1064–1072.

Decaporale-Ryan, L., Warren, A. R., & Steffen, A. M. (in press). Interprofessional teams and psychology. In G. Asmundson (Ed.), *Comprehensive clinical psychology* (2nd ed.). Elsevier.

Dennis, J. P., & Brown, G. K. (2011). Suicidal older adults: Suicide risk assessments, safety planning, and cognitive behavioral therapy. In K. H. Sorocco & S. Lauderdale (Eds.), *Cognitive behavior therapy with older adults: Innovations across care settings* (pp. 95–123). Springer.

Diedrich, A., Hofmann, S. G., Cuijpers, P., & Berking, M. (2016). Self-compassion enhances the efficacy of explicit cognitive reappraisal as an emotion regulation strategy in individuals with major depressive disorder. *Behaviour Research and Therapy, 82,* 1–10.

DiGiuseppe, R., David, D., & Venezia, R. (2016). Cognitive theories. In J. C. Norcross, G. R. VandenBos, & D. K. Freedheim (Eds.), *APA handbook of clinical psychology: Theory and research* (pp. 145–182). American Psychological Association.

Dimidjian, S., Barrera, M. Jr., Martell, C., Muñoz, R. F., & Lewinsohn, P. M. (2011). The origins and current status of behavioral activation treatments for depression. *Annual Review of Clinical Psychology, 7*, 1–38.

Edelstein, B. A., & Segal, D. L. (2011). Assessment of emotional and personality disorders in older adults. In K. W. Schaie & S. L. Willis (Eds.), *Handbook of the psychology of aging* (7th ed., pp. 325–337). Elsevier Academic Press.

Epstein-Lubow, G., Gaudiano, BA, Hinckley, M., Salloway, S., & Miller, I. W. (2010). Evidence for the validity of the American Medical Association's Caregiver Self-Assessment Questionnaire as a screening measure for depression. *Journal of the American Geriatrics Society, 58*(2), 387–388.

Etxeberria, I., Salaberria, K., & Gorostiaga, A. (2020). Online support for family caregivers of people with dementia: A systematic review and meta-analysis of RCTs and quasi-experimental studies. *Aging & Mental Health*. https://doi.org/10.1080/13607863.2020.1758900

Fernandez, E., Salem, D., Swift, J. K., & Ramtahal, N. (2015). Meta-analysis of dropout from cognitive behavioral therapy: Magnitude, timing, and moderators. *Journal of Consulting and Clinical Psychology, 83*(6), 1108–1122.

Fishman, D. B. (2016). Behavioral theories. In J. C. Norcross, G. R. VandenBos, & D. K. Freedheim (Eds.), *APA handbook of clinical psychology: Theory and research* (pp. 79–115). American Psychological Association.

Fiske, A., Wetherell, J. L., & Gatz, M. (2009). Depression in older adults. *Annual Review of Clinical Psychology, 5*, 363–389.

Folke, F., Kanter, J. W., & Ekselius, L. (2016). Integrating behavioural activation into acute inpatient services. *Journal of Psychiatric Intensive Care, 12*(2), 109–118.

Freund, A. M., & Baltes, P. B. (2007). Toward a theory of successful aging: Selection, optimization, and compensation. In R. Fernández-Ballesteros (Ed.), *Geropsychology: European perspectives for an aging world* (pp. 239–254). Hogrefe & Huber Publishers.

Fried, E. I., Epskamp, S., Nesse, R. M., Tuerlinckx, F., & Borsboom, D. (2016). What are "good" depression symptoms? Comparing the centrality of DSM and non-DSM symptoms of depression in a network analysis. *Journal of Affective Disorders, 189*, 314–320.

Friedman, B., Heisel, M. J., & Delavan, R. L. (2005). Psychometric properties of the 15-item Geriatric Depression Scale in functionally impaired, cognitively intact, community-dwelling elderly primary care patients. *Journal of the American Geriatric Society, 53*(9), 1570–1576.

Fruzzetti, A. E., & Ruork, A. K. (2019). Validation principles and practices in dialectical behaviour therapy. In M. A. Swales (Ed.), *Oxford handbook of dialectical behaviour therapy* (pp. 325–344). Oxford University Press.

Galatzer-Levy, I. R., & Bonanno, G. A. (2012). Beyond normality in the study of bereavement: Heterogeneity in depression outcomes following loss in older adults. *Social Science & Medicine, 74*(12), 1987–1994.

Gallagher, D. E., & Thompson, L. W. (1982). Treatment of major depressive disorder in older adult outpatients with brief psychotherapies. *Psychotherapy: Theory, Research and Practice, 19*(4), 482–490.

Gallagher-Thompson, D., Arean, P., Rivera, P., & Thompson, L. W. (2001). A psychoeducational intervention to reduce distress in Hispanic family caregivers: Results of a pilot study. *Clinical Gerontologist, 23*(1/2), 17–32.

Gallagher-Thompson, D., Bilbrey, A. C., Apesoa-Varano, E. S., Ghatak, R., Kim, K. K., & Cothran, F. A. (2020a). Conceptual framework to guide intervention research across the trajectory of dementia caregiving. *The Gerontologist, 60*(S1), S29–S40.

Gallagher-Thompson, D., Bilbrey, A. C., Cassidy-Eagle, E. L. & Thompson, L. W. (2020b). Late-life depression. In L. B. Dunn & E. L. Cassidy-Eagle (Eds.), *Practical strategies in geriatric mental health: Cases and Approaches* (pp. 1–14). American Psychiatric Association.

Gallagher-Thompson, D., Coon, D. W., Solano, N., Ambler, C., Rabinowitz, Y., & Thompson, L. W. (2003). Change in indices of distress among Latina and Anglo female caregivers of elderly relatives with dementia: Site-specific results from the REACH national collaborative study. *The Gerontologist, 43*(4), 580–591.

Gallagher-Thompson, D., Gray, H. L., Dupart, T., Jimenez, D., & Thompson, L. W. (2008). Effectiveness of cognitive/behavioral small group intervention for reduction of depression and stress in Non-Hispanic White and Hispanic/Latino women dementia family caregivers: Outcomes and mediators of change. *Journal of Rational-Emotive and Cognitive-Behavior Therapy, 26*, 286–303.

Gallagher-Thompson, D., Gray, H., Tang, P., Pu, C.-Y., Tse, C., Hsu, S., Leung, L., Wang, P., Kwo, E., Tong, H.-Q., Long, J., & Thompson, L. W. (2007). Impact of in-home intervention versus telephone support in reducing depression and stress of Chinese caregivers: Results of a pilot study. *American Journal of Geriatric Psychiatry, 15*, 425–434.

Gallagher-Thompson, D., Hanley-Peterson, P., & Thompson, L. (1990). Maintenance of gains versus relapse following brief psychotherapy for depression. *Journal of Consulting and Clinical Psychology, 58*(3), 371–374.

Gallagher-Thompson, D., Steffen, A., & Thompson, L. W. (Eds.). (2008). *Handbook of behavioral and cognitive therapies with older adults.* Springer.

Gallagher-Thompson, D., & Thompson, L. W. (2010). Effectively using cognitive/behavioral therapy with the oldest old: Case examples and issues for consideration. In N. A. Pachana, K. Laidlaw, & B. Knight (Eds.), *Casebook of clinical geropsychology: International perspectives on practice* (pp. 227–241). Oxford University Press.

Gallagher-Thompson, D., & Thompson, L. W. (2021). Working successfully with older persons on the dementia continuum, and their informal caregivers. In N. Pachana, V. Molinari, L. W. Thompson, & D. Gallagher-Thompson (Eds.), *Psychological assessment and treatment of older adults* (pp. 123–138). Hogrefe.

Gallagher-Thompson, D., Tzuang, Y., Au, A., Brodaty, H., Charlesworth, G., Gupta, R., Lee, S. E., Losada, A., & Shyu, Y.-I. (2012). International perspectives on nonpharmacological best practices for dementia family caregivers: A review. *Clinical Gerontologist, 35*(4), 316–355.

Gallagher-Thompson, D., Wang, P-C., Liu, W., Cheung, V., Peng, R., China, D., & Thompson, L. W. (2010). Effectiveness of a psychoeducational skill training DVD program to reduce stress in Chinese American dementia caregivers. *Aging and Mental Health, 14*(3), 263–273.

Galvin, J. E., Roe, C. M., Powlishta, K. K., Coats, M. A., Muich, S. J., Grant, E., Miller, J. P., Storandt, M., & Morris, J. C. (2005). The AD8: A brief informant interview to detect dementia. *Neurology, 65*(4), 559–564.

Gentry, M. T., Lapid, M. I., & Rummans, T. A. (2019). Geriatric telepsychiatry: Systematic review and policy considerations. *American Journal of Geriatric Psychiatry, 27*(2), 109–127.

Georgakis, M. K., Papadopoulos, F. C., Protogerou, A. D., Pagonari, I., Sarigianni, F., Biniaris-Georgallis, S.-I., Kalogirou, E. I., Thomopoulos, T. P., Kapaki, E., Papageorgiou, C., Papageorgiou, S. G., Tousoulis, D., & Petridou, E. T. (2016). Comorbidity of cognitive impairment and late-life depression increase mortality: Results from a cohort of community-dwelling elderly individuals in rural Greece. *Journal of Geriatric Psychiatry and Neurology, 29*(4), 195–204.

Gerolimatos, L. A., Gregg, J. J., & Edelstein, B. A. (2014). Interviewing older adults. In N. A. Pachana & K. Laidlaw (Eds.), *Oxford handbook of clinical geropsychology* (pp. 163–183). Oxford University Press.

Gilbert, P. (2010). An introduction to compassion focused therapy in cognitive behavior therapy. *International Journal of Cognitive Therapy, 3*(2), 97–112.

Gilbert, P. (Ed.). (2017). *Compassion: Concepts, research and applications.* Taylor & Francis.

Glover, J. A., & Srinivasan, S. (2017). Assessment and treatment of late-life depression. *Journal of Clinical Outcomes Management, 24*(3).

Glueck, D., Myers, K., & Turvey, C. L. (2013). Establishing therapeutic rapport in telemental health. In K. Myers & C. L. Turvey (Eds.), *Telemental health: Clinical, technical and administrative foundations for evidence-based practice* (pp. 29–46). Newnes Press.

Gould, C. E., Karna, R., Jordan, J., Kawai, M., Hirst, R., Hantke, N., Pirog, S., Cotto, I., Schussler-Fiorenza Rose, S. M., Beaudreau, S. A., & O'Hara, R. (2018). Subjective but not objective sleep is associated with subsyndromal anxiety and depression in community-dwelling older adults. *American Journal of Geriatric Psychiatry, 26*(7), 806–811.

Greenwald, P., Stern, M. E., Clark, S., & Sharma, R. (2018). Older adults and technology: In telehealth, they may not be who you think they are. *International Journal of Emergency Medicine, 11*(1), 2–4.

Gregg, J. J., Fiske, A., & Gatz, M. (2013). Physicians' detection of late-life depression: The roles of dysphoria and cognitive impairment. *Aging & Mental Health, 17*(8), 1030–1036.

Haber, D. (2016). *Health promotion and aging: Practical applications for health professionals* (7th ed.). Springer.

Haigh, E. A. P., Bogucki, O. E., Sigmon, S. T., & Blazer, D. G. (2018). Depression among older adults: A 20-year update on five common myths and misconceptions. *American Journal of Geriatric Psychiatry, 26*(1), 107–122.

Harerimana, B., Forchuk, C., & O'Regan, T. (2019). The use of technology for mental healthcare delivery among older adults with depressive symptoms: A systematic literature review. *International Journal of Mental Health Nursing, 28*(3), 657–670.

Harvey, A. G., Lee, J., Williams, J., Hollon, S. D., Walker, M. P., Thompson, M. A., & Smith, R. (2014). Improving outcome of psychosocial treatments by enhancing memory and learning. *Perspectives in Psychological Science, 9*, 161–179.

Hawley, L. L., Padesky, C. A., Hollon, S. D., Mancuso, E., Laposa, J. M., Brozina, K., & Segal, Z. V. (2017). Cognitive-behavioral therapy for depression using *Mind Over Mood*: CBT skill use and differential symptom alleviation. *Behavior Therapy, 48*(1), 29–44.

Hayes, S. C., & Hofmann, S. G. (Eds.). (2018). *Process-based CBT: The science and core clinical competencies of cognitive behavioral therapy.* New Harbinger Publications.

Hays, P. A. (2012). *Connecting across cultures: The helper's toolkit*. Sage Publications.

Hays, P. A. (2016). *Addressing cultural complexities in practice: Assessment, diagnosis, and therapy* (3rd ed.). American Psychological Association.

Hershenberg, R. (2017). *Activating happiness: A jump-start guide to overcoming low motivation, depression, or just feeling stuck*. New Harbinger Publications.

Hinrichsen, G. A. (2020). *Assessment and treatment of older adults: A guide for mental health professionals*. American Psychological Association.

Hofmann, S. G. (2016). *Emotion in therapy: From science to practice*. Guilford Press.

Holland, J. M., Klingspon, K. L., Lichtenthal, W. G., & Neimeyer, R. A. (2020). The Unfinished Business in Bereavement Scale (UBBS): Development and psychometric evaluation. *Death Studies, 44*(2), 65–77.

Holsinger, T., Plassman, B. L., Stechuchak, K. M., Burke, J. R., Coffman, C. J., & Williams, J. W. Jr. (2012). Screening for cognitive impairment: Comparing the performance of four instruments in primary care. *Journal of the American Geriatric Society, 60*(6), 1027–1036.

Hope, D. A., Heimberg, R. B., & Turk, C. L. (2019a). *Managing social anxiety, workbook: A cognitive-behavioral therapy approach* (3rd ed.). Oxford University Press.

Hope, D. A., Heimberg, R. B., & Turk, C. L. (2019b). *Managing social anxiety, therapist guide: A cognitive-behavioral therapy approach* (3rd ed.). Oxford University Press.

Ince, B. Ü., Riper, H., van't Hof, E., & Cuijpers, P. (2014). The effects of psychotherapy on depression among racial-ethnic minority groups: A metaregression analysis. *Psychiatric Services, 65*(5), 612–617.

Ivey, K., Allen, R. S., Liu, Y., Parmelee, P. A., & Zarit, S. H. (2018). Immediate and lagged effects of daily stress and affect on caregivers' daily pain experience. *The Gerontologist, 58*(5), 913–922.

Iwamasa, G. Y., & Hays, P. A. (Eds.) (2019). *Culturally responsive cognitive behavior therapy: Practice and supervision* (2nd ed.). American Psychological Association.

James, I. A., Blackburn, I. M., & Reichelt, F. K. (2001). *Manual of the Revised Cognitive Therapy Scale (CTS-R)*. Newcastle Cognitive and Behavioural Therapies Centre, Newcastle, UK.

Jobes, D. A. (2016). *Managing suicidal risk: A collaborative approach* (2nd ed.). Guilford Press.

Jordan, J. R., & McGann, V. (2017). Clinical work with suicide loss survivors: Implications of the US Postvention Guidelines. *Death Studies, 41*(10), 659–672.

Judd, L. L., & Akiskal, H. S. (2002). The clinical and public health relevance of current research on subthreshold depressive symptoms to elderly patients. *American Journal of Geriatric Psychiatry, 10*(3), 233–238.

Kaiser, A. P., Cook, J., Glick, D., & Moye, J. (2019). Posttraumatic stress disorder in older adults: A conceptual review. *Clinical Gerontologist, 42*(4), 359–376.

Kane, K. D., Yochim, B. P., & Lichtenberg, P. A. (2010). Depressive symptoms and cognitive impairment predict all-cause mortality in long-term care residents. *Psychology and Aging, 25*(2), 446–452.

Kanfer, F. H., & Schefft, B. K. (1988). *Guiding the process of therapeutic change*. Research Press.

Kanter, J. W., Manos, R. C., Bowe, W. M., Baruch, D. E., Busch, A. M., & Rusch, L. C. (2010). What is behavioral activation? A review of the empirical literature. *Clinical Psychology Review, 30*, 608–620.

Kanter, J. W., & Puspitasari, A. J. (2016). Global dissemination and implementation of behavioural activation. *Lancet, 388*(10047), 843–844.

Karlin, B. E., Trockel, M., Brown, G. K., Gordienko, M., Yesavage, J., & Taylor, C. B. (2015). Comparison of the effectiveness of cognitive behavioral therapy for depression among older versus younger veterans: Results of a national evaluation. *Journals of Gerontology, 70*(1), 3–12.

Karpiak, C. P., Norcross, J. C., & Wedding, D. (2016). Evolution of theory in clinical psychology. In J. C. Norcross, G. R. VandenBos, & D. K. Freedheim (Eds.), *APA handbook of clinical psychology: Theory and research* (pp. 3–17). American Psychological Association.

Kaufer, D. I., Cummings, J. L., Ketchel, P., Smith, V., MacMillan, A., Shelley, T., Lopez, O. L., & DeKosky, S. T. (2000). Validation of the NPI-Q, a brief clinical form of the Neuropsychiatric Inventory. *Journal of Neuropsychiatry and Clinical Neurosciences, 12*(2), 233–239.

Kay, D. B., Dombrovski, A. Y., Buysse, D. J., Reynolds, C. F., III, Begley, A., & Szanto, K. (2016). Insomnia is associated with suicide attempt in middle-aged and older adults with depression. *International Psychogeriatrics, 28*(4), 613–619.

Kazantzis, N., Whittington, C., & Dattilio, F. (2010). Meta-analysis of homework effects in cognitive and behavioral therapy: A replication and extension. *Clinical Psychology: Science and Practice, 17*, 144–156.

Kazdin, A. E., & Blase, S. L. (2011). Rebooting psychotherapy research and practice to reduce the burden of mental illness. *Perspectives on Psychological Science, 6*(1), 21–37.

Kimerling, R. E., Zeiss, A. M., & Zeiss, R. A. (2000). Therapist emotional responses to patients: Building a learning-based language. *Cognitive and Behavioral Practice, 7*(3), 312–321.

Knight, B. G., & Pachana, N. A. (2015). *Psychological assessment and therapy with older adults.* Oxford University Press.

Koerner, K. (2012). *Doing dialectical behavior therapy: A practical guide.* Guilford Press.

Koerner, K., & Linehan, M. M. (2004). Validation principles and strategies. In W. T. O'Donohue & J. E. Fisher (Eds.), *Cognitive behavior therapy: Applying empirically supported techniques in your practice* (p. 456–462). Wiley.

Krause, N., Pargament, K. I., Hill, P. C., & Ironson, G. (2019). Exploring religious and/or spiritual identities: Part 2—A descriptive analysis of those who are at risk for health problems. *Mental Health, Religion & Culture, 22*(9), 892–909.

Kraus-Schuman, C., Wilson, N. L., Amspoker, A. B., Wagener, P. D., Calleo, J. S., Diefenbach, G., Hopko, D., Cully, J. A., Teng, E., Rhoades, H. M., Kunik, M. E., & Stanley, M. A. (2015). Enabling lay providers to conduct CBT for older adults: Key steps for expanding treatment capacity. *Translational Behavioral Medicine, 5*(3), 247–253.

Kroenke, K., Spitzer, R. L., & Williams, J. B. (2001). The PHQ-9: Validity of a brief depression screening measure. *Journal of General Internal Medicine, 16,* 606–613.

Laidlaw, K. (2015). *CBT for older people: An introduction.* Sage Publications.

Laidlaw, K., & Thompson, L. W. (2014). *Cognitive-behaviour therapy with older people.* In N. A. Pachana & K. Laidlaw (Eds.), *Oxford handbook of clinical geropsychology* (pp. 603–621). Oxford University Press.

Laidlaw, K., Thompson, L. W., Gallagher-Thompson, D., & Dick-Siskin, L. (2003). *Cognitive behaviour therapy with older people.* John Wiley & Sons.

Lau, A. W., & Kinoshita, L. M. (2019). Cognitive behavior therapy with culturally diverse older adults. In G. Y. Iwamasa & P. A. Hays (Eds.), *Culturally responsive cognitive behavior therapy: Practice and supervision* (pp. 231–256). American Psychological Association.

Lawton, M. P., & Brody, E. M. (1969). Assessment of older people: Self-maintaining and instrumental activities of daily living. *The Gerontologist, 9*(3, Part 1), 179–186.

Levy, S. R. (2018). Toward reducing ageism: PEACE (Positive Education about Aging and Contact Experiences) model. *The Gerontologist, 58*(2), 226–232.

Lewinsohn, P. M., Hoberman, H., Teri, L., & Hautzinger, M. (1985). An integrative theory of depression. In S. Reiss & R. R. Bootzin (Eds.), *Theoretical issues in behavior therapy* (pp. 331–359). Academic Press.

Lewinsohn, P. M., Munoz, R. F., Youngren, M. A., & Zeiss, A. M. (1986). *Control your depression: Revised and updated* (2nd ed.). Prentice Hall.

Li, M. J., Kechter, A., Olmstead, R. E., Irwin, M. R., & Black, D. S. (2018). Sleep and mood in older adults: Coinciding changes in insomnia and depression symptoms. *International Psychogeriatrics, 30*(3), 431–435.

Lichtenberg, P. A. (Ed.). (2010). *Handbook of assessment in clinical gerontology* (2nd ed.). Elsevier Academic Press.

Lichtenberg, P. A., Mast, B. T., Carpenter, B. D., & Loebach Wetherell, J. (Eds.). (2015). *APA handbook of clinical geropsychology, Vol. 2: Assessment, treatment, and issues of later life*. American Psychological Association.

Linehan, M. M. (1997). Validation and psychotherapy. In A. C. Bohart & L. S. Greenberg (Eds.), *Empathy reconsidered: New directions in psychotherapy* (pp. 353–392). American Psychological Association.

Linehan, M. M. (2015). *DBT® skills training manual* (2nd ed.). Guilford Press.

Livingston, G., Huntley, J., Sommerlad, A., Ames, D., Ballard, C., Banerjee, S., Brayne, C., Burns, A., Cohen-Mansfield, J., Cooper, C., Costafreda, S.G., Dias, A., Fox, N., Gitlin, L.N., Howard, R., Kales, H.C., Kivimäki, M., Larson, E.B., Ogunniyi, A., Orgeta, V., et al. (2020). Dementia prevention, intervention, and care: 2020 Report of the Lancet Commission. *Lancet, 396*(10248), 413–446.

Livingston, G., Sommerlad, A., Orgeta, V., Costafreda, S. G., Huntley, J., Ames, D., Ballard, C., Banerjee, S., Burns, A., Cohen-Mansfield, J., Cooper, C., Fox, N., Gitlin, L.N., Howard, R., Kales, H.C., Larson, E.B., Ritchie, K., Rockwood, K., Sampson, E.L., Samus, Q., et al. (2017). Dementia prevention, intervention, and care. *Lancet, 390*, 2673–2734.

Llorente, M. (Ed.). (2018). *Culture, heritage, and diversity in older adult mental health care*. American Psychiatric Association.

Lorig, K., Laurent, D., Schreiber, R., Gecht-Silver, M., Gallagher-Thompson, D., Minor, M., Gonzalez, V., Sobel, D., & Lee, D. (2018). *Building better caregivers*. Bull Publishing.

Lutz, J., & Fiske, A. (2018). Functional disability and suicidal behavior in middle-aged and older adults: A systematic critical review. *Journal of Affective Disorders, 227*, 260–271.

Lutz, J. A., Gallegos, J. V., & Edelstein, B. A. (2018). Assessment of psychopathology in older adults. In J. N. Butcher & J. M. Hooley (Eds.), *APA handbook of psychopathology: Psychopathology: Understanding, assessing, and treating adult mental disorders, Vol. 1* (pp. 273–299). American Psychological Association.

Luxton, D. D., Nelson, E. L., & Maheu, M. M. (2016). *A practitioner's guide to telemental health: How to conduct legal, ethical, and evidence-based telepractice.* American Psychological Association.

Lynch, T. R., Cheavens, J. S., Cukrowicz, K. C., Thorp, S. R., Bronner, L., & Beyer, J. (2007). Treatment of older adults with co-morbid personality disorder and depression: A dialectical behavior therapy approach. *International Journal of Geriatric Psychiatry, 22*(2), 131–143.

Lyon, A. R., & Koerner, K. (2016). User-centered design for psychosocial intervention development and implementation. *Clinical Psychology: Science and Practice, 23*(2), 180–200.

Maragakis, A., & O'Donohue, W. T. (Eds.) (2018). *Principle-based stepped care and brief psychotherapy for integrated care settings.* Springer.

Martell, C. R., Dimidjian, S., & Herman-Dunn, R. (2010). *Behavioral activation for depression: A clinician's guide.* Guilford Press.

Mazzucchelli, T. G., Kanter, J. W., & Martell, C. R. (2016). A clinician's quick guide of evidence-based approaches: Behavioural activation. *Clinical Psychologist, 20*(1), 54–55.

McCrae, C. S., Petrov, M. E., Dautovich, N., & Lichstein, K. L. (2016). Late-life sleep and sleep disorders. In K. W. Schaie & S. L. Willis (Eds.), *Handbook of the psychology of aging* (pp. 429–445). Academic Press.

McCrae, C. S., Roth, A. J., Zamora, R., Dautovich, N. D., & Lichstein, K. L. (2015). Late-life sleep and sleep disorders. In P. A. Lichtenberg, B. T. Mast, B. D. Carpenter, & J. Loebach Wetherell (Eds.), *APA handbook of clinical geropsychology, Vol. 2: Assessment, treatment, and issues of later life* (pp. 369–394). American Psychological Association.

McKay, M., Davis, M., & Fanning, P. (2018). *Messages: The communication skills book* (4th ed.). New Harbinger Press.

Meeks, S., Looney, S. W., Van Haitsma, K., & Teri, L. (2008). BE-ACTIV: A staff-assisted behavioral intervention for depression in nursing homes. *The Gerontologist, 48*(1), 105–114.

Meeks, S., Van Haitsma, K., Schoenbachler, B., & Looney, S. W. (2015). BE-ACTIV for depression in nursing homes: Primary outcomes of a randomized clinical trial. *Journals of Gerontology Series B: Psychological Sciences and Social Sciences, 70*(1), 13–23.

Meeks, S., Van Haitsma, K., & Shryock, S. K. (2019). Treatment fidelity evidence for BE-ACTIV: A behavioral intervention for depression in nursing homes. *Aging & Mental Health, 23*(9), 1192–1202.

Meeks, T. W., Vahia, I. V., Lavretsky, H., Kulkarni, G., & Jeste, D. V. (2011). A tune in "A minor" can "B major": A review of epidemiology, illness course, and public health implications of subthreshold depression in older adults. *Journal of Affective Disorders, 129*(1–3), 126–142.

Mitchell, A. J., Bird, V., Rizzo, M., & Meader, N. (2010). Diagnostic validity and added value of the Geriatric Depression Scale for depression in primary care: A meta-analysis of GDS30 and GDS15. *Journal of Affective Disorders, 125*(1), 10–17.

Monson, E., Lonergan, M., Caron, J., & Brunet, A. (2016). Assessing trauma and posttraumatic stress disorder: Single, open-ended question versus list-based inventory. *Psychological Assessment, 28*(8), 1001–1008.

Moshier, S. J., & Otto, M. W. (2017). Behavioral activation treatment for major depression: A randomized trial of the efficacy of augmentation with cognitive control training. *Journal of Affective Disorders, 210*, 265–268.

Moye, J., Marson, D. C., & Edelstein, B. (2013). Assessment of capacity in an aging society. *American Psychologist, 68*(3), 158–171.

Muir, H. J., Coyne, A. E., Morrison, N. R., Boswell, J. F., & Constantino, M. J. (2019). Ethical implications of routine outcomes monitoring for patients, psychotherapists, and mental health care systems. *Psychotherapy, 56*(4), 459–469.

Myers, K., & Turvey, C. (Eds.). (2012). *Telemental health: Clinical, technical, and administrative foundations for evidence-based practice*. Newnes.

Nadorff, M. R., Drapeau, C. W., & Pigeon, W. R. (2018). Psychiatric illness and sleep in older adults: Comorbidity and opportunities for intervention. *Sleep Medicine Clinics, 13*(1), 81–91.

Neff, K., & Germer, C. (2018). *The mindful self-compassion workbook: A proven way to accept yourself, build inner strength, and thrive*. Guilford Publications.

Neimeyer, R. A., & Holland, J. M. (2015). Bereavement in later life: Theory, assessment, and intervention. In P. A. Lichtenberg, B. T. Mast, B. D. Carpenter, & J. Loebach Wetherell (Eds.), *APA handbook of clinical geropsychology, Vol. 2: Assessment, treatment, and issues of later life* (pp. 645–666). American Psychological Association.

Neimeyer, R. A., Kazantzis, N., Kassler, D. M., Baker, K. D., & Fletcher, R. (2008). Group cognitive behavioural therapy for depression outcomes predicted by willingness to engage in homework, compliance with homework, and cognitive restructuring skill acquisition. *Cognitive Behaviour Therapy, 37*, 199–215.

Nelson, E.-L., & Duncan, A. B. (2015). Cognitive behavioral therapy using televideo. *Cognitive and Behavioral Practice, 22*(3), 269–280.

Ngandu, T., Lehtisalo, J., Solomon, A., Levälahti, E., Ahtiluoto, S., Antikainen, R., Bäckman, L., Hänninen, T., Jula, A., Laatikainen, T.,

Lindström, J., Mangialasche, F., Paajanen, T., Pajala, S., Peltonen, M., Rauramaa, R., Stigsdotter-Neely, A., Strandberg, T., Tuomilehto, J., Soininen, H., & Kivipelto, M. A. (2015). A 2-year multidomain intervention of diet, exercise, cognitive training, and vascular risk monitoring versus control to prevent cognitive decline in at-risk elderly people (FINGER): A randomised controlled trial. *Lancet, 385*, 2255–2263.

Officer, A., & de la Fuente-Núñez, V. (2018). A global campaign to combat ageism. *Bulletin of the World Health Organization, 96*(4), 295–296.

Okamoto, A., Dattilio, F. M., Dobson, K. S., & Kazantzis, N. (2019). The therapeutic relationship in cognitive–behavioral therapy: Essential features and common challenges. *Practice Innovations, 4*(2), 112–123.

O'Malley, K. A., & Qualls, S. H. (2016). Development and preliminary examination of the psychometric properties of the Behavior Problem Checklist. *Clinical Gerontologist, 39*(4), 263–281.

Pachana, N. A., Mitchell, L. K., & Knight, B. G. (2015). Using the CALTAP life span developmental framework with older adults. *Geropsychology, 28*(2), 77–86.

Padesky, C. A., & Mooney, K. A. (2012). Strengths-based cognitive–behavioral therapy: A four-step model to build resilience. *Clinical Psychology & Psychotherapy, 19*(4), 283–290.

Pargament, K. I. (2011). *Spiritually integrated psychotherapy: Understanding and addressing the sacred.* Guilford Press.

Pearce, M. J., Koenig, H. G., Robins, C. J., Nelson, B., Shaw, S. F., Cohen, H. J., & King, M. B. (2015) Religiously integrated cognitive behavioral therapy: A new method of treatment for major depression in clients with chronic medical illness. *Psychotherapy, 52*(1), 56–66.

Petkus, A. J., Lenze, E. J., & Wetherell, J. L. (2013). Anxious depression: Application of a unified model of emotional disorders to older adults. In H. Lavretsky, M. Sajatovic, & C. F. Reynolds III (Eds.), *Late-life mood disorders* (pp. 144–163). Oxford University Press.

Petrik, A. M., Kazantzis, N., & Hofmann, S. G. (2013). Distinguishing integrative from eclectic practice in cognitive behavioral therapies. *Psychotherapy, 50*(3), 392–397.

Pocklington, C., Gilbody, S., Manea, L., & McMillan, D. (2016). The diagnostic accuracy of brief versions of the Geriatric Depression Scale: A systematic review and meta-analysis. *International Journal of Geriatric Psychiatry, 31*(8), 837–857.

Poole, L., & Jackowska, M. (2018). The epidemiology of depressive symptoms and poor sleep: Findings from the English Longitudinal Study of Ageing (ELSA). *International Journal of Behavioral Medicine, 25*(2), 151–161.

Pot, A. M., Gallagher, T. D., Xiao, L. D., Willemse, B. M., Rosier, I., Mehta, K. M., Zandi, D., & Dua, T. (2019). iSupport: A WHO global online intervention for informal caregivers of people with dementia. *World Psychiatry, 18*(3), 365–366.

Powers, D. V., Thompson, L. W., & Gallagher-Thompson, D. (2008). The benefits of using psychotherapy skills following treatment for depression: An examination of "afterwork" and a test of the skills hypothesis in older adults. *Cognitive and Behavioral Practice, 15*, 194–202.

Prescott, D. S., Maeschalck, C. L., & Miller, S. D. (2017). *Feedback-informed treatment in clinical practice: Reaching for excellence.* American Psychological Association.

Qualls, S. H. (2016). Caregiving families within the long-term services and support system for older adults. *American Psychologist, 71*(4), 283–293.

Qualls, S. H., & Williams, A. A. (2013). *Caregiver family therapy: Empowering families to meet the challenges of aging.* American Psychological Association.

Ranjan, R., Priyamvada, R., Jha, G. K., & Chaudhury, S. (2017). Neuropsychological deficits in elderly with depression. *Industrial Psychiatry Journal, 26*(2), 178–182.

Rapsey, C. M., Scott, K. M., & Patterson, T. (2019). Childhood sexual abuse, poly-victimization and internalizing disorders across adulthood and older age: Findings from a 25-year longitudinal study. *Journal of Affective Disorders, 244*, 171–179.

Reis, M., & Nahmiash, D. (1995). Validation of the Caregiver Abuse Screen (CASE). *Canadian Journal on Aging/La Revue Canadienne Du Vieillissement, 14*(S2), 45–60.

Reiser, R. P., Thompson, L. W., Johnson, S. L., & Suppes, T. (2017). *Bipolar disorder* (Vol. 1, 2nd ed.). Hogrefe Publishing.

Reynolds, C. F., Lenze, E., & Mulsant, B. H. (2019). Assessment and treatment of major depression in older adults. *Handbook of Clinical Neurology, 167*, 429–435.

Richards, D. A., Ekers, D., McMillan, D., Taylor, R. S., Byford, S., Warren, F. C., Barrett, B., Farrand, P.A., Gilbody, S., Kuyken, W., O'Mahen, H., Watkins, E.R., Wright, K.A., Hollon, S.D., Reed, N., Rhodes, S., Fletcher, E., &Finning, K. (2016). Cost and outcome of behavioural activation versus cognitive behavioural therapy for depression (COBRA): A randomised, controlled, non-inferiority trial. *Lancet, 388*(10047), 871–880.

Rider, K. L., Thompson, L. W., & Gallagher-Thompson, D. (2016). California Older Persons Pleasant Events Scale: A tool to help older adults increase positive experiences. *Clinical Gerontologist, 39*(1), 64–83.

Riper, H., & Cuijpers, P. J. (2016). Telepsychology and eHealth. In J. C. Norcross, G. R. VandenBos, D. K. Freedheim, & R. Krishnamurthy (Eds.), *APA handbook of clinical psychology: Applications and methods* (Vol. 3, pp. 451–463). American Psychological Association.

Roth, D. L., Brown, S. L., Rhodes, J. D., & Haley, W. E. (2018). Reduced mortality rates among caregivers: Does family caregiving provide a stress-buffering effect? *Psychology and Aging, 33*(4), 619–629.

Rowe, J. R., & Kahn, R. L. (1998). *Successful aging.* Pantheon Books.

Sachs-Ericsson, N., Corsentino, E., Moxley, J., Hames, J. L., Rushing, N. C., Sawyer, K., & Steffens, D. C. (2013). A longitudinal study of differences in late- and early-onset geriatric depression: Depressive symptoms and psychosocial, cognitive, and neurological functioning. *Aging & Mental Health, 17*(1), 1–11.

Sachs-Ericsson, N. J., Rushing, N. C., Stanley, I. H., & Sheffler, J. (2016). In my end is my beginning: Developmental trajectories of adverse childhood experiences to late-life suicide. *Aging & Mental Health, 20*(2), 139–165.

Samarina, V., Suresh, M., Picchiello, M., Lutz, J., Carpenter, B., & Beaudreau, S. (2021). Assessment approaches for psychiatric and cognitive syndromes. In N. Pachana, V. Molinari, L. Thompson & D. Gallagher-Thompson (Eds.), Psychological assessment and treatment of older adults (pp. 15–42). Hogrefe Press.

Satterfield, J. M. (2008). *A cognitive-behavioral approach to the beginning of the end of life, "Minding the Body": Facilitator guide.* Oxford University Press.

Schaie, K. W., & Willis, S. L. (Eds.). (2015). *Handbook of the psychology of aging* (8th ed.). Elsevier Academic Press.

Schulz, R., & Eden, J. (Eds.). (2016). *Families caring for an aging America.* National Academies Press.

Scogin, F., & Shah, A. (Eds.). (2012). *Making evidence-based psychological treatments work with older adults.* American Psychological Association.

Sheikh, J. I., & Yesavage, J. A. (1986). Geriatric Depression Scale (GDS): Recent evidence and development of a shorter version. *Clinical Gerontologist, 5*(1–2), 165–173.

Sheline, Y. I., Barch, D. M., Garcia, K., Gersing, K., Pieper, C., Welsh-Bohmer, K., Steffens, D. C., & Doraiswamy, P. M. (2006). Cognitive function in late life depression: Relationships to depression severity, cerebrovascular risk factor and processing speed. *Biological Psychiatry, 60*(1), 58–65.

Smarr, K. L., & Keefer, A. L. (2011). Measures of depression and depressive symptoms: Beck Depression Inventory-II (BDI-II), Center for

Epidemiologic Studies Depression Scale (CES-D), Geriatric Depression Scale (GDS), Hospital Anxiety and Depression Scale (HADS), and Patient Health Questionnaire-9 (PHQ-9). *Arthritis Care Research*, *63*(S11), 454–466.

Solomonov, N., Bress, J. N., Sirey, J. A., Gunning, F. M., Flückiger, C., Raue, P. J., Arean, P. A., & Alexopoulos, G. S. (2019). Engagement in socially and interpersonally rewarding activities as a predictor of outcome in "engage" behavioral activation therapy for late-life depression. *American Journal of Geriatric Psychiatry*, *27*(6), 571–578.

Sorocco, K. H., & Lauderdale, S. (Eds.). (2011). *Cognitive behavior therapy with older adults: Innovations across care settings*. Springer Publishing Company.

Spencer, J., Goode, J., Penix, E. A., Trusty, W., & Swift, J. K. (2019). Developing a collaborative relationship with clients during the initial sessions of psychotherapy. *Psychotherapy*, *56*(1), 7–10.

Stanley, M. A., Wilson, N., Shrestha, S., Amspoker, A. B., Armento, M., Cummings, J. P., Evans-Hudnall, G., Wagener, P., & Kunik, M. E. (2016). Calmer life: A culturally tailored intervention for anxiety in underserved older adults. *American Journal of Geriatric Psychiatry*, *24*(8), 648–658.

Steffen, A. M., Gallagher-Thompson, D., Arenella, K., Au, A., Cheng, S. T., Crespo, M., Cristancho-Lacroix, V., López, J., Losada Baltar, A., Márquez-González, M., Nogales-González, C., & Romero-Moreno, R. (2019). Validating the Revised Scale for Caregiving Self-Efficacy: A cross-national review. *The Gerontologist*, *59*(4), e325–e342. https://doi.org/10.1093/geront/gny004

Steffen, A. M., Gallagher-Thompson, D., & Thompson, L. W. (2021). Theoretical support and practical strategies for CBT with depressed older adults. In N. Pachana, V. Molinari, L. W. Thompson, & D. Gallagher-Thompson (Eds.), *Psychological assessment and treatment of older adults* (pp. 45–71). Hogrefe Press.

Steffen, A. M., & Gant, J. R. (2016). A telehealth behavioral coaching intervention for neurocognitive disorder family carers. *International Journal Of Geriatric Psychiatry*, *31*(2), 195–203.

Steffen, A. M. & Schmidt, N. E. (in press). The CBTs in Later Life. In G. Asmundson (Ed.), Comprehensive clinical psychology, 2nd edition. Oxford, UK: Elsevier.

Steffen, A. M., & Zeiss, A. M. (2017). Interprofessional health care teams in geriatrics. In *Reference Module in Neuroscience and Biobehavioral Psychology*, Elsevier, ISBN 9780128093245. https://doi.org/10.1016/B978-0-12-809324-5.05142-7

Steffen, A. M., Zeiss, A. M. & Karel, M. (2015). Interprofessional geriatric health care: Competencies and resources for teamwork. In N. Pachana & K. Laidlaw (Eds.), *Oxford handbook of clinical geropsychology: International perspectives* (pp. 733–752). Oxford University Press.

Stirman, S. W., Baumann, A. A., & Miller, C. J. (2019). The FRAME: An expanded framework for reporting adaptations and modifications to evidence-based interventions. *Implementation Science, 14*(1), 1–10.

Stott, R., Mansell, W., Salkovskis, P., & Lavender, A. (2010). *Oxford guide to metaphors in CBT: Building cognitive bridges.* Oxford University Press.

Swift, J. K., & Greenberg, R. P. (2015). *Premature termination in psychotherapy: Strategies for engaging clients and improving outcomes.* American Psychological Association.

Swift, J. K., Greenberg, R. P., Tompkins, K. A., & Parkin, S. R. (2017). Treatment refusal and premature termination in psychotherapy, pharmacotherapy, and their combination: A meta-analysis of head-to-head comparisons. *Psychotherapy, 54*(1), 47–57.

Szanton, S. L., Wolff, J. W., Leff, B., Thorpe, R. J., Tanner, E. K., Boyd, C., Xue, A., Guralnik, J., Bishai, D., & Gitlin, L. N. (2014). CAPABLE trial: A randomized controlled trial of nurse, occupational therapist and handyman to reduce disability among older adults: Rationale and design. *Contemporary Clinical Trials, 38*(1), 102–112.

Te Pou (2015). Scope it right: Working to top of scope literature review. https://www.tepou.co.nz/uploads/files/resource-assets/scope-it-right-literature-review.pdf

Thoma, N. C., & McKay, D. (Eds.). (2014). *Working with emotion in cognitive-behavioral therapy: Techniques for clinical practice.* Guilford Publications.

Thompson, L. W. (1996). Cognitive-behavioral therapy and treatment for late-life depression. *Journal of Clinical Psychiatry, 57*(Suppl. 5), 29–37.

Thompson, L. W., Coon, D. W., Gallagher-Thompson, D., Sommer, B., & Koin, D. (2001). Comparison of desipramine and cognitive behavioral therapy in the treatment of elderly outpatients with mild to moderate depression. *American Journal of Geriatric Psychiatry, 9*(3), 225–240.

Thompson, L. W., & Gallagher, D. (1984). Efficacy of psychotherapy in the treatment of late-life depression. *Advances in Behaviour Research and Therapy, 6*(2), 127–139.

Thompson, L. W., Gallagher, D., & Breckenridge, J. S. (1987). Comparative effectiveness of psychotherapies for depressed elders. *Journal of Consulting and Clinical Psychology, 55*(3), 385–390.

Thompson, L. W., Kaye, J. L., Tang, P. C. Y., & Gallagher-Thompson, D. (2004). Bereavement and adjustment disorders. In D. Blazer, D. Steffens & E. Busse (Eds.), *Textbook of Geriatric Psychiatry, 3rd ed.* (Chapter 19, pp. 319–338). Washington, D.C.: American Psychiatric Press.

Thompson, L. W., McGee, J. S., & Gallagher-Thompson, D. (2005). Cognitive behavioral therapy. In B. J. Sadock & V. A. Sadock (Eds.), *Comprehensive textbook of psychiatry* (Vol. II, 8th ed., pp. 3758–3763). Lippincott Williams & Wilkins.

Thompson, L. W., Powers, D. V., Coon, D. W., Takagi, K., McKibbin, C., & Gallagher-Thompson, D. (2000). Older adults. In J. R. White & A. S. Freeman (Eds.), *Cognitive-behavioral group therapy for specific problems and populations* (pp. 235–261). American Psychological Association.

Thompson, L. W., Spira, A. P., Depp, C. A., McGee, J. S., & Gallagher-Thompson, D. (2006). The geriatric caregiver. In M. E. Agronin & G. J. Maletta (Eds.), *Principles and practice of geriatric psychiatry* (pp. 37–48). Lippincott Williams & Wilkins.

Thorn, B. E. (2017). *Cognitive therapy for chronic pain: A step-by-step guide.* Guilford Publications.

Tighe, C. A., Dautovich, N. D., & McCrae, C. S. (2016). Daily social contact in relation to sleep: The role of age. *Behavioral Sleep Medicine, 14*(3), 311–324.

Tolin, D. F. (2016). *Doing CBT: A comprehensive guide to working with behaviors, thoughts, and emotions.* Guilford Publications.

Tompkins, M. A. (2004). *Using homework in psychotherapy: Strategies, guidelines, and forms.* Guilford Press.

Törneke, N. (2017). *Metaphor in practice: A professional's guide to using the science of language in psychotherapy.* New Harbinger Publications.

Uher, I., & Liba, J. (2017). Correlation between functional fitness of older people and environmental and accommodation conditions. *Journal of Physical Education and Sport, 17*(4), 2365–2371.

Van Orden, K. A., Bower, E., Lutz, J., Silva, C., Gallegos, A. M., Podgorski, C. A., Santos, E. J., & Conwell, Y. (2020). Strategies to promote social connections among older adults during "social distancing" restrictions. *American Journal of Geriatric Psychiatry.* https://doi.org/10.1016/j.jagp.2020.05.004

Van Ryckeghem, D. M. L., Van Damme, S., Eccleston, C., & Crombez, G. (2018). The efficacy of attentional distraction and sensory monitoring in chronic pain patients: A meta-analysis. *Clinical Psychology Review, 59*, 16–29.

van't Veer-Tazelaar, P. J., van Marwijk, H. W. J., van Oppen, P., van Hout, H. P. J., van der Horst, H. E., Cuijpers, P., Smit, F., & Beekman, A.

T. F. (2009). Stepped-care prevention of anxiety and depression in late life: A randomized controlled trial. *Archives of General Psychiatry, 66*(3), 297–304.

Varker, T., Brand, R., Ward, J., Terhaag, S., & Phelps, A. (2019). Efficacy of synchronous telepsychology interventions for people with anxiety, depression, posttraumatic stress disorder, and adjustment disorder: A rapid evidence assessment. *Psychological Services, 16*(4), 621–635.

Verplanken, B. (Ed.). (2018). *The psychology of habit.* Springer.

Videler, A. C., van Alphen, S. P. J., van Royen, R. J. J., van der Feltz-Cornelis, C. M., Rossi, G., & Arntz, A. (2018). Schema therapy for personality disorders in older adults: A multiple-baseline study. *Aging & Mental Health, 22*(6), 738–747.

Vieten, C., Scammell, S., Pierce, A., Pilato, R., Ammondson, I., Pargament, K., & Lukoff, D. (2016). Competencies for psychologists in the domains of religion and spirituality. *Spirituality in Clinical Practice, 3*(2), 92–114.

Wang, S., & Blazer, D. G. (2015). Depression and cognition in the elderly. *Annual Review of Clinical Psychology, 11*, 331–360.

Warren, A. R., & Steffen, A. M. (2020). Development of a transgender and gender nonconforming language self-efficacy scale for social service providers working with older adults. *Journal of Applied Gerontology, 39*(5), 555–560.

Webb, C. A., Cui, R., Titus, C., Fiske, A., & Nadorff, M. R. (2018). Sleep disturbance, activities of daily living, and depressive symptoms among older adults. *Clinical Gerontologist, 41*(2), 172–180.

Wei, J., Hou, R., Zhang, X., Xu, H., Xie, L., Chandrasekar, E. K., Ying, M., & Goodman, M. (2019). The association of late-life depression with all-cause and cardiovascular mortality among community-dwelling older adults: Systematic review and meta-analysis. *British Journal of Psychiatry, 215*(2), 449–455.

Wenzel, A., Brown, G. K., & Beck, A. T. (2009). *Cognitive therapy for suicidal patients: Scientific and clinical applications.* American Psychological Association.

Wild, B., Eckl, A., Herzog, W., Niehoff, D., Lechner, S., Maatouk, I., Schellberg, D., Brenner, H., Müller, H., & Löwe, B. (2014). Assessing generalized anxiety disorder in elderly people using the GAD-7 and GAD-2 scales: Results of a validation study. *American Journal of Geriatric Psychiatry, 22*(10), 1029–1038.

Wilkinson, P., & Izmeth, Z. (2016). Continuation and maintenance treatments for depression in older people. *Cochrane Database of*

Systematic Reviews. https://doi.org/10.1002/14651858.CD006727. pub3

Wilt, J. A., Stauner, N., Harriott, V. A., Exline, J. J., & Pargament, K. I. (2019). Partnering with God: Religious coping and perceptions of divine intervention predict spiritual transformation in response to religious–spiritual struggle. *Psychology of Religion and Spirituality, 11*(3), 278–290.

Wood, W., & Rünger, D. (2016). Psychology of habit. *Annual Review of Psychology, 67,* 289–314.

Wright, J. H., Brown, G. K., Thase, M. E., & Basco, M. R. (2017). *Learning cognitive-behavior therapy: An illustrated guide.* American Psychiatric Publishing.

Wuthrich, V. M., Johnco, C. J., & Wetherell, J. L. (2015). Differences in anxiety and depression symptoms: Comparison between older and younger clinical samples. *International Psychogeriatrics, 27*(9), 1523–1532.

Yaffe, M. J., Weiss, D., & Lithwick, M. (2012). Seniors' self-administration of the Elder Abuse Suspicion Index (EASI): a feasibility study. *Journal of Elder Abuse & Neglect, 24*(4), 277–292.

Yeo, G., Gerdner, L., & Gallagher-Thompson, D. (2019). *Ethnicity and the dementias* (3rd ed.). Routledge Press.

Yesavage, J., Brink, T. L., Rose, T. L., Lum, O., Huang, V., Adey, M., & Leirer, V. O. (1983). Development and validation of a geriatric depression screening scale: A preliminary report. *Journal of Psychiatric Research, 17*(1), 37–49.

Zabihi, S., Lemmel, F. K., & Orgeta, D. V. (2020). Behavioural activation for depression in informal caregivers: A systematic review and meta-analysis of randomised controlled clinical trials. *Journal of Affective Disorders, 274,* 1173–1183.

Zarit, S. H., & Heid, A. R. (2015). Assessment and treatment of family caregivers. In P. A. Lichtenberg, B. T. Mast, B. D. Carpenter, & J. Loebach Wetherell (Eds.), *APA handbook of clinical geropsychology, Vol. 2: Assessment, treatment, and issues of later life* (pp. 521–551). American Psychological Association.

Zeiss, A. M., & Steffen, A. (1996). Treatment issues with elderly clients. *Cognitive and Behavioral Practice, 3*(2), 371–389.

Zietemann, V., Kopczak, A., Müller, C., Wollenweber, F. A., & Dichgans, M. (2017). Validation of the Telephone Interview of Cognitive Status and Telephone Montreal Cognitive Assessment against detailed cognitive testing and clinical diagnosis of mild cognitive impairment after stroke. *Stroke, 48*(11), 2952–2957.